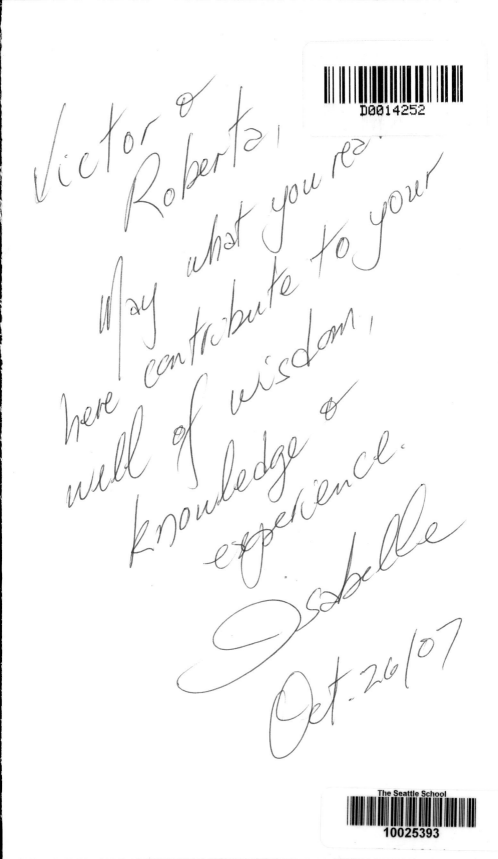

Victor &
Roberta,
May what you rea
here contribute to your
well of wisdom,
knowledge &
experience.

Isabelle

Oct. 26/07

# Einstein's Business
## Engaging Soul, Imagination, and Excellence in the Workplace

edited by
# DAWSON CHURCH, PH.D.

associate editors
Courtney Arnold
Jeanne House
Isabelle St-Jean
Barbara Stahura

Elite Books

Santa Rosa, CA 95403

www.EliteBooksOnline.com

Cataloging-in-Publication Data:

Einstein's business : engaging, soul, imagination, and excellence in the workplace / edited by Dawson Church, Courtney Arnold, Jeanne House, Isabelle St. Jean, Barbara Stahura. 1st ed.

p. cm.

Includes bibliographical references.

ISBN-10: 1-60070-015-2
ISBN-13: 978-1-60070-015-6

1. Organizational change. 2. Social responsibility of business. 3. Sustainable development. 4. Human ecology. I. Church, Dawson 1956- II. Arnold, Courtney III. House, Jeanne, IV. St. Jean, Isabelle IV. Stahura, Barbara.

Cover Design by Victoria Valentine
Typesetting by Maria Ayala Cirner
Copyedited by Courtney Arnold
Proofreading by Melissa Mower
Printed by Bang Printing
Typeset in Mona Lisa and Book Antiqua
First Edition

10   9   8   7   6   5   4   3   2   1

This book is dedicated to all the
warriors of the heart who are living out
their values in the workplace
and revolutionizing organizations
and the world through their fearless
thoughts, words, and actions.

# CONTENTS

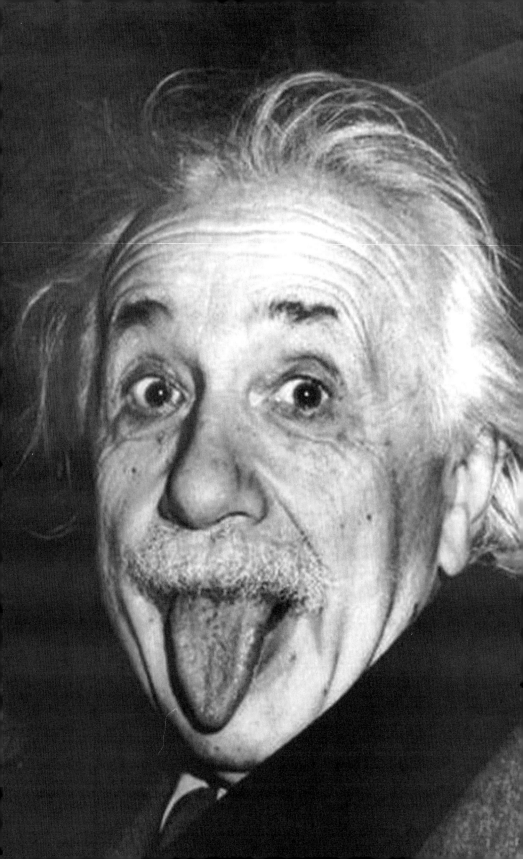

# Introduction

# Isabelle St-Jean

Be warned: You are entering a treacherous terrain, a portal of alchemy! This unprecedented anthology simmers up years of powerful collective insights, research, experience, and actionable ideas about doing business and working together. As you join us in this inquisitive journey, you're likely to become infected with the virus of inspiration, the buzz of "Aha!" moments, and the thrill of renewed creativity. A tantalizing proposition at the end of a hard working day, you say? Come along as we point the way to engaging soul and imagination as we stand for excellence in our working communities.

Einstein was a bit like a sorcerer, incubating new theories and inventing revolutionary ideas out of the cauldron of his brilliant mind. Like a sorceress, I ignited the fire under the cauldron of this anthology by conceiving the idea in early 2005 at a conference I attended with publisher Dawson Church. The final creation, however, turned out to be much more potent than I had anticipated. I was setting out to execute my favorite recipe and choose only my preferred ingredients. But then, along the way, unexpected flavors and spices turned up in the pot. I became inspired to write my own manuscript, and Dawson put on the editorial apron. With ingredients from the two of us, plus several contributing editors, the end result will stir up your synapses as a delightful concoction would stir up your taste buds. Perhaps, like us, you have also strayed from your recipes, only to find, in the end, an exciting richness of flavors beyond the reach of your earlier imagination!

As my preconceived notions for this project gradually gave way to a more spacious and engaging endeavor, I've come to see that this anthology is a celebration of inclusiveness. In fact, the book you are holding resembles a microcosm of the typical workplace today. With the different personalities, areas of expertise, and experiences behind these varied authors, we are honoring diversity rather than uniformity. What's more, I've come to see that diversity and inclusiveness are absolutely essential values in the process of orchestrating our continuity on this planet while we work. Without prioritizing these values, we cannot reverse the dangerous patterns of divisiveness entrenched in our world.

As you read you'll be provoked, informed, and challenged — as well as finding affirmation of your innermost cherished values. At this particular threshold of our evolution, all kinds of people are asking themselves the same questions and holding the same concerns that you have. Much of it boils down to this: How do we work and prosper in harmony and integrity, while co-creating the socially and ecologically sustainable world we need?

Quite simply, at this point on our planet Earth, we can no longer deny that the old "business as usual" approach is taking us straight down the road to our own extinction. In these pages, we are joining the momentum away from the dead end of the status quo. As audacious pioneers, we're running at the pace of the new paradigms emerging in the workplace. Some of the coauthors in this book offer innovative solutions from the macro perspective, revealing imbalances and misguided perceptions that have lead to fragmentation in our organizations and institutions. Other contributors, myself included, have taken the micro end of the lens, generating insights about the largely unconscious zone wedged between our personal and professional selves.

One of the questions we have pondered is: What will it take for integrity to prevail in our workplaces? The scandals that have come to light in recent years are just the tip of the iceberg of corporate crime. In her chapter, Riane Eisler reminds us that the business executives responsible for these scandals were able to accomplish their arrogant feats "because of the system under which most of society functions." Following her 30 years of research, Eisler has identified an alternative approach that simultaneously resolves many of the problems that threaten our existence on this planet. Through her study of relational dynamics, she leads us away from the dualistic mode of our current social and economic frameworks to provide an alternative, a larger, compelling perspective. From this vantage point she invites us into a novel system of partnership. This system offers new social categories to help us make the changes in the social and economic rules that govern our lives so that we can access a more secure, equitable, and sustainable future. In a brilliant analysis of human personality types, Sandra Seagal, another visionary thinker, shows that huge companies like IBM can thrive when they are structured to accommodate human differences.

Julie Gerland is another of several coauthors who address the issue of integrity. Her passionate plea to listen to the voice of conscience, and the conviction that the ends don't justify the means, are an inspired reminder to heed the still, small voice within. Tuning into our soul's wisdom and acting from that place yields an integration of spirit, mind, and body that produces integrity in the workplace. Mandy Ellis Voisey's exuberant description of how she built her global company, Junction 18, using her own moral compass (her colleagues jokingly referred to her as the "Moral Director" of the company), is an example of how an ethical bottom line can reinforce the financial bottom line.

The present flow toward integrity and sustainability in our endeavors has intensified largely because of the increasing influence of women in the workplace. Women in business often bring a perspective that supports the shift toward a more equitable society and away from the patriarchal vestiges of our Western society. And the feminine psyche provides a great counter-balance to the left-brain-dominant, rationally focused tendencies of the masculine mind. In her chapter, Lynne Twist wisely points out that women have a natural inclination toward life-affirming values. This predisposes them to taking a stance for the preservation of their moral principles and integrity. A current example is that of Sherron Watkins who, supported by her mother, had the courage to blow the whistle on the wrongdoings of the Enron Corporation. Bonnie Sarkisian's delightful chapter using gardening as a metaphor emphasizes the power of nurturing when applied to work teams, and Fionnuala Herder-Wynne's eloquent intertwining of her personal and business journeys gives an example of how heart, family, and work can interact in a dynamic, complementary weave of growth and self-understanding.

Yet there's a trap in this growth process, as bestselling author of *Care of the Soul*, Thomas Moore, points out in his chapter "Joyful Ethics." Change agents like you or I can be perceived as a "white knight full of ideals" and alienate colleagues by coming across as holier-than-thou. Instead, he reminds us, we are more effective when we approach people in business with respect, acknowledging their strengths — while skillfully bringing our vision to their attention. "Trying to implant a new vision on them while denigrating their established ways of doing things will never work," Moore warns us. If we lead with an overly intense fervor of idealism ungrounded in current realities, we will only trigger more skepticism and cynicism, thus reinforcing the duality of "us" versus "them."

Aside from ethical issues, our present working society is strained by many factors, including a continuing perception that fierce competition is the only way for a company to prosper. In his fascinating chapter on what he calls "leapfrogging," Dawson Church demonstrates that innovation and leaps of consciousness propel some organizations ahead of others. He suggests practical ways to cultivate the consciousness and conditions conducive to leapfrogging. When put into practice, these ways of thinking and behaving also serve to promote the well-being of individuals, not just the company in which they work.

Across any cityscape, office towers are filled with people whose health and energies are being depleted because of increasing demands on them. From corporate take-over to budget restraints and lay offs, more and more employees are doing the work that was once done by several people. Numerous studies indicate that people at work are overly stressed and are working longer hours than they used to. In a 2005 survey of senior Fortune 500 male executives, 84 percent said they'd like to have more time for their personal lives while continuing to pursue their professional aspirations.

In my own coaching practice I have witnessed the pain of professionals working frantically for wealth and financial security, only to realize in mid-life that they've become alienated from their authentic selves and life purpose. Ultimately, it is not sustainable to be overly consumed with work while severed from our inner self and soul. This kind of alienation puts us at risk of burning out, having a health crisis, or resigning ourselves while we just hold on until retirement. But rather than dreaming of resting on the beach, we would be wise to take on the inner journey that can lead us to renewal and real engagement. Wholeheartedness is a powerful antidote to exhaustion because it generates energy and motivation. In these pages, you will be inspired to follow your inner guidance, recommit, or make new choices to recover a sense of balance in your personal and professional life.

Quality of life and well-being in a society are the true measure of human development and social progress, not the numbers on the GNP figures (Gross National Product), affirms Hazel Henderson. In her chapter, "Gross National Happiness," Henderson points out the entrenched bias of economics: "Rather than being a science, it is a political ideology, pure and simple." With her compelling arguments she brings us to the reality that the field of economics is neither gender-neutral nor value-free. She also turns our attention to the little Buddhist country of Bhutan, where the well-being of its people has been measured through the Gross National Happiness index. This is a reflection of this country's priorities to promote prosperity while ensuring that it is shared across their society and balanced with the protection of environment and preservation of cultural traditions.

While at the Quest for Global Healing conference in Bali in May 2006, I delighted in the presence of one of Bhutan's Ministers, the Honorable Lyonpo Jigmi Thinley. He spoke of the joys and challenges of measuring people's perception of their happiness through the surveys that were used to arrive at the Gross National Happiness figures. I was moved by Jigmi Thinley's most gracious way of speaking and inspired by his authentic leadership. He delivered an important message about the heart of happiness, the spirit of interdependence, and about redefining wealth.

While I participated in this conference I also got to know some Balinese people and witnessed the strong bonds that connect them together. It appeared to me that in this culture, every action is taken with the well-being of family and community foremost in heart and mind. Although many Balinese live in material poverty, their inner richness and generosity abounds. Without knowing it, these people are leading the way to embrace Einstein's suggestion: "Try not to be a person of success, but, rather, a person of value."

Leadership is another strong theme that we have embraced in this anthology. We've tackled the thorny issue of bad leaders — people who have great leadership abilities, but use them to take their followers down the garden path — as well as looking at the characteristics of a good leader. Partly since the field of coaching has spread and influenced the culture in workplaces, the top-down, dictate and control, mechanical style of leadership is no longer seen as appropriate or effective. Moreover, the level of complexity and speed of change in our world have demanded a new worldview along with new ways to lead. As you will read, the authors assembled here bring you their own ideas about inspired leadership, collective leadership, and leadership styles we are best to avoid. But as co-authors we join in one narrow place of certainty: that true leadership arises from within. Stephen Covey concludes in his chapter about influence that "There is no such thing as organizational behavior," and instead, "There is only individual behavior and everything else flows out of that."

It's not just the CEO who has the power to change an organization; we all influence people daily in ways of which we are barely aware. When we create changes within ourselves, they manifest as outer change, and when we take 100 percent responsibility for our inner climate, we develop immense leverage to change the outer climate. Donald Trump describes how, when he's feeling down, he makes a conscious decision to "change his altitude," his perspective. The enormous power we all have to create change is a persistent theme of this book. Hunter Arnold gives surprising examples of how people can catalyze significant change in organizations even without resources additional to those they already have, and Tom Peters points out many concrete ways in which employees on low rungs of the organizational ladder can produce creative shake-ups.

Several coauthors apply the breakthroughs of quantum physics to the business world in practical ways. While we think of the external world as fixed and immutable, the remarkable perspective offered by quantum physics now indicates to us that what happens "out there" is influenced by the observer, as scientist Jeffrey Schwartz and coach David Rock make plain in their chapter. Psychologist Gabriele Hilberg shows how we can use these quantum effects to make changes effortlessly using the quantum field—an approach that's a far cry from the effort and struggle associated with building the Newtonian business—while consultants Noel McInnis and Douglas Yeaman demonstrate that acting from an absolutely clear outcome conditions every aspect of the intervening reality.

I believe that the best leaders are those who not only "walk the talk" but who have also relinquished their own blocks to greatness within themselves. This requires taking on the arduous journey of moving beyond the limitations that most of us were conditioned to perceive in ourselves. Paradoxically, as we become freer to tap our deepest strengths, we come to peace with the places in ourselves where we often feel challenged. From that inner place of acceptance and humility we can best nourish the relationships that become conduits for a unifying force field that promotes a culture of respect, trust, and innovation. Self-knowledge is a theme of many contributors. Matthew Gilbert's "Now Thyself," about developing self-understanding that transcends the sterile classifications of the HR department, is a masterpiece of clarity. Francine Ward, Wally Amos, and Robert Kiyosaki stress the importance of allowing yourself the leeway of making mistakes in the course of the adventure of self-discovery.

In my own chapter about the "Circle Being," I focus on interdependence and collective intelligence. These values provide an antidote to being overwhelmed and submerged by the enormity of the tasks and problems we often surmount individually at work and in life. As you are witness to an experience of collective intelligence, you will also read about what is conducive to its occurrence in dialogue groups and meetings. You will see that tapping this higher level of wisdom enables us to innovate and be linked together into one masterful mind operating from a more purposeful consciousness.

As we reap the benefits of collective intelligence in the workplace, we can trail-blaze our way into areas that artificial intelligence will never reach.

Margaret Wheatley reminds us, in her chapter, that "no single person or school of thought has the answer, because what's required is far beyond isolated answers." As we inquire together here in this book, we reveal bold new perspectives. We can find new ways to live and work in the heat of the cauldron that holds existing challenges and arising possibilities.

This book is ultimately about alchemy, because it has the power to transform apathy into fierce resolve, to shift cynical attitudes into renewed enthusiasm, and to transform denial into consciousness-in-action. With the stimulating flavors you will taste, you are urged to contribute your own special ingredients in the cauldron of your own endeavors. Then we can participate together in the great turning toward the functional global community and the richly imagined future we so yearn for. As Margaret Wheatley suggests, let us "turn to one another as our best hope for inventing and discovering the worlds we are seeking." Albert Einstein would concur with this suggestion, and I hope you do, too.

# Part One

Thriving Through Change

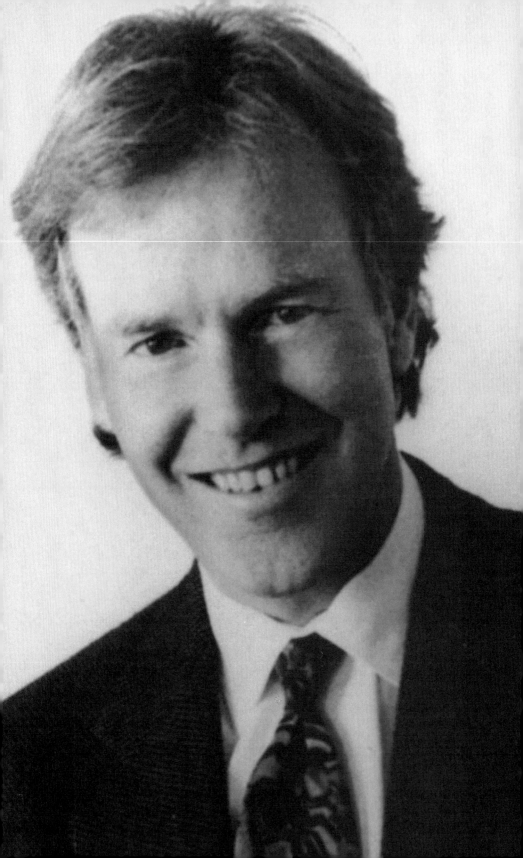

# PETER SENGE:

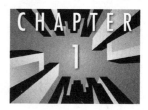

# The Feedback Loop in Living Systems

M eeting the challenges of profound change does not represent a set of separate tasks, a sort of checklist of problems to be solved by aspiring leaders. Rather, these challenges—of initiating, of sustaining, and of redesigning and rethinking—arise and present formidable barriers because the world in which we are seeking to sustain profound change is a living world.

We tend not to see it that way. Our personal history in institutions, starting with school, has conditioned most of us to see a mechanical world—a world of measures, plans, and programs, a world of people "in control" and leaders who "drive" change. This leads us to be blind to critical features of the living world that shape whether or not we ever have any success in actually sustaining change.

## The Nature of the Challenges

The 10 challenges of profound change are dynamic, nonlinear, and interdependent. They are dynamic because they arise from balancing processes that naturally "push back" against efforts to produce change. They are "nonlinear," in the sense that you cannot extrapolate reliably from one experience to another. In a different setting, with only a few small distinctions, a given challenge may play out entirely differently. Last, they are interdependent. Addressing one

Peter Senge is a senior lecturer at the Massachusetts Institute of Technology, chairman of the Society for Organizational Learning, and author of the bestselling *The Fifth Discipline* (Currency, 2006), named by the *Harvard Business Review* as one of the five "key business books" of the past two decades. He is a recognized pioneer, theorist, and writer in the field of management innovation in business, education, health care, and government. The *Journal of Business Strategy* named him a "Strategist of the Century," one of 24 people who have had the greatest influence on business strategy in the last 100 years.

can increase the challenge of addressing another. Or, in other cases, make it easier.

## Appreciating Balancing Processes and Compensating Feedback

Self-proclaimed "change agents" often complain that "people resist change." But the people or groups typecast as resistant rarely see themselves that way. Often, instead, they believe themselves to be quite open. From a systems viewpoint, it is not the people "who are resisting" — rather, it is a system functioning to maintain its internal balances, as all living systems function. Just as all growth in nature is achieved through self-reinforcing growth processes, "homeostasis" — maintaining balances critical to survival — is accomplished through balancing processes.

"History is a process of transformation through conservation," according to biologist Humberto Maturana. In our efforts to produce change, we often forget how important it is to pay attention to what is being conserved. Balancing processes are not the enemy. They are neither inherently good nor bad. Whether or not we value a particular balancing process depends on how much we value *what it conserves*. Balancing processes that conserve financial cash balances, adequate production capacity, technological know-how and innovation, or committed customers are not problems. Indeed, many of the change strategies at the heart of developing learning organizations hinge on conservation of personal purposefulness, honesty, love of inquiry, and the quality of relationships. But, balancing processes that conserve inflexible cultures, outmoded centralized styles of management, defensive routines that stifle innovation, misleading metrics, organizational "stovepipes" that thwart knowledge diffusion, high levels of stress, and fragmented ways of thinking are problems.

The flaw in most leadership strategies stems from fighting blindly against balancing processes, rather than seeking to understand what is being conserved. When this happens, leaders of all types become the victims of "compensating feedback."

Compensating feedback arises when people attempting to produce change do not see the balancing processes that are conserving the status quo. When they encounter difficulties, they "naturally" work harder to overcome them. But "the harder they push, the harder the system pushes back."

Compensating feedback is what happens when a person enters a room with no knowledge of the thermostatic heating system in place.

Imagine that the thermostat is set at 90 degrees. You open a window to cool down the room. It works for a short while, until the heater comes on and it starts getting warmer again. You then open another window, with the same results. After a while you have opened every window there is and you can't understand why the room will not cool off. In this case, there is no leverage in opening the windows. Achieving lasting change requires understanding the thermostatic balancing process in operation; You need to either alter the balancing process (for example by turning off the furnace) or reset the thermostat.

## Nonlinearity

Understanding limiting processes and principles like compensating feedback is very different from having a list of "how to's." Yet many managers seek just these types of answers, and many management books endeavor to provide them. The only problem is that most "how to" books are not very practical.

Generalizing from one situation to the next can be logically sound in a system like the solar system. If you know the location of Pluto today, you can extrapolate its position for the next 2,000 years. This is because the laws of motion that govern the planets are linear laws, where each incremental change in one variable causes a constant incremental change in another. But extrapolation is a fool's occupation in a nonlinear world, where even "perfect knowledge" leads to highly imperfect predictions.

Effective leaders know this intuitively. They know that it is tempting to say, "This is how we did it over there and it worked. So, we should follow the same rules here." But "here" and "there" are never identical and even small differences can alter the outcome of so-called "tried and true" formulas. If you have ever worked for a manager who knows "exactly how things should be done," you know what I mean. He or she is trapped in a futile struggle to make today's reality fit yesterday's answers, and everyone suffers as a consequence. This does not imply that there is no learning from experience, but real learning is more subtle than can ever be captured in simple formulas or rules.

This is why we repeatedly emphasize intuitive appreciation of the different challenges to profound change, and reflection on their meaning in your own context. Only through deep understanding of these issues can you lay a foundation for real learning. Only through practice, and continuing reflection, will practical know-how develop. There are no answers. But there are ways of looking at reality that are higher leverage than others.

## Interdependences Among the Challenges

There are three different types of interdependencies, each presenting both problems and opportunities.

1. Shifting dominance: when efforts to address one challenge shift pressures to others, so that they require more attention. This is akin to compensating feedback; only here the interaction among different limiting processes generates the difficulties. The more that any one limit is relaxed, the more that others come into play.

Shifting dominance is important to understand because it is easy for leaders to feel like "I've fixed the problem that was holding people back; now we'll really make progress." Given this attitude, it is easy to be surprised when new problems arise. But those new problems are suddenly evident precisely because an earlier problem was fixed. Conversely, leaders who understand shifting dominance continually guard against this sort of complacency and are always strategizing about the next challenges, even before they arise.

2. Related capacities exist when different constraints underlying different limiting processes stem from similar capabilities. Where there are related capacities, progress with one challenge can carry over to benefit another.

For example, the challenge of fear and anxiety arises to the extent that candor and openness develop more rapidly than a group's capacity for openness. The key in addressing this challenge lies in building "capacity for openness," the ability to hear one another and tolerate multiple views.

Leaders who understand related capacities can see how some developments are more fundamental than others because they can benefit multiple challenges. Those who do not understand related capacities see each challenge as unrelated to the others. This is one reason that effective leaders continue to emphasize the core learning capabilities of aspiration, reflective conversation, and understanding complexity.

3. Last, there are also "fractal relationships" among particular challenges. In these cases, local challenges constitute microcosms of more global challenges, and local successes may establish a foundation for global change.

For example, the experience of developing time flexibility in a pilot group will be very useful in the complex time coordination that goes into, say, a governance structure based on increased local responsibilities and lateral organizational processes. In this increasingly "networked world," goals, work tasks, and time deadlines are not handed down from bosses and then controlled by traditional management control systems. People continually form and reform working groups to meet emerging market opportunities and organizational needs. Their skills in prioritizing and coordinating their efforts grow directly from learning to increase time flexibility in pilot groups.

Similarly, coaching skills, the ability to mentor and guide others' development in the context of facing practical issues, can prove foundational for designing learning infrastructure for community building.

One last fractal relationship has to do with authenticity and "walking the talk." Line leaders who inquire effectively into their own values and behaviors at the pilot group level become more reflective and credible. In effect, they become models for the integrity and interpersonal trust needed to explore a host of organizationwide issues. These qualities can help other pilot groups become more open to learning from one another and can be invaluable when the time comes to explore potentially volatile countercultural approaches to governance and strategic dilemmas.

## Communities of Leaders or No Leadership at All

It would take a genuine flight of fantasy to both take seriously the multiple, interdependent challenges involved in sustaining profound change and still hold the view that change happens because great men "drive" change from the top.

Undoubtedly, the diversity of people who lead in addressing these forces exceeds the simple categorization: local line leaders, executive leaders, and internal networkers. But these three types of leaders still represent a good place to begin in thinking about the constituents of a healthy "leadership ecology," an interdependent human community commensurate in diversity and robustness to the challenges of profound change.

▪ **Local line leaders.** These leaders are vital to initiating significant change. The four challenges of initiating: "no time," "no help," "not relevant," and "walking the talk"—constitute a litmus test for the effectiveness of local line leaders. Unless they deal successfully with all four of these challenges, they will not create conditions where the growth processes of personal results, networks of committed people, and business results can develop momentum. Likewise, local line leaders are vital in addressing the challenges of sustaining change, which play out both within innovative pilot groups, such as the challenge of "fear and anxiety," and between those pilots and the larger organization. Experience has shown again and again that without committed and talented local line leaders, little significant change ever gets initiated and takes root. Value is actually created at the front lines of all organizations, where products and services are designed, produced, marketed, and sold, where customers are served, and where the practical problems impeding these processes are addressed. In a fundamental sense, organizational learning involves the enhancement of capacity to generate value—hence, all organizational learning, ultimately, involves front line people and core business processes where value is created. This is why local line leadership is so essential.

But the strengths of great local line leaders are also their limitations. They are vitally committed to their units or teams, but they tend to pay much less attention to how others might learn from their efforts, or how they might learn from others. They can easily develop disdain for other groups less innovative than theirs. They can run afoul of organizational measurement processes and cultural taboos. They often disregard how their innovations affect other groups. By themselves, they can do little about the challenges of redesigning and rethinking. They depend on internal networkers for mentoring and to connect them to other, like-minded leaders within the larger organization. They depend on executives to develop an overall organizational environment conducive to innovation, and often for mentoring as well. By themselves, effective local line leaders generate tremendous energy, but more energy will ultimately produce more frustration without effective partnerships with internal networkers and executive leaders.

▪ **Executive leaders.** The real role of executive leadership is not in "driving people to change," but in creating organizational environments that inspire, support, and leverage the imagination and initiative that exists at all levels.

Executive leaders do this in at least three ways.

They are designers in the sense of having unique responsibilities around the formal structures within organizations—such as the infrastructures of performance measurement, assessment, and reward, formal governance structures, and the infrastructures that support learning communities. Good design will not create commitment and innovation, but poor design will surely thwart them. If executive leaders do not help in meeting the challenges of formal design, the possibilities for emergence will be limited, and innovators throughout the enterprise will be continually frustrated.

As teachers, executive leaders mentor local line leaders, especially guiding them in their interactions with those outside their teams. This is vital in dealing with the potential power clashes that the challenge of governance can bring.

Last, effective executive leaders serve as role models. They can embody genuine commitment to change through their example of "walking the talk," through their efforts to transform the functioning of top management teams, and to demonstrate genuine commitment to values and purpose. In these ways, the symbolic role of executives as stewards for the organization's long-term contribution can be as important as what they do. This stewardship extends to being convey-ors of strategic conversations. The real work of strategy, we believe, is less about setting "the strategy" than creating forums, both formal and informal, for addressing deep strategic issues that otherwise would become undiscussable, and for cultivating the collective capacity to rethink and re-create.

In general, as you progress from the challenges of initiating and sustaining to the challenges of redesigning and rethinking, executive leadership becomes more and more important. But, redesigning and rethinking always require initiating and sustaining, and it is always important to remember how limited executive leaders are in their abil-ity to genuinely initiate change. They can encourage. They can provide a compelling business case for change. They can continually work to reduce barriers to change, but they depend critically on committed local line leaders to integrate new ideas into business practices and on effective internal networkers to support and interconnect those line leaders. Likewise, their ability to really understand the "current real-ity" of the organization—how people are thinking and feeling about difficult issues and challenges—is limited. Hierarchies distort informa-tion, and they have limited usefulness in spreading new knowledge and practices. On the other hand, information that travels laterally tends to be less distorted, and most knowledge sharing occurs through informal networks. These are domains where effective network lead-ers are vital allies to executives in organization-wide learning.

▪ **Network leaders.** Many of the most crucial issues that determine the long-term course of organizational change occur at interfaces— between pilot groups and the larger organization, across functional boundaries, and between the organization and its surrounding envi-ronment. If anything, learning across such interfaces is becoming increasingly important in an increasingly interconnected world. This is why the role of internal networkers is growing in importance.

Internal networkers play critical support roles in facing the chal-lenges of initiating and sustaining within pilot teams. They are guides, advisors, active helpers, and "accessors" in the sense of helping pilot group members access resources outside the team. In challenges of sustaining they help connect local line leaders to one another, thereby reducing the isolation and misperceptions that fuel "believers and nonbelievers," as well as lead to power clashes. Since the challenges of design are as much about "enacted designs" as formal designs, internal networkers are vital at bringing new organization-wide structures, like improved community-building processes and more effective governance processes, to life.

But because they have little formal power or business accountability, they only provide leadership in partnership with line managers at all levels—local, middle, and senior managers. In this sense, the internal networkers are the penultimate example of the community of leadership that fuels all profound change. They can ill afford to live under the illusion that "they are doing it." They know they depend upon others. They know that they must develop genuine partnerships in order to be effective. Ironically, those with the least formal organizational authority may hold many of the keys to better understanding the leadership communities that will determine organizational vitality in the future.

Organizations will enter a new domain of leadership development when we stop thinking about preparing a few people for "the top" and start nurturing the potential for leaders at all levels to participate in shaping new realities. There is no real option. The re-creation of industrial-age enterprises can only happen through countless actions of thousands, indeed millions, of people.

## Creating the Future

The core leadership challenge of our era lies in addressing core issues for which hierarchical authority is inadequate. Contemporary society is afflicted with deep problems like environmental destruction, decline of community and family structures, deterioration of systems of public education, and inequity. None of these problems will be "fixed" by a few great leaders. They have arisen, or been exacerbated, as a by-product of the industrialization process. The primary agents of the industrialization process are us, our collective decision making, mediated through the large institutions of the industrial era—in particular, corporations, school systems, and governmental institutions.

It is easy for individuals to feel powerless when we confront such global problems. Perhaps this is one reason we feel that we need to wait for leaders to emerge. It is pointless, we feel, to start on our own.

But organizations, and pilot groups within them, provide a way to start together. Learning to build and sustain momentum in the face of challenges will build confidence and practical know-how. Eventually it may build momentum beyond individual organizations.

Laying at the root of the profound inventions ahead will be a slow, gradual process of rediscovering how the natural world, the living world, operates, and reorienting our institutions to embody this knowledge. The guiding image might be that of the Earth itself, as the living system which is our home.

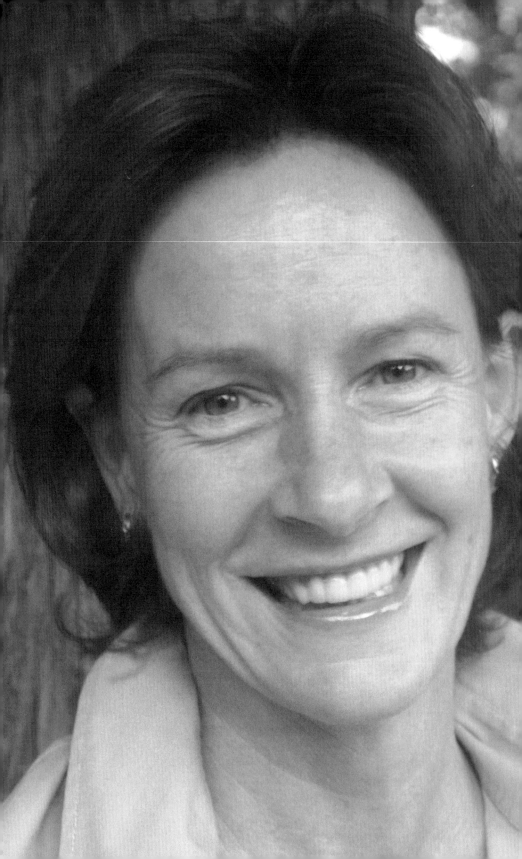

# FIONNUALA HERDER-WYNNE:

## Calling in the Magic

"**W**e stand at a critical moment in Earth's history, a time when humanity must choose its future. A future that at once holds great peril and great promise." These words, taken from the preamble to the Earth Charter, echo throughout my entire being. Everywhere I look I see the need for humankind to choose. I see it in the ruins of New Orleans; I see it in the eyes of children dying because of famine or war; I see it in the devastation our shortsightedness has exacted on the environment. And I ask myself what kind of world I have brought my son into. This is how I felt a year ago, deeply connected with the pain of this world and deeply saddened—too much change needed, not enough time.

Much has shifted for me in this last year, at all levels: on my own personal journey, the steps I take in work, the people that I have deeply connected to, and that which I see happening in the world. There is now in me a deep certainty that transformation is possible, a deep trust and joy that we can do it. And this has brought with it a powerful commitment to walk the path of my purpose and take my part in making it happen. We have to see in the world around us that it is possible for the butterfly to emerge from the caterpillar—that, in fact, the butterfly has always been present within the energy field of the caterpillar—because it is transformation that is needed. Linear change is not enough.

The challenge facing us is not that of sustainability; sustainability is

Fionnuala Herder-Wynne, Ph.D., has been active in business for more than 20 years as a new business development manager, director of innovation, and coach. She holds a doctorate in genetics, is a certified transformation consultant, and a certified energy reader and healer. She is co-founder of the Global Leadership Academy, an international network research and facilitation organization, and an active supporter of the Earth Charter business dialogue. Fionnuala and her family live in the Netherlands; she consults with companies and leaders throughout Europe. Visit www.globalleadersacademy.com and www.earthcharter.org.

not sufficient. The shift that needs to happen lies in our consciousness. It lies in our minds. It lies in how we think and our ability to re-perceive our world and ourselves. And therein lie both the great promise and the great peril. It is we who are the magic wand. It is we who can shape a new covenant with God and this earth. Only we can do it.

As leaders in business, each of us must walk the path of self-transformation. Though we have heard the call to be authentic, it is not easy to live our life's purpose. We try to avoid the tough work by creating beautiful models and conceptual frameworks for the process of transformation. Don't get me wrong, these are a necessary part of understanding the landscape, the possible paths that we can choose to travel. But an enormous fire awakens in me when I sense that we are forgetting the blood and guts of being human, because that is where we must go. We have to dive on in there and surrender to full intimacy with ourselves, with each other, with this Earth, with God. Only then can we design and enact the transformation agenda — only then will transformation be possible.

I recently spoke with a CEO for whom I care dearly, a man who has done an enormous amount of transformational work on both himself and his company, and who is preparing to play his part on the world stage. This powerful man was almost in tears as he admitted to being "scared mindless" by the realization that the universe was asking him to really understand and live the meaning of the word intimacy, the meaning of trust. And I hear the words of my dearly beloved husband, whose company is fighting for survival: "You cannot know how often I have wished to be in my power. You cannot know how it feels, to know that it is there, to have blips of it now and then, but to have no real access. To know that whatever problems I or my company and its people face, my real problem is that I am fighting myself."

So, what does transformation really mean — and what could it mean for these men? How does it connect to our daily reality, within our relationships, our organizations, and the world? What possibilities does it awaken, and how does it help to connect us with our deep power? Does it really apply to each and every one of us, or is it only possible for those able to sit on a mountain somewhere and meditate for years? What is this paradigm shift that is being talked about, what will guide us, and what can we practically use?

The paradigm in which most of us in the West grew up held that the world was linear and rational, predictable, and full of things that could be measured. This is reflected in all of our frames of reference: our economic and educational systems; the way our businesses compete with each other; the way countries and cultural and religious groups go to war over their worldviews. We live in a world where the most powerful man on this earth feels called to respond to the 9/11 tragedy by threatening that "you are either with us or against us." What kind of fear calls forth that response? The old paradigm, based on separation, was supported by a science that emphasized the duality of object and subject and told us that only those things that could be measured by an impartial observer were real. This worldview led us into technical mastery and spiritual poverty. As recently as the 1950s, B. F. Skinner pronounced that nothing without physical attributes exists. Thus, he argued, feelings do not exist; love does not exist. Even consciousness, as it has no physical basis, does not exist. Just imagine that for one moment — a world without feelings, a world without even the wherewithal to realize that it *is* a world without feelings.

But there has been a paradigm shift. Insights from fields as diverse as quantum physics, neuroscience, and consciousness studies are converging with the wisdom of the great spiritual traditions. We now know that at the most elementary level we are not just building blocks made up of matter interacting through chemical reactions. Instead, each of us, every "thing" in this universe is a concentration of energy, deeply connected to everything else in the universe by an energy field. We are not and cannot be alone; we are embedded in and embraced by the field. We make it. We are part of it. Matter, life, thinking, and consciousness emerge from it. And it is here that we make magic happen.

We literally create matter (order) from energy through our attention. The stronger and more concentrated our attention, the more powerful and deliberate we become as creators. Attention bundles and focuses the waves of consciousness that resonate between the energy field and this material world. We become the magic wand along which that energy travels. Matter emerges through us; we are the co-creators. Moreover, when we share purpose with others, we touch a deep pulse in the universe, causing the energy to resonate and form a pattern of alignment, a strange attractor[1], which inspires and motivates those it touches. So, transformation of our consciousness is both necessary and possible. It does not matter where we begin, which strand — self, organization, or society — we pay attention to, because they weave in and out of each other.

My journey has been just that, an interweaving. I move into being in this field of divine magic and get whammed back into "reality" by what is happening with those closest to me. At times I wonder what in the name of God is the point of knowing all this about magic, transformation, and being if I am totally unable to hold it with those closest to me. Having just returned from bringing my son, Benjamin, to school, I sit down to my computer and scream my head off, throat raw.

*"You put my stuff into the locker," he commands.*

*"No sweetheart—just watch the other children, they do it themselves. Other mums don't do it for them." Silence. "Do you remember where to put your fruit and juice?"*

*He stalks off, hands over his ears, and I retort, "Okay, go into school by yourself." He does. The highly enlightened me storms back to the car, gets in...and realizes, I can't do this. I rush back to kiss him.*

Transition to greater independence is difficult for my usually oh-so-loving boy—and I have not helped, entangled in my own expectations that by now I should have created a home filled with divine magic. And here I am, scheduled to visit the UK to speak about global transformation with business partners and thought leaders who consider me to be deeply intuitive and wise, and with whom I have a soul relationship. I had so wanted to be able to engage with them at that level—to be Fionnuala in her power—but I feel like a phoney. Who am I to talk about transformation when I can't even get it right at home?

So, with an enormous migraine, I do the only thing possible and tell them honestly about where I am, how I feel, and how I got here. And from this honesty emerges the magic of the trust circle.

I was a child full of energy, passion, and love, born to the tropical thunderstorms of Kumasi. But a difficult labour triggered my mother's regression into childhood schizophrenia and I lost her. Throughout my childhood I continued to lose her again and again, as eyes that were one moment filled with love shifted into a cold anger that delighted in causing pain. My father, with whom I shared a deeply intuitive love, disintegrated into alcoholism and then manic depression. We returned to Ireland, leaving the warmth of Africa far behind. Madness and delusions remained hidden behind the "happy Catholic" family front door. The burden of lies and truths untold, atmospheres you could choke in, kept us separated from family and friends and we became isolated. I was 12 years old when Dad had a total mental breakdown and fled. Financial nightmares crystallized and we left Northern Ireland as refugees with only the clothes on our back. The house and all its contents were auctioned off to pay our debts, and we arrived in Dublin homeless and unwanted. My childhood long over, I started to work and to steal in order to survive.

But there is also another story: I was conceived in joy and passion—even now I can feel my parents' happiness and energy before my birth. I have been blessed with a deep knowing, an utter trust in the world, a deep relationship with God, and the people who have come into my life. And then there has been my fire, always so very present, my passion to explore nature, science, business, and my own inner world.

All of this I shared with my colleagues as I was guided through once again feeling what it was like to be the child Fionnuala, not knowing what mood my asking would trigger: rage or coldness, the shame of asking, the rawness of still daring. I told them that the energy of my childhood experiences had closed into a circle of control around me—and the sharing itself opened up the possibility for new intimacy and trust.

Like so many others, I have exhausted myself trying to sense the danger or safety behind the masks of others; I have fearfully turned inwards, gone it alone, become caught up in perfection. But now that I have been given this gift of trust I find myself playing with it all day long, reflecting on the different kinds of magic that I have known.

There is the magic of love, which flows and heals our past and our present, opening our eyes afresh. In August 2001, Mum phoned to let me know that Dad wasn't feeling well. My intuition told me to fly to Chester immediately, and yet that whole journey was a struggle: What was I doing? Why was I going? I didn't want to get involved, couldn't forgive him for all that had happened. I told myself that there was nothing especially wrong—he'd been talking about dying for the last year and was just looking for attention. My heart hardened and closed in self-protection. But then, in my mind's eye, I saw Benjamin looking at me that morning, eyes shining with love, and I wished that I could feel that way again toward my father. On the radio, a song— *tell him that you love him...love will be the gift you give yourself*—and my heart broke.

He reached out to me in the hospital, locking both arms around my neck as I knelt in front of him. There were tears, but there was also gladness as we looked into each other's eyes. I had found my way back to loving him, the greatest gift I could give myself. Dad died peacefully in his sleep that night.

And then there is the magic of shared purpose bubbling up unstoppable, laughing and delighting to connect. It opens our being to how the world could be. In my business life I have felt this often. At the Earth Charter meeting in Amsterdam in November 2005, young and old from all over the planet came together to declare their responsibility to build a sustainable global society founded on respect for nature and the magnificent diversity of cultures and life forms. Though the business community was under-represented, one man shone. Herman Mulder, VP of ABN AMRO, had been asked to give a keynote speech on the topic of how the Earth Charter could contribute to sustainable development and economic and social justice. He stood at the podium and asked simply, "Why am I here?" And then he was still. The presence of everyone in that room was enormous. We were fully engaged with this man, who was willing to stand before us and ask himself this most basic of questions. He explained that because of what he had experienced during the meeting, he had thrown his prepared speech into the bin. He spoke to the absence of the business community, of his own personal experience, and of the role that business can and should play. He spoke to the need for deep listening and learning. The energy and magic of shared purpose was vibrantly alive, the sense of possibility resonating through the room and out into the world.

At a different scale, I have seen how the power of shared purpose can transform belief in what is possible even within long-established industry. This story opens in 2002 with a worldwide recession. Dutch paper and board companies were facing incredible challenges: strong competition, investment going elsewhere, capacity allocation decisions over which Dutch managers had no say, and the resulting sense of a lack of control over their own destiny. Fears shared at board level only strengthened the general feeling that the tide had turned against the industry.

The limit of their vision in early 2003 was "better usage of raw materials and wastage in the paper chain"—not very exciting and unlikely to awaken much creative spirit. But then the Dutch Government introduced the "transition initiative" where, via stakeholder partnerships, industry was encouraged to shoot for "man on the moon targets" to create sustainable energy balance. Literally within months the vision had dramatically shifted. The new shared intention was to become world champions, ensuring survival today and sustainability into the future. They set a target of 50 percent energy reduction by 2012! Magic had happened: a radical re-envisioning of their world, a shift in consciousness. Transition provided the vehicle for the vision of industry and government to come together and resonate with a deep pulse of purpose.

So, there is work to be done—the work of transformation. It will allow us to reclaim our birthright, to be the conduit for the divine into this world of matter. This work requires our total commitment and dedication. As my husband said, trust is the channel and honesty is the torch. Trust is the energy connection between God and ourselves; honesty is the torch by which we can see what is in the way. You see, there are different kinds of intention: conscious, unconscious, and manifest. Our thoughts are powerful forms of energy that, when focused, act like laser beams—literally magic wands—connecting this world of matter to the world of quantum possibility. But our subconscious is also sending a stream of messages that often contradict or cancel out our conscious intentions. We have to clear that channel of whatever blocks the flow. The key is to recognize that the same fear that stands in our way is also a signpost. In the Jewish tradition all obstacles are called *klippot*; they block the path of the divine. In *The Way of Flame* Avram Davis writes, "It is said that the energy of the klippot, the trickster, the Adversary—is actually a helpful angel. Its purpose is to draw us out and help us bloom." It is in the engagement that we reach for our power, that our consciousness expands and we regain our birthright. And I realize that we have created exactly the conditions under which our collective human consciousness can— and must—make the next great leap. This is our klippot, and on the other side is the Promised Land.

But the shift will also require attention and focus—what the Buddhists call mindfulness. If our thoughts are scattered across our daily worries and concerns, if we are unable to take a moment to pause and reconnect, to gather our thoughts and choose where to place our attention, we cannot become powerful creators. To be the magic wand we must bundle and focus our energy and create the bridge. But—here is the deepest magic—we don't have to do it alone. All we have to do is to *be aware* of the energy field that nurtures and nourishes us, and allow ourselves to step back into its embrace. When we can trust in this way, we are able to be and do with grace and ease, knowing that we can shape reality as necessary. The more we act from this understanding, the stronger the strange attractor pulling us into the new world.

Many of us have had to struggle spiritually in order to clear the channel and reclaim our birthright. Sometimes it feels as if all of humanity is struggling with God. Everything that we care enough to fight for will be an ingredient in the future that we are creating, for only those things that we are willing to have burned in the sacred flame can belong to the eternal. And right now that is what each of is being called to do: to find our life's purpose, to find that which arouses all our passion, to heal ourselves and others, and by doing so to manifest the divine.

What do I care passionately for? Joy, tears, courage, honesty, healing, the smiles of loved ones, eyes alight, hearts open, relationship—at all levels of being: in the home, within my community, in my business life. In the last year I have worked together with some amazing people on issues that matter to the world. I have wondered: *"Who am*

*I to aim so high and strike out so boldly?"* But wise and forthright friends have challenged me, asking, "Who are you not...?" and reminding me that the grand work is made up of small steps along the path. I am now deeply certain that transformation is possible. With this trust, the commitment to hard work is infused with joy.

We stand at the brink of the unknown. The challenges are great and the stakes high, but as we walk the path of our purpose a new world unfolds ahead of us. It is we who are the magic wand, and only we can make the change. As my father lay in his hospital bed, staring death in the face, he finally opened himself to the field of intimacy and forgiveness. We wept, the three of us, but it was as much for the beauty of coming together as for the pain of our grief. Looking back, I repeat the prayer that my mother read to us all that night:

Come as you are
That's how I want you
Don't run away shamed and disheartened
Nothing can change the love that I bear you
All will be well
Just come as you are

---

1. An attractor is like a gravitational field. A strange attractor is an energy field that pulls otherwise chaotic behavior into complex and beautiful patterns. We cannot see it, but we can feel it. It "tugs" our behaviour into its pattern; we become aligned to a certain way of being. The paradigm in which we live today is one where the attractors are based around fear, scarcity, and competition. Those coming into being are attractors based on love, compassion, and abundance.

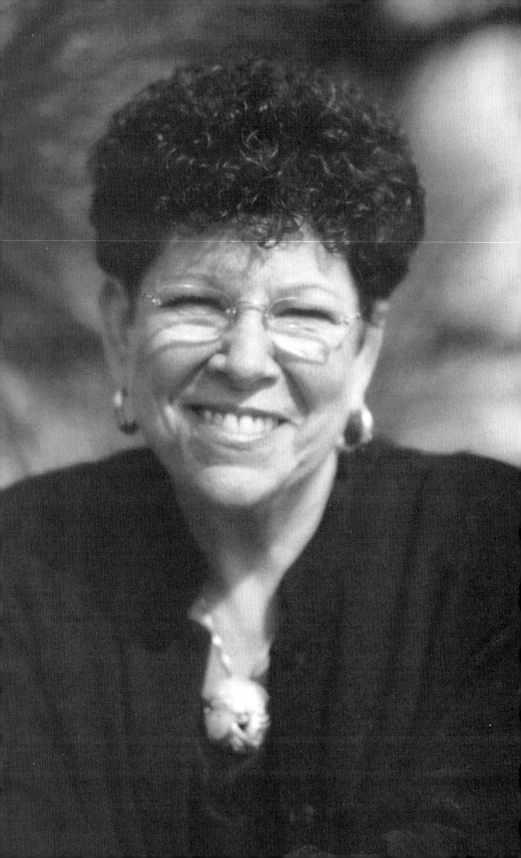

# MARGARET WHEATLEY:

# The Creative Force of Chaos

A cross the valley, the last colors of this day warm the horizon. Two dimensions move across the land, removing all contours, smoothing purple mountains flat against a rose-radiant sky. Whenever natural forces of destruction are active anywhere in Asia, the skies of Utah light up. At every twilight, visiting dust shimmers red in the air, intensifying the colors of an always-intense sky. I sit bathed in strange light, anchored by dark magenta mountains.

I move differently in the world these days since traveling in the realms of new science. The world has become a strange and puzzling place that keeps insisting I give up what I thought I knew. I don't expect to ever again feel secured by intellectual confidence. But I find life much more interesting now, living with not knowing, trying to stay curious rather than certain. In the process of playing with certain ideas for a number of years and then making the observations that have informed the core of my work, a few things about the journey stand out.

I was in this work a few years before I was able to identify its real nature. I realized that I and others weren't asking people simply to adopt some new approaches to leadership or to think about organizations in a few new ways. What we were really asking, and what was also being asked of us, was that we change our thinking at the most fundamental level: that of our worldview. The dominant worldview of Western culture — the world as machine — doesn't help us to live well in this world any longer. We have to see the world differently if we are to live in it more harmoniously.

**Margaret Wheatley is an internationally renowned speaker, consultant, educator, and co-founder and President Emerita of the Berkana Institute, a global foundation dedicated to serving life-affirming leaders. She has served as graduate faculty at Cambridge College in Cambridge, Massachusetts, and The Marriott School of Management at Brigham Young University. Among her books are *Leadership and the New Science* (Berrett-Koehler, 2006), and *Finding Our Way: Leadership for an Uncertain Time* (Berrett-Koehler, 2005). Visit www.margaretwheatley.com.**

Once I understood the nature of the work, it helped me relax and be more generous. I learned that people get frightened if asked to change their worldview. And why wouldn't they? Of course people will get defensive; of course they might be intrigued by a new idea but then turn away in fear. They are smart enough to realize how much they would have to change if they accepted that idea. I no longer worry that if I could just find the right worlds or techniques, I could instantly convince people. I no longer expect a new worldview to be embraced quickly; I don't know if I'll see it take root in my lifetime. I also know that people are being influenced from sources far beyond anyone's control. I know many people who've been changed by events in their lives, not by words they read in a book.

These people have been changed by life's great creative force, chaos. One of the gifts offered by this new worldview is a clearer description of life's cyclical nature. The mechanistic worldview promised us lives of continual progress. Since we were in control and engineering it all, we could pull ourselves straight uphill, scarcely faltering. But life doesn't work that way, and this new worldview confirms what most of us knew—no rebirth is possible without moving through a dark passage. Dark times are normal to life; there's nothing wrong with us when we periodically plunge into the abyss.

Over the past years, nudged by the science, I have come to know personally that the journey of newness is filled with the black potholes of chaos. The science has restrained me from trying to negotiate my way out of dark times with a quick fix. But even though I know the role of chaos, I still don't like it. It's terrifying when the world I so carefully held together dissolves. I don't like feeling lost and emptied of meaning. I would prefer an easier path to transformation. But even as I experience their demands as unreasonable, I know I am in partnership with great creative forces. I know that chaos is a necessary place for me to dwell occasionally. So I have learned to sit with these dark moments—confused, overwhelmed, only faintly trusting that new insights will appear. I know that this is my only route to new ways of being.

The more I contemplate these times, when we truly are giving birth to a new worldview, the more I realize that our culture is presently journeying through chaos. The old ways are dissolving, and the new has not yet shown itself. If this is true, then we must engage with one another differently, as explorers and discoverers. I believe it will make the passage more fruitful if we can learn how to honor each other in these roles. We can realize that no single person or school of thought has the answer, because what's required is far beyond isolated answers. We can realize that we must inquire together to find the new. We can turn to one another as our best hope for inventing and discovering the worlds we are seeking.

In the past, exploration was easier. We could act as patrons and pay somebody to do it for us. *They* would set sail and bring the answers and riches back to us. We still want it to work this way; we still look to take what others have discovered and adopt it as our own. But we have all learned from experience that solutions don't transfer. These failures have been explained by quantum physics. In a quantum world, everything depends on context, on the unique relationships available in the moment. Since relationships are different from place to place and moment to moment, why would we expect that solutions developed in one context would work the same in another?

So we can no longer act as patrons, waiting expectantly for the right solution. We are each required to go down to the dock and begin our individual journeys. The seas need to be crowded with explorers, each of us looking for our answers. We *do* need to be sharing what we find, but not as models. From each other, we need to learn what's possible. Another's success encourages us to continue our own search for treasure.

This need to discover for ourselves is unnerving. I keep hoping I'm wrong and that someone, somewhere, really *does* have the answer. But I know we don't inhabit that universe any longer. In this new world, you and I have to make it up as we go along, not because we lack the expertise or planning skills, but because this is the nature of reality. Reality changes shape and meaning as we're in it. It is constantly new. We are required to be there, as active participants. It can't happen without us, and nobody can do it for us.

If we take seriously the role of explorer and inventor, we will realize that we can't do this alone. It's scary work, trying to find a new world, hoping we won't die in the process. We live in a time of chaos, as rich in the potential for disaster as for new possibilities. How will we navigate these times?

The answer is, together. We need each other differently now. We cannot hide behind our boundaries, or hold onto the belief that we can survive alone. We need each other to test out ideas, to share what we're learning, to help us see in new ways, to listen to our stories. We need each other to forgive us when we fail, to trust us with their dreams, to offer their hope when we've lost our own.

I crave companions, not competitors. I want people to sail *with* me through this puzzling and frightening world. I expect to fail at moments on this journey, to get lost—how could I not? And I expect that you too will fail. Even our voyage is cyclical; we can't help but move from old to new to old. We will vacillate, one day doing something bold and different, excited over the progress, the next day, back to old behaviors, confused about how to proceed. We need to expect that we will wander off course and not make straight progress to our destination. To stay the course, we need patience, compassion, and forgiveness. We should require this of one another. It will help us be bolder explorers; it might keep us from going mad.

This is a strange world, and it promises only to get stranger. Niels Bohr, who engaged with Heisenberg in those long, nighttime conversations that ended in despair, once said that great ideas, when they appear, seem muddled and strange. They are only half-understood by their discoverer and remain a mystery to everyone else. But if an idea does not appear bizarre, he counseled, there is no hope for it.[1] So we must live with the strange and the bizarre, directed to unseen lands by faint glimmers of hope. Every moment of this journey requires that we be comfortable with uncertainty and appreciative of chaos's role. Every moment requires that we stay together. After all is said and done, we have the gift of each other. We have each other's curiosity, wisdom, and courage. And we have life, whose great ordering powers, if we choose to work with them, will make us even more curious, wise, and courageous.

For me, poetry is a way of awakening leaders and people to the deeper realms of human experience, to the mysterious, complex, paradoxical, and the spiritual.

---

1. Wilber 1985, 20.

# The True Professional
## Margaret Wheatley

*This is a "found" poem. All phrases were taken from — found — in Parker Palmer's book* The Active Life. *I then played with them and extended them beyond Parker's original prose. I wrote this in tribute to Parker Palmer for the profound influence he has had on my work.*

"The true professional is a person whose action points beyond his or herself to that underlying reality,
that hidden wholeness, on which we all can rely."

— Parker Palmer

## Illusion

Too much of our action is really reaction. Such doing does not flow
from free and independent hearts
but depends on external provocation.

Such doing does not flow
it depends on external provocation.

It does not come from our sense of
who we are and what we want to do, but from
our anxious reading of how others define us
     our anxious reading of how others define us
        our anxious reading of how others define us

and of what the world demands.

      When we react in this way we do not act humanly.

The true professional is one
who does not obscure grace
with illusions of technical prowess,
the true professional is one
who strips away all illusions to reveal

a reliable truth
a reliable truth in which
the human heart can rest.

     Can rest.

## Unveil the illusions

unveil the illusions that
      masquerade
the illusions that masquerade
as reality and reveal
    the reality
    behind the masks.

    Catch the magician
deceiving us
    get a glimpse
        a glimpse of the
truth behind the trick.

    A glimpse.
Contemplation happens anytime we get a glimpse of the truth.

## Action

Action, like a sacrament,
is the visible form of an invisible spirit
an outward manifestation of
an inward power.

    An expressive act is not to achieve a goal outside myself
    but to express a conviction
    a leading, a truth that is within me.

An expressive act is one taken
because if I did not
if I did not
if I did not take it
I would be denying
my own insight, gift, nature.

Action, like a sacrament, is the visible form of an invisible spirit
an outward manifestation of
an inward power. But as we act,
we not only express what is in us
and help give shape to the world.

We also receive what is outside us
and we reshape
    our inner selves.

When we act, the world acts back.

The world acts back
and we and the world,
we and the world are
co-created.

Right action is a process of birthing that cannot be forced
but only followed.


## Surrender

When God's love for the world pierces our armor of fear
it is an awesome experience of calling and accountability.
When God's love pierces our armor of fear
it is awesome
it is awesome to be pierced by God
to be called to accountability
to be called by God's love
for the world.

The true professional is one
who does not obscure grace
with illusions of technical prowess,
the true professional is one
who strips away all illusions to reveal
a reliable truth in which
the human heart can rest.

Reveal a reliable truth.

Let our human hearts rest.

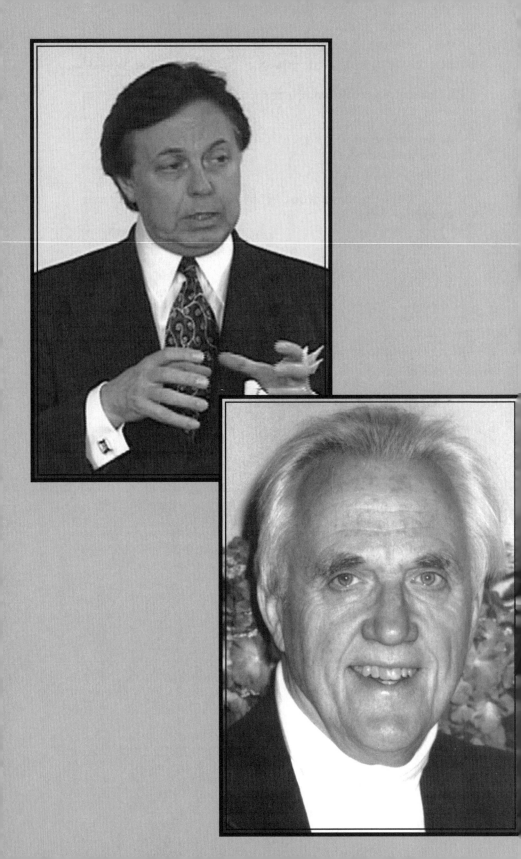

# DOUGLAS YEAMAN & NOEL McINNIS:

# The Science of Causing Outcomes

One morning when single parent Susan Bradford entered her kitchen to make breakfast for herself and her three-year-old daughter, Amanda, she found the child lying semi-conscious on the floor. Amanda had been awakened by a now subsiding storm, and had come to the kitchen to play. An open, empty pill bottle lying beside her told the rest of the story.

Susan quickly read the bottle's label, which warned that death from an overdose could occur within half an hour of loss of consciousness. Though Susan was still dressed in her negligé and her hair was in curlers, she scooped Amanda into her arms and ran to her car with the empty bottle in hand.

When the car would not start, Susan dashed back to the house to call a neighbor. The phone line was dead, as service had been disrupted by a fallen tree. Rather than lose precious time by going to her neighbor's house, Susan raced back to the car, grabbed her now unconscious child, and ran to the nearby freeway. Despite being so

Douglas M. Yeaman, founder and CEO of Quantum Management Systems, is a management consultant and trainer. He has trained over 155,000 management and sales professionals in executive effectiveness, employee performance, and corporate productivity and profitability. His training programs are in use by Coldwell Banker, Prudential, and others. He has led a national Masters group of the top 2 percent of individuals in their related industries.

Noel Frederick McInnis is an educator, author, editor, and minister. He is academically trained as a journalist and historian of ideas, and self-educated in cosmology, consciousness, subtle energetics, self-dominion, and organizational and self-transformation. He was a principal co-founder of the North American environmental education movement in the 1960s and 1970s, and managing editor of Marilyn Ferguson's *Brain/Mind Bulletin* in the 1980s.

Douglas Yeaman and Noel McInnis co-authored *The Power of Commitment* (Science of Mind, 1990). Examples of their Quantum Management Model appear at www.ProveItToYourself.com.

scantily clad, she was unconcerned about either the chilly and still blustery weather or her semi-naked appearance. She stepped onto the freeway to wave down a car, and immediately got a ride. Amanda was at the nearest hospital emergency room in just a few minutes.

Susan Bradford's masterful demonstration of the science of causing outcomes stands in stark contrast to the two million persons who undergo coronary bypasses and angioplasties each year—only one in nine of whom make subsequent lifestyle changes consistent with maintaining a healthy heart. Those who are fortunate enough not to have a heart attack before another intervention is required must nevertheless undergo additional bypass or angioplasty procedures, and often a continued series thereof.

-§-
Experience is not what happens to us, it is ratherwhat we do with what ahppens to us.
—Aldous Huxley
-§-

Why do some people act consistently in their own self-interest, as Susan Bradford did, while so many others do not? Why do some people manage to cause positive outcomes, while others persist in causing outcomes that are inconsistent with and often directly contrary to their deepest self-interest? Why, when the science of causing outcomes is the same for everyone, do so many apply it dysfunctionally? What accounts for the success of those who do choose to cause self-empowering and life-enhancing outcomes? How may those committed to life-diminishing outcomes become empowered to cause life-enhancing outcomes instead?

Answering these questions requires an understanding of how the science of causing outcomes works. This understanding begins with the realization that every outcome is caused, that all self-outcomes are self-caused, and that every person is at all times causing his or her own outcomes, whether consciously or unconsciously. With this comes the realization that all causation of outcomes is from within, which means that all power of causation is within. The potency of this realization was cited by Rudolph Steiner:

> If it depends on something other than myself whether I should get angry or not, I am not master of myself...I have not yet found the ruler within myself. I must develop the faculty of letting the impressions of the outer world approach me only in the way in which I myself determine.

It seldom occurs to most people that they have the power of personal authority to determine how the impressions of the outer world approach them. Yet this is precisely how Susan Bradford arrived at the ER in time to save her daughter's life, as evidenced in her answer to the question of what went through her mind as she read the warning label on the empty pill bottle. "I saw myself in the emergency room with Amanda," she replied. Thus guided by her intention of being in the ER, she never entertained the thought of not arriving in time. Non-divertibly programmed with an outcome, her mindset moved her to take every possible step until it was accomplished. She managed her journey to the ER from her projected outcome of already being there. Her trajectory was managed from the perspective of its already successful accomplishment.

Had Susan's mind instead been set on getting to the ER, rather than on being there, the stalled vehicle and dead phone might have impeded her progress with persistent attempts to start the car or to reach a neighbor. It was her mindset of already being at the ER that got her there so efficiently and effectively in spite of all impediment to her doing so. It was the accomplished presence-in-mind of her intended outcome—the state of already being at the ER in her own mind's eye—that assured her getting there while sensitizing her to every pertinent detail, such as carrying in her purse the pill bottle required to inform the ER doctors.

-§-
We don't see things as they are. We see things as we are.
–The Talmud
-§-

When Susan was further asked during one of our management trainings what she would have done had passing motorists ignored her, she declared, "I'd have undressed and laid down naked on the freeway—or whatever else it took—until someone did stop." Her mindset of being at the ER prevailed over all obstacles and reasons not to succeed. By thus exercising her personal authority (Steiner's "inner ruler") over her outcome, she succeeded in making the outer world's impressions approach her in the way that she herself determined.

# Reality Is an Inside Job

Access to our personal authority is via our perception, which integral psychologist Ken Wilber warns is susceptible to what he calls "the myth of the given." This myth is our belief that the world as it appears in our consciousness is the equivalent of the real thing, even though what our awareness delivers to us is deeply embedded in cultural, linguistic, and other contexts that structure our perceptions prior to their reaching our awareness. Accordingly, Wilber concludes, "what we call real or what we think of as *given* is actually *constructed*." In other words, what we assume to be presented to us as "reality" is actually fabricated by our perception, and is thus an estimate rather than a full reproduction of reality.

Nineteenth century American humorist Artemus Ward acknowledged the impact of our self-constructed givens in his proclamation that "It ain't so much the things you don't know that get you in trouble. It's the things you know that just ain't so." Our ability to perceive things that "just ain't so" is revealed by optical illusions like the one below.[1]

In the checkered board on the left, the center square is perceived as being of a shade intermediate between those of the dark and light squares surrounding it, because of the shadow cast by the pillar. Yet when it is bracketed between two columns of the same shade as

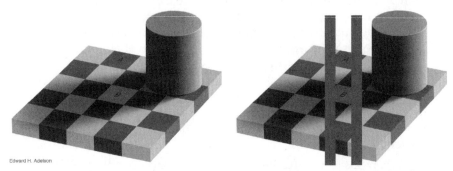

Edward H. Adelson

the dark squares, the center square appears to be equally dark. This discrepancy of viewpoints is made up entirely in our own minds, as technically explained on Adelson's website.

Optical illusions deceive us because our perceptual faculties are hardwired to see them a certain way. Similarly, as we grow up we become hardwired to see things from the perspectives of the family, social, political, and other contexts that construct our perceptions of what is given. Professor of cognitive science and linguistics George Lakoff calls our perceptual constructs "frames," which he characterizes as arbitrary "mental structures that shape the way we see the world," and signifies their alteration as "reframing." Princeton University scientist Dean Radin adds in an interview:

Our perception of the world is our own construction. We don't see the world the way the world actually is, we see the world the way we construct the world. Yet numerous experiments have demonstrated that the way we experience the world, both in time and in space, really is a construction, and that when you make very slight changes in your expectations of what you are going to see you will see completely different things.

Steiner, Wilber, Adelson, Lakoff, and Radin are just a few of legions of scholars and scientists who know that causing outcomes is a science of managing one's perceptions. It was Susan Bradford's successful self-management of her own perceptions that caused her timely arrival at the ER. As her commitment to being there overrode all barriers and obstacles to her getting there, she perceived neither the stalled car, the dead phone, nor her physical appearance as an impediment to her progress. Constructing them as such would have been the equivalent of being tricked by an optical illusion. Instead of that she exercised her personal authority to pursue alternative solutions. In doing so she epitomized the science of managing one's perceptions to accomplish an outcome.

Another example of the application of this science was demonstrated by Tim Atkins, a father who likewise participated in our management training. Tim was a skilled and competent manager who worked with hundreds of employees every day. Yet he was plagued by an ongoing conflict with his son over the boy's "horribly messy and constantly dirty room." No amount of reasoning, persuasion, or reasonable punishment had succeeded in motivating the boy to keep a neat, clean room. The resulting chronic stress was making their relationship just as messy, even though neither of them wanted their relationship to be stressful.

Father and son were caught up in the conflict or stress that occurs whenever dissonance exists between what one expects (*expectations*) and what one accepts (*acceptations*). All relationships are managed in either accordance or discordance with their participants' standards of expectation and acceptance, and dissonance prevails whenever anyone's expectations are out of alignment with his or her acceptations. This is because our standards of expectation are among the "constructs" with which we create our estimate (rather than full reproduction) of reality, and the failure of our estimated reality to meet our standards leaves us with only three choices: to let go of our standards, to let go of those who don't meet our standards, or to continue living with both our standards and those who don't meet them in stress, struggle, and conflict.

Accordingly, as long as Tim's standard of a neat, clean room was not being met by his son, and Tim continued to accept his son's presence in their home, Tim was committed to a relationship based on stress, struggle, and conflict in which he perceived the boy to be bad, wrong, and awful and therefore in need of fixing. Yet it was Tim and not the son who was the cause of their stress, by holding on simultaneously to a standard of expectation and to a person who wasn't meeting that standard.

So we told Tim several things: that having his son's room neat and clean was entirely his own standard; that the room's messiness was therefore entirely his problem and not the boy's; and that until he resolved his standard in his own mind rather than continue to project it outward on the son by trying to fix him, their relationship would continue to be conflicted. Finally, we told him that it was *his* commitment to being in conflict that was stressing his relationship with his son. Tim became quite angry at this, denying that he was committed to their ongoing conflict, declaring that the only option we were giving him was to clean the room himself and defiantly exclaiming "I most certainly won't do that!"

We all have both standards and people in our lives, but we cannot have both our standards and people who are noncompliant with them at the same time and not have conflict as well. The source of the conflict is the experience of resistance to either the standard or to the person. We must either lower our standard while keeping the person(s) in conflict with the standard or, or else let go of the person(s) while maintaining the standard.

Still angry when he got home from the training, Tim busied himself in the garage with repairing some broken furniture. While he was thus distracted, it occurred to him that his actual problem with the son's room was seeing the mess whenever he walked by it, rather than (as we had told him) the messy room itself. As soon as this was clear to him, he devised a solution. He removed the door from his son's room and sawed off the lower third. He nailed the upper two-thirds into the doorway so it would be permanently closed, then remounted the doorknob in the lower third of the door so that his son could still enter and leave the room. He then explained to his son that since he would never again see the mess it wouldn't bother him, and that the room would no longer be the occasion of constant contention in their relationship.

Many weeks later his son came to him and said, "Dad, we've got to talk. When I bring friends home from school, it is so embarrassing to have to get down on our hands and knees to crawl into my room. I'll keep my room in order if you'll fix the door."

The "first law" of causing outcomes is that all causation is internal. Accordingly, every expectation is internal to and causal from the person who has the expectation, in keeping with causation's "first law." As soon as Tim fully owned the fact that the stress in relationship to his son was a product of his own inner causation, and was being driven by his not wanting to see the messy room rather than by the outer symptom of the messy room itself, he was empowered to adopt a workable solution. He did this by managing his standard for their relationship instead of attempting to manage his son.

## Principles and Standards

The "second law" of causing outcomes is that our actions must be consistent with the principles that govern our outcomes. As defined by twentieth-century polymath R. Buckminster ("Bucky") Fuller, principles govern outcomes by causing the conditions that generate life and experience. All actions that are inconsistent with the principles that govern our outcomes therefore tend to be degenerative and unworkable.

Life-enhancing outcomes are accomplished only when the ends and means of our actions, as well as our expectations and acceptations, are aligned in mutual consistency with the principle that governs all workability:

§ Nourish spiritual values in yourself and others.

§ Doing what doesn't work does not work.

§ Doing more of what doesn't work does not work.

§ Trying harder at what doesn't work does not work.

§ Improving what doesn't work does not work.

§ Getting better at what doesn't work does not work.

§ Mastering what doesn't work does not work.

§ Committing to what doesn't work does not work.

§ The only thing that works is what does work.

The workability of action whose expectations, acceptations, ends (projected outcomes), and means (of getting there) are mutually consistent with the principles that govern outcomes is demonstrated in the science of airborne navigation, which allows little margin for error. Flight is governed by the Bernoulli principle's effect of "lift" in cooperation with the gravitational principle's effect of "fall." The projected outcome of flight is a safe and harmless landing at a predetermined destination, or elsewhere if necessitated by mechanical problems or weather conditions. The means to this outcome consist of actions that are consistent with its governing principles: impeccable equipment maintenance, traffic control, and aircraft piloting. When a flight's projected outcome and the means thereto are consistent with the principles that govern flying, a safe landing is correspondingly accomplished.

-§-
In matters of style,
swim with the current;
in matters of principle,
stand like a rock.
–Thomas Jefferson
-§-

So is it likewise with the "safe landing" of any intended outcome, be it a geographical destination, a vocational accomplishment, or the completion of some task. Acting consistently with governing principles, while keeping our actions (expectations, acceptations, ends, and means) mutually consistent with these principles and with one another, is the foundation of all life-enhancing outcomes.

Governing principles do not require that we be consciously aware of our actions in order that the principles work, they require only that we act consistently with them, although the more we are aware of them the more we can exert our personal authority over them. Our greatest problem with determining outcomes is action that is inconsistent with governing principles.

Maintaining one's expectations, acceptations, ends, and means in constructive mutual alignment is a function of the standards that govern the *quality* of our outcomes. A dramatic example of establishing such alignment is physician and professor of medicine Dean Ornish's success in getting heart-bypass and angioplasty patients to adopt life-enhancing lifestyles rather than continue with their life-diminishing habit patterns. seventy-seven percent (rather than a mere one in nine) of his patients made this change, as a result of his introduction of changes of expectation (á la Dean Radin's comment above). Expectation of longer life is insufficient to motivate changes of behavior in patients who associate a longer life with additional years to be lived in fear of dying. So Dr. Ornish persuaded them to reframe their expectations by convincing them to focus on the quality of their life by extending it for the sake of their family or by realizing that they could feel better while living longer. Ornish gave them a chance to prove this to themselves by adopting new lifestyle practices of eating, exercise, and recreation that immediately increased their experience of well-being.

Establishing constructive alignment of expectations, acceptations, ends, and means that are in organizational chaos is a daunting yet achievable task, as demonstrated by a real estate firm that was struggling to survive during America's severe 1990 housing market slump. The firm's sales force was totally entranced by the prevailing perception of a "bad market," and its co-owners were blaming each other for the downward spiral of the firm's sales productivity. I (Yeaman) convinced the firm's employees that they could outperform the sales forces of rival firms by resuming the work habits they had observed during good times, leaving behind competitors who continued to be entranced by their perception of bad times. I also mediated the co-owners' conflict by channeling its energy into a commitment to pursue the same "good times" strategy. By 1999 the firm had reframed its 250-employee culture of mediocrity into a 4,000-employee culture of excellence, thus becoming the largest privately owned firm in the industry.

When we manage our outcomes from the perspective of their already being accomplished, as Susan Bradford did, while also maintaining standards that align our expectations, acceptations, ends, and means, we are practicing the most powerful of all principles: the principle of commitment.

# The Heart of the Matter: Maintaining Commitment

Because our lives can be lived only forward, being alive is the equivalent of navigating into a headwind. Successful outcomes therefore become possible only as we act in ways that successfully engage such life-challenging headwinds as a medical emergency or a severe market slump. No matter what our current outcome may be—arriving at an ER or obsessing about a messy room—it is the result of either a conscious or unconsciousness commitment for it to be however it actually is.

Being committed to an outcome consists of pursuing it without being deterred by obstacles and barriers to its accomplishment—which we define as "maintaining a non-divertible intention." *Every* accomplished outcome is the end result of maintaining a non-divertible intention. No matter what outcome we are experiencing, it has been produced by a non-divertible intention (not always conscious) to experience it just as it is. When we are unsure of what our non-divertible intentions actually are, we can determine this by considering our current outcomes and asking, "What kind of intentions does one have to maintain in order to end up with the outcome I presently have?"

-§-
Life can only be understood backwards. It must be lived forwards.
–Soren Kierkegaard
-§-

This doesn't mean that persons committed to life-enhancement are never off course toward their intended outcome. It rather means that they conduct their lives the way a pilot flies an airplane. Since airborne vehicles tend to be drifting off course as much as 98 percent of the time, the job of a pilot (whether human or automatic) is full-time course correction. As the foregoing examples have all demonstrated, a consistent conscious commitment to continually return to a course from which we are being diverted is essential to the accomplishment of every intended outcome.

A major scientific precedent for managing our outcomes was set by quantum physicists who, when seeking to determine whether light consists of particles or waves, discovered that light invariably behaves in compliance with their experimental expectations. Light always and only behaves like waves in experiments designed to detect waves, yet just as consistently shows up as particles in experiments designed to detect particles. In both cases, experimental outcomes conform to the experimenters' expectations.

The consistent correlation between expected and accomplished outcomes led quantum physicist Werner Heisenberg to postulate, "What we observe is not nature itself, but nature exposed to our method of questioning." In other words, the questions we ask about the world determine the answers we get from the world in return. The world shows up for us by mirroring the way we choose to experience it, because our outcomes conform to the expectations that structure *and* give them substance. In other words, we manage the world of our experience from the perspective of our expected outcomes. This realization holds equally true for our unconscious expectations as it does for our conscious ones. Armed with this awareness, we realize our immense ability to shape the world to create the life-enhancing outcomes we choose.

---

1. Used by permission. A neuroscientific explanation of this illusion's deceptive dynamics is provided on the website of its creator, MIT Vision Science Professor Edward H. Adelson: http://web.mit.edu/persci/people/adelson/checkershadow_illusion.html.

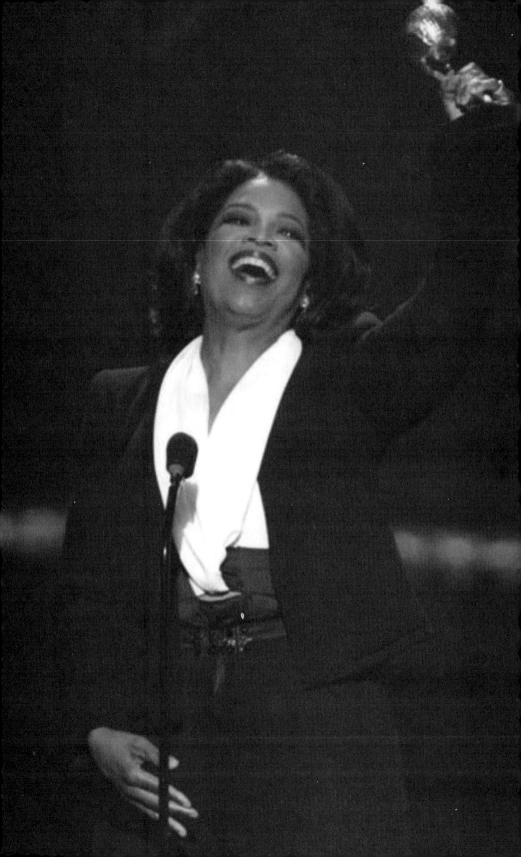

# OPRAH WINFREY:

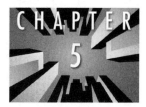

# Living the Church Inside

As the first African-American woman to become a billionaire—and to do so without pillaging her competitors or exploiting the planet—Oprah Winfrey surely deserves a place in business history. The role of the TV talk show host is traditionally that of focusing attention on the show's guests. Oprah has inverted the equation, becoming the focus of her show from her first day on the air. She has become more famous than most of her guests will ever be. An episode of her TV show is as much about Oprah as it is about the subject. Viewers and readers ask, "What is Oprah thinking? What is she interested in? What personal journey is she going through?" Though she is far from an everywoman, hundreds of millions of fans worldwide identify with Oprah, so she has become a cultural touchstone, a barometer of the emotional psyche of our society.

Oprah's family origins were not promising. Her mother, Vernita, left her with her grandmother, Hattie May, when she was four years old. Hattie Mae lived on a Mississippi farm, without indoor plumbing. One of Oprah's chores was to carry water from a well twice a day. Hattie Mae taught Oprah to read and encouraged her to memorize Bible passages—though one of Hattie Mae's favorite Bible sayings was "To spare the rod is to spoil the child." Oprah began reciting Bible passages in church, and at home to anyone who would listen. After two years with Hattie Mae, Oprah's mother took her back, but was dismissive of her daughter's desire to read. When she was seven

> **Oprah Winfrey may be the best-known woman in the world. In addition to her long-running talk show, her media empire extends into movies, books, and magazines. The Oprah Winfrey show is one of the primary arbiters of global dialog, being broadcast in over 100 countries, and including her magazines and other media, Oprah reaches hundreds of millions of people each week. Disclaimer: This chapter has not been prepared, endorsed, or licensed by Oprah Winfrey or any person or entity affiliated with Oprah Winfrey, Harpo Productions, Inc., or related properties. Her site, www. Oprah.com, receives over a million visitors a day.**

years old, Oprah went to live in Nashville with her father, Vernon, whom she had hardly ever seen. One of the first things her father did was take her to get a library card. Oprah remembers, "Getting my library card was like citizenship."[1]

At age 17, while still in high school, she got her first job as a news reader with radio station WVOL in Nashville. The following year she won three beauty pageants, including Miss Black Tennessee, and at the age of 19 she was hired as a news anchor by Nashville's WTVF-TV, at an annual salary of $15,000.

She moved to a larger station, WJZ-TV in Baltimore. Soon the station asked her move from her news anchor slot to co-host a new show called *People Are Talking*. After the first show, Oprah says, "I came off the air thinking, 'This is what I should have been doing.' Because it was...like breathing to me."[2] The TV station's management was nervous because *People Are Talking* aired in the same slot as the largest national talk show, *The Phil Donahue Show*. But within a few weeks, the Nielsen audience size ratings showed that Oprah's show was more popular in the region, due to her more personal style. When Phil Donahue interviewed a very short actor, Dudley Moore, he asked him about his forthcoming movies. When Oprah interviewed the same actor, she asked him about how it felt to date tall women, Moore's usual choice. Oprah's choice of topic was much more interesting to audiences—and her warm personal style made her guests feel relaxed enough to open up about their private lives and problems.

To critical acclaim, Oprah starred in the movie *The Color Purple* in 1985, and the following year, King World Productions bought the rights to air the Chicago-based Oprah Winfrey Show nationally, making her the first African American host of a national show. The income allowed Oprah to start a TV and movie production business, Harpo Productions, and within a couple of years she bought back the rights to her show. By the late 1980s, an appearance on Oprah could make a guest an overnight national celebrity, as Deepak Chopra and Marianne Williamson discovered.

Ophrah's Book Club, an on-air book circle, was launched in 1996; the first title discussed was Jaqueline Michard's *The Deep End of the Ocean*. The club immediately became a vehicle that could make a title a bestseller overnight. When she launched *O-The Oprah Magazine* in 2000, the first issue sold 1.1 million copies, perhaps the most auspicious magazine launch in history. Oprah starts each day with meditation and exercise, and shares her own personal journey with her viewers. She writes a column for the magazine, talking about therapies she's discovered, charities she endorses, and dispensing food as well as fashion and diet tips. Her fans talk back to Oprah, too: some 25,000 letters and emails arrive at Harpo Productions each week.

While she's the interviewer, and not the interviewee, Oprah has written and said a great deal that illuminates her values and beliefs. Here's a selection of her quotes about her journeys and discoveries that reflect some facets of this genuinely intriguing human being.

"I learned to read at age three and soon discovered there was a whole world to conquer that went beyond our farm in Mississippi.[3] Books showed me there were possibilities in life, that there were actually people like me living in a world I could not only aspire to but attain. Reading gave me hope. For me, it was the open door."[4]

"For every one of us that succeeds, it's because there's somebody there to show you the way out. The light doesn't necessarily have to be in your family; for me it was teachers and school."[5]

"If you grow up a bully and that works, that's what you do. If you're the class clown and that works, that's what you do. I was always the smartest kid in class and that worked for me—by third grade I had it figured out. So, I was the one who would read the assignment early and turn the paper in ahead of time. That makes everyone else hate you, but that's what worked for me."[6]

"If I wasn't doing this, I'd be teaching fourth grade. I'd be the same person I always wanted to be, the greatest fourth-grade teacher, and win the Teacher of the Year award. But I'll settle for 23 Emmies and the opportunity to speak to millions of people each day and, hopefully, teach some of them."[7]

"As I peeled away the layers of my life, I realized that all my craziness, all my pain and difficulties, stemmed from me not valuing myself. And what I now know is that every single bit of pain I have experienced in my life was a result of me worrying about what another person was going to think of me."[8]

"I understand that many people are victimized, and some people certainly more horribly than I have been. But you have to be responsible for claiming your own victories, you really do. If you live in the past and allow the past to define who you are then you never grow."[9]

"I am a woman in progress. I'm just trying, like everyone else. I try to take every conflict, every experience, and learn from it. All I know is that I can't be anybody else. And it's taken me a long time to realize that"[10]

"To me, one of the most important things about being a good

manager is to rule with a heart. You have to know the business, but you also have to know what's at the heart of the business, and that's the people. People matter."[11]

"I don't invest in anything that I don't understand—it makes more sense to buy TV stations than oil wells."[12]

"I'm trying to create more balance, spend more time with my boyfriend and concentrate on the things that are important. Because all the money in the world doesn't mean a thing if you don't have time to enjoy it."[13]

"I go into the closet in my makeup room and I just close the door. Here, standing among the shoes, I'll just close my eyes and pause for a minute to re-center myself. Because after I tape two shows, I know that there will be six people outside my office wanting to see me about one thing or another."[14]

"Before it was just a view [of Lake Michigan from my Chicago apartment]. And from season to season I would never see daylight. I'd come in to work at 5:30 in the morning when it was dark, and leave at 7:00 or 8:00 when it was dark. I went from garage to garage. This morning, I actually took time to enjoy the sun rising over the lake while I was drinking my cup of coffee. I actually allowed myself to see the sun reflected off the water and make it look like glass."[15]

"I've realized it's very simple things that make me happy, but that I have to be open to happiness. I have to want to be happy rather than just busy. And once I am more willing to be happy, it becomes easier for me to feel the happiness."[16]

"People have this fear of success. They're afraid if they get it, they can't keep it. I don't have a fear of it at all. Everything you do in life indicates how your life goes. I don't want to go all spiritual on you, but I just have always had this sense of connection. I was always a very eloquent child, and when I was 12 years old, I was paid $500 to speak at a church. I was visiting my dad and I remember coming home that night and telling him that was what I wanted to do for a living—to be paid to talk. I told my daddy then and there that I planned to be very famous."[17]

"For me, greatness isn't determined by fame. I don't know if you want to be famous. I don't know if you want to go to the bathroom and have people say, 'Is that you in there?' 'What is she doing?' That is the price of fame—and then reading about it in the tabloids. I don't know if you want that for yourselves, but I do believe that what you want is a sense of greatness. What Dr. King says, greatness is determined by service."[18]

"I'd like to set the record straight and let people know I really am not defined by dollars. I would do what I'm doing even if I weren't getting paid And I was doing this when I was getting paid much, much less. At my first job in broadcasting, my salary was $100 a week. But I was just as excited about making that amount of money and doing what I love to do as I am now."[19]

"The external part of my life—where I live and what I drive, and what kind of panty hose I wear and can afford, and that kind of stuff—none of that stuff in the end means anything. The thing I'm most proud of is that I have acquired a lot of things, but not one of those things defines me...it feels like something outside of myself. It doesn't feel like me. It doesn't feel like who I am."[20]

"I remember when I was four, watching my Grandma boil clothes in a huge iron pot. I was crying and Grandma asked, 'What the matter with you, girl?' 'Big Mammy,' I sobbed, 'I'm going to die someday.' 'Honey,' she said, 'God doesn't mess with His children. You gotta do a lot of work in your life and not be afraid. The strong have got to take care of the others.'

"I soon came to realize that my grandma was loosely translating from the Epistle to the Romans in the New Testament—'We that are strong ought to bear the infirmities of the weak.' Despite my age, I somehow grasped the concept I knew I was going to help people, that I had a higher calling, so to speak."[21]

"What I now feel is reenergized by a vision of empowerment in the ability to use television in a way that I know can be even more profound. To use the connection that I have established over the years with the viewers in such a way that lets them think about themselves differently, be moved to their own personal greatness."[22]

"I have church with myself: I have church walking down the street I believe in the God force that lives inside all of us, and once you tap into that, you can do anything."[23]

"Because I'm so connected to the bigger picture of what God is, I realize I'm just a particle in the God chain. I see God as the ocean, and I'm a cup of water from the ocean."[24]

"Everything that happens to you happens for a reason— everything you do in your life comes back to you. I call it 'Divine Reciprocity.' That's why I try to be kind to people—more for my sake than theirs."[25]

"What I try to do is get God on the whisper. He always whispers first. Try to get the whisper before the earthquake comes because the whisper is always followed by a little louder voice, then you get a brick, I say, and then sometimes a brick wall, and then the earthquake comes. Try to get it on the whisper."[26]

"I believe we are all given the power to use our lives as instruments. What we think is what manifests in reality for all of us. If all of us would only strive for excellence in our own backyards, we would bring that excellence to the rest of the world. Yes, we would."[27]

1. Katherine Krohn, *Just the Facts Biographies: Oprah Winfrey* (Minneapolis: Lerner Publications Co., 2005), p. 16.
2. Katherine Krohn, *Just the Facts Biographies: Oprah Winfrey* (Minneapolis: Lerner Publications Co., 2005), p. 52.
3. "Oprah Donates $100,000 to Harold Washington Library," *Jet*, Oct. 7, 1991, p. 18.
4. Alan Ebert, "Oprah Winfrey Talks Openly About Oprah," *Good Housekeeping*, Sept. 1991, p. 62.
5. Stedman Graham, *You Can Make It Happen Every Day* (New York: Simon & Schuster, 1988), p. 136.
6. Marcia Ann Gillespie, "Winfrey Takes All," *Ms.*, Nov. 1988, p. 54.
7. Oprah Winfrey, Interview, America Online, Oct. 3, 1995.
8. Laura B. Randolph, "Oprah Opens Up About Her Weight, Her Wedding, and Why She Withheld the Book," *Ebony*, Oct. 1993, pl. 131.
9. Lyn Torrnabene, "Here's Oprah, " *Woman's Day*, Oct. 1, 1996, p. 59.
10. Miriam Kanner, "Oprah at 40: What She's Learned the Hard Way," *Ladies' Home Journal*, Feb. 1994, p. 96.
11. Gretchen Reynolds, "A Year to Remember: Oprah Grows Up." *TV Guide*, Jan. 7, 1995, p. 15.
12. "Oprah Winfrey, Media Magnate," *Esquire*, Dec. 1989, p. 114.
13. Linden Gross, "Oprah Winfrey, Wonder Woman," *Ladies' Home Journal*, Dec. 1988, p. 40.
14. Melina Gerosa, "Oprah: Fit for Life," *Ladies' Home Journal*, Feb. 1996, p. 108.
15. Joanna Powell, "I Was Trying to Fill Something Deeper," *Good Housekeeping*, Oct. 1996, p. 80.
16. Pearl Cleage, "Walking in the Light," *Essence*, June 1991, p. 48.
17. Judy Markey, "Brassy, Sassy Oprah Winfrey," *Cosmopolitan*, Sep. 1986, p. 96.
18. Oprah Winfrey, Graduation Address, Wesleyan University, Middletown, Connecticut, May 1998.
19. Susan Taylor, "An Intimate Talk With Oprah," *Essence*, Aug. 1987, p. 57.
20. J. Randy Taraborrelli, "The Change That Has Made Oprah So Happy," *Redbook*, May 1997, p. 94.
21. Leslie Rubinstein, "Oprah! Thriving on Faith," *McCall's*, Aug 1987, p. 140.
22. *Broadcast and Cable* magazine, Jan. 24, 2005, quoted in Bednarski, P. J. *All About Oprah Inc.*
23. "Upfront Goes to Zip-A-Dee-Doo-Dah Lunch With Oprah," *Chicago*, Nov 1985, p. 16.
24. Melina Gerosa, "What Makes Oprah Run," *Ladies' Home Journal*, Nov. 1994, p. 200.
25. Chris Anderson, "Meet Oprah Winfrey," *Good Housekeeping*, Aug. 1986, p. 52.
26. Oprah Winfrey, Commencement Address, Wellesley College, Wellesley, Massachusetts, May 30 1997.
27. Julia Cameron, "Simply Oprah," *Cosmopolitan*, Feb. 1989, p. 215.

# PART TWO

Heart-Centered Leadership

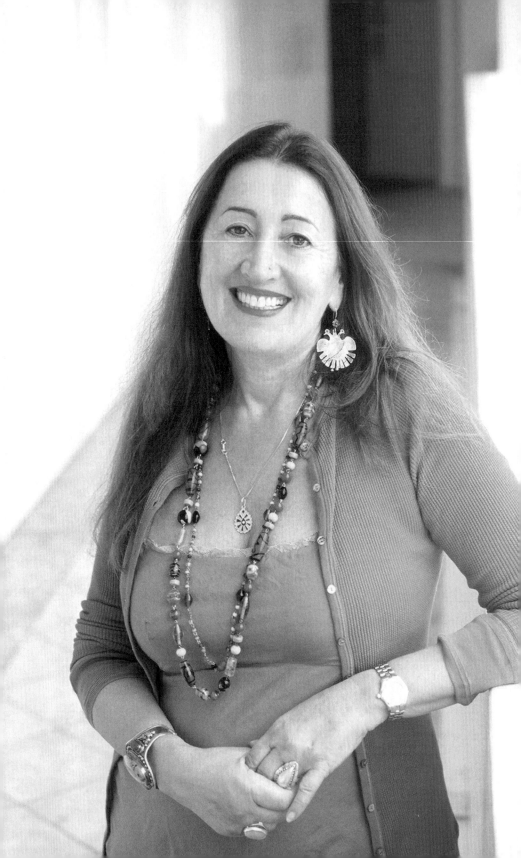

# LYNNE FRANKS:

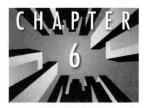

# Can Corporations Save the World?

M y vision of the world is for the creation of a new type of conscious society, where we can live and behave in a way that will bring peace, harmony, and long-term security to this planet and all its inhabitants. In order to realize this vision, one of our biggest challenges is to redefine our ideas of success.

Recently, in the context of a spiritual environment, I heard success defined as "how we can benefit others." This is a profound idea, but what struck me most was that it is the complete opposite of our traditional way of thinking about success in business. In fact, it feels far more connected to what we think of as the old ways, to the things that we have left behind in our rush forward to so-called "civilized" living.

When we think about the old ways, we think of things like agriculture and tribal community structures that seem far removed from much of our present experience. But these are actually the very things that we need to reconnect to. Technology, and the way we communicate in general, is literally shifting by the day. We continue to develop incredible tools, and yet we can learn from our indigenous people, from our own connection with what I believe is a global memory. For me, the future will have to be about combination. It cannot be about only the newest things, but about the best things. The future that I envision depends upon our ability to combine technology with ancient wisdom and a deepened connection with the Earth, with community, with each other, and with very strong spiritual values.

**Lynne Franks**—businesswoman, author, broadcaster, and speaker, described by the world's media as a lifestyle guru and visionary—is an acclaimed international spokesperson on the changes in today's and tomorrow's world. Her public- and private-sector consulting experience, global work with women's enterprise, and gift as a "futurist" have given her considerable insight into the way forward for modern individuals and society. She is the founder of SEED—Sustainable Enterprise and Economic Dynamics. Her books include *The SEED Handbook* (Hay House, 2005) and *Grow* (Hay House, 2004). Visit www.lynnefranks.com.

Of course, I wouldn't go into a consulting job with a big company and talk about spiritual values, particularly — although more and more companies in the UK are incorporating meditation into the workplace, offering quiet rooms, for instance, and yoga. But there is really no need to get caught up in the language, because spiritual or otherwise, we are talking about values. Labels don't matter when people are saying that they want to run their businesses with integrity.

The shift that is occurring involves community, and it is very much being led by women. Whether they are involved in nonprofits or entrepreneurs starting small businesses that in and of themselves will benefit the community, women in the UK are building a movement of social enterprise that is becoming a very important part of the economy. It is similar to the cooperatives in America, which are actually based on an expanded idea of the old agricultural model. In the original context, the form of doing business was very small and self-contained; but the concept has become much bigger, and we have developed a whole language and applied values that are based in the metaphor of growing things.

Large or small, a business won't stay in business if it doesn't make some form of profit. It has to be commercially viable. But what happens with this profit? How can we restructure our businesses so that they are more in line with the values of the cooperative, tribal, old ways? Women's-led small business has been working actively with this dynamic, but I think it will spread out. Things like cause-related marketing and socially responsible business practices are being adopted by all the big international conglomerates. It used to be only people like Ben and Jerry, before they sold their company, and other small entrepreneurs who were socially conscious. But their strategies are now being taken on board by a lot of large companies. They will always be concerned with making profits — that is never going to change — but they are coming to understand. Even within the context of being responsible to shareholders, it is becoming increasingly important that they work together with the resources of people and the environment.

I am on the advisory board for McDonald's in the UK. They are currently looking at how to turn their chip oil into bio-diesel. And they have just launched a huge program, which I have been involved with, to empower and educate their 16-to-24-year-old staff members. They are one of the biggest employers in the world and they are working to benefit the young people who work for them, even those who intend to move on to other companies further down the line. They are using the technology of the Internet in very interesting ways to support this education initiative. Instead of looking for the quickest, cheapest way of doing business, they are really considering the long-term situation, which will benefit the world we live in.

I've also been working with Starbucks in the UK on a six-week community project that they developed through my SEED program. Their goal has been to create empowering community initiatives for the young mothers that make up a good part of their customer base. It is the aim of any business to increase its market, but I get the sense that the intentions are quite genuine.

At the moment there are huge drives among both manufacturers and retailers to rethink packaging in order to be as environmentally friendly as possible. In addition to reducing the amount of packaging materials used, many are also beginning to switch to bio-degradables. They have to—it's market driven. One of our fastest-growing supermarket chains, which happens to be cooperative, has also been putting all their marketing energy into educating people about fair trade and organics. Yes, it's good for business, but they also want to be concerned citizens.

The shift is occurring faster here in the UK than in many places; but then, we're a little island. Information moves along here faster. And the media are actively involved, because our challenging political party has taken on the environment as one of their main platforms. Suddenly, the Labor Party—the government—is waking up to it, so now everyone is talking about the environment. There used to be an eight- or nine-month waiting list to purchase a hybrid car, but now they're coming in all the time. In the city, it's no longer considered socially acceptable to have four-wheel drive.

We're living in a changing world, from a business perspective, and some very influential companies are taking this into account. But it is really the small business owners that are leading the shift, because they have the entrepreneurial freedom to run their businesses according to their own values. And when they scale up, they are able to maintain a good deal of their vision. You can see this even in major corporations such as Microsoft, where so much money has been directed back into a foundation. Whether their philanthropy is the result of vision or clever PR, valuable, life-affirming work is being done.

Still, it isn't enough. I always considered myself an optimist, but that is no longer necessarily true. We've done irreparable damage to the environment—the glaciers melting, all those species are not coming back. In order to truly change, we will need to adopt a very different lifestyle. Those of us in the wealthiest countries of the industrialized world are kidding ourselves if we thing we're doing our part. We're sticking our heads in the sand if we think that life in the future is going to be a continuation of the way we're living now. We won't be able to travel the way we have been, driving gas-fueled cars and flying on airplanes at a whim. That is why it is so important that we use technology in the service of our true values. We need to seriously look at alternative resources like solar and wind energy, not only to get around, but also in manufacturing and operations. This is crucial, and I don't know whether we'll be able to change our habits quickly enough.

Consider the fact that in new, emerging markets such as India and China—which are already creating a huge demand for resources such as energy and water—people want what they see that we have. How do you tell someone who has finally seen their family elevate themselves from dire poverty that they are destroying the planet by buying the things we have been enjoying for so long? How do you tell them? These emerging markets are not going to go backward, and they're not going to curb their growth. But we may be forced into thinking differently. We may be forced to change our entire lifestyle.

We are living in a very unhealthy time, but if we can truly learn to live in a different way, we can rebuild a healthier society. I think about the earthquake in Pakistan, the fact that people are still living in tents one year later, and give thanks every day for my well-being and the wellbeing of my family and friends. I pray. But that is really personal growth, personal responsibility. I see everything that way. I cannot divorce business from the rest of life, so I look at my own life and think about where I need to concentrate my energy right now. The program I started, SEED, is wonderful. It is helping lots of people and it has huge potential for growth—but do I really want to put my energy and attention into that? Or do I want to work in a smaller way? How sustainable do I want to be?

The idea of sustainability is incredibly important, and yet it is so often used flippantly, without any clear definition. Even the word "value" has become devalued, because we apply it intellectually without really knowing what it means to us, or what responsibilities it imparts. Sustainability, for me, suggests a situation that supports itself and its community. Nature sustains itself, taking only what it needs. But this idea can apply to individuals, as well, and to business.

As my spiritual teachers tell me, instead of looking outward we must first look within. We must each become as aware as possible in every aspect of the way we live our lives. And if we, as individuals, can find a more peaceful interior, a more spacious way of being, then we will inspire others to do the same. Find that space inside.

Meditate; spend time in nature or with your loved ones—whatever works for you. We can affect our outward environment, but we must begin with the self.

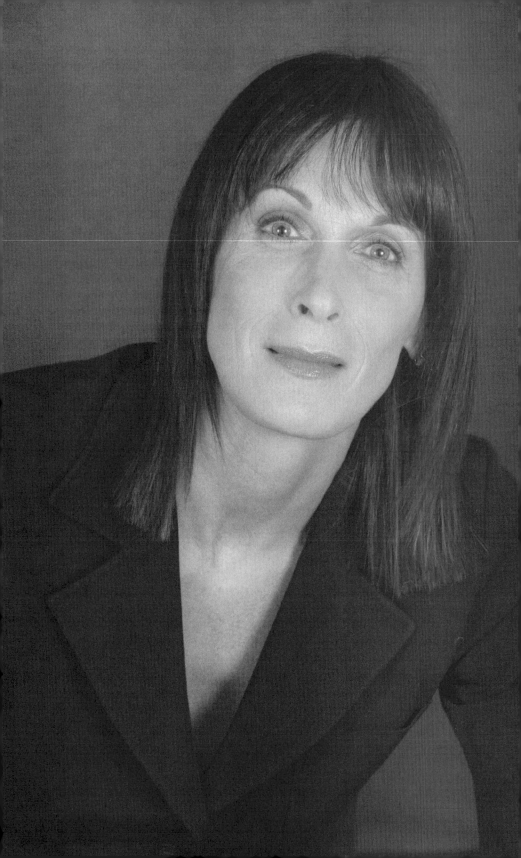

# Áine Maria Mizzoni:

CHAPTER 7

# Strength in Vulnerability

"The results show abnormal cell activity," said the Master of the National Maternity Hospital Dublin. "We'd like to operate straight away. I will personally perform the hysterectomy before I go on holidays."

I could barely get the question out, "Are you saying I have cancer?"

"Well, the tests show it's invasive, but cancer is such a broad term..."

"It's cancer, isn't it?"

"Yes. I'm sorry, it is, Áine Maria. Can you come in tomorrow?"

And I whispered "I can," but wanted to run. Instead, I headed back to the office.

From as early as I can remember, I wanted to lead and change my world—a desire birthed by the choices of my parents, a gifted teacher and an ambitious nurse and full-time mother, who spent the early years of their marriage "on the missions" in Africa, followed by time in Northern Ireland during my father's short political career at the start of nearly 40 years of armed conflict known as "The Troubles." He, too, had wanted to change the world using his repertoire of teaching, poetry, and politics.

While gifted, my parents were also deeply vulnerable people who

Áine Maria Mizzoni, MSc, CPA, is Managing Director of Grafton ESP Ireland, an international employment solutions agency. She is the immediate Past President of the Dublin Chamber of Commerce, a former member of the National Competitive Council and the Institute of Directors, a member of the North/South Joint Business Council. Her passion lies in co-creating and realizing visions of organizational transformation. She is dedicated to self-development. Her life experience has made her a committed practitioner and advocate of ethical and sustainable business. She lives in Dublin, Ireland, and shares her life with her partner, four daughters, close family, and friends.

struggled to cope with the challenging lessons and realities of life — so much so that, by the age of 12, my elder sister and I were helping to manage the household budget, problem solving for the family, negotiating the upheavals of eviction, and precariously setting up home again — only for the pattern to repeat itself. To cope as a child, I put on a hard mask and being strong and taking responsibility became a way of life.

As an adult, I became a manic, driven, task-focused woman concerned with getting my needs met in relationships. I was successful in a male-dominated corporate world, where business was "the Art of War." We eliminated the competition, drove out costs, right-sized organizations, outsourced non-core activities, and left anyone who couldn't keep up behind. We weren't vicious, just ruthlessly efficient in what I now see as a very masculine paradigm.

Then, at 34, came cancer, and I took it on in the same way. It was another battle to fight: shields up, coping, and getting on with it. After my hysterectomy, I returned to full-time work in less than six weeks, to an expanded role at a more senior level in an enlarged organization. To the outside world, all was well; my mask of invulnerability was still beautifully intact. Inside my heart and soul were breaking.

Despite the internal conflict, there was no immediate change in my goal-directed behavior. I launched into the following decade convinced that I could cope with anything and succeed at any cost. I gathered directorships and non-executive public service roles, attained a postgraduate degree and other qualifications, and attempted to be a successful mother and wife. At the same time I sought space for a journey of deep personal exploration and development. And as the insights took shape and form, the disparity between my external self and the stranger on the inside came into focus.

I struggled to invest in my relationships with my children, weighed down by my trepidations and external commitments. And while I sought more intimacy in my marriage, it was not met with a similar desire and finally the marriage ended, soulfully and in friendship.

I learned firsthand that childhood and family leave a deep imprint on our lives. To a large extent, these experiences shape our relationship with ourselves and, in turn, our relationships with those we come to know and love, as well as with the world at large.

There is a fatalistic Irish truism: What's meant for you doesn't pass you by. In another context this might be interpreted as karma. At some point the opportunity emerges to experience more inner reconciliation and peace. Within the world of work, that opportunity came to me through a job in which I took the risk of abandoning my assumptions about leadership, which had grown from years of copying macho role models, to express my authentic self while leading a business.

Grafton ESP, an international staffing organization headquartered in Belfast, was recruiting for a managing director of its Irish business. I clipped the ad and sat on it. Although the business and career opportunity appealed to me, I hesitated, fearing I would repeat past patterns and pay the price with my health and my children. Still, friends were encouraging, and always one to "feel the fear and do it anyway," I soon found myself as their new managing director.

As I stepped into this leadership role, I was determined to do this one differently. This time I would bring all of myself—my life knowledge as well as nearly 25 years of business know-how, network, and experience—to the task at hand.

Staffing is a highly competitive service industry. It attracts driven people motivated to succeed by meeting targets. They love the financial reward and they love being recognized for their successes. The culture is big on self-interest and self-exposure, and less focused on team or corporate goals. The predominant leadership style tends to be that of carrot and stick: wrap your arms around those individuals who succeed, and beat up on those who are underperforming.

My task seemed fairly straightforward at the outset: I was to take this business to the next level. Specifically, that meant putting together a business strategy to build shareholder value, professionalize the organization, provide leadership to a young team, and shape the business on an all-Island basis: both Northern Ireland, or "the North," and the Republic of Ireland, "the South."

We were a geographically dispersed staffing agency, with a tendency to operate in silos and stark differences between the success and underlying business performance of the northern and southern companies. Flying in the face of sustained economic growth, the southern business was a substantial loss maker while our northern business, in a much smaller, predominately public sector-dependant market, returned excellent market share and above average profitability.

Our strengths lay in a network providing local access for clients and candidates, a strong team of human resource experts, and the passion, commitment, and energy of many managers and recruiters who knew the agency business inside out.

The vision was to transform the business into an all-Island employment solutions agency. Our aim was to deliver a consistent, high quality candidate and client experience. In market terms, we sought to focus on emerging, growing, and profitable sectors of the Island economy and align our brands with these sectors. We also wanted to become an employment solutions outsourcer, to whom companies could turn to when they chose to outsource not only recruitment, but also their nonstrategic human resource requirements.

From where we stood, it was a significant leap forward.

To realize the strategy, we needed to build our internal capability with a substantial change program that addressed people, process, and technology issues and opportunities. There was no person or part of the organization untouched by the change program. We also needed to transition the culture from a "sales at all costs" foundation, to a wider focus on profitability, cash flow, and performance, measured against a comprehensive range of interrelated indicators.

Up until then, the business had grown very successfully by a heavy reliance on a small number of people who held "the crown jewels," some driving the heavy sales focus, others busy with control. However, this was an inadequate basis to hold the business together at its current size and complexity, never mind facilitating the levels of growth and diversity we wanted to accommodate in the future.

One of the most challenging things we were trying to transition was the predominant leadership style of "telling and selling" to each other. This entrepreneurial style was well embedded, having delivered much historic success. However, while the inheritance carried many successful dynamics like the idea that "success breeds success," it also inculcated some self-defeating ones too, such as our predisposition for apportioning blame. This was brought home to me one day when a member of my management team said, "Success has many fathers in this business, but failure is an orphan!" In other words, if a business venture, idea, or project was not successful, there was likely to be lack of ownership and a tendency toward pointing the finger of blame. Consequently, upward delegation and a lack of true ownership were gathering momentum, from the grassroots of the organization through to the top. The stress this placed on our fast-growing and increasingly more complex business was becoming unbearable.

Unsurprisingly, therefore, the management team felt that leadership and cultural development was an incredibly important part of the change program. Intuitively they knew that a coaching program that would encourage people to facilitate the performance of others, to share best practices, and to take personal responsibility for problem solving and leveraging opportunities, was paramount to the success of the strategy. And they were right.

Boards and shareholders are hungry for short-term results, and Grafton ESP was no different. So while there was an understanding that the change agenda was significant, there was also anxiety that the new strategy not only made sense on paper but proved itself in practice. They needed quick wins to build their confidence.

Conflicts began to arise as we pushed forward with implementation. While everyone was enthusiastic, the substantial resources, commitment, and investment required placed heavy demands on young and relatively inexperienced business managers. For a period of time, it caused us to turn our focus inwards and away from sales and quality of service. In addition, in an effort to turn the South around, we redeployed some strong managers and training resources away from the North. And the strategy introduced an array of concepts and jargon into a world of people and chemistry that had grown from a bottom-up (local market, entrepreneurial focus) to a top-down strategic visionary approach.

Two quarters into the change program the inevitable happened: the northern sales and profit numbers started to slide, while the South showed insufficient liftoff.

Some parts of the strategy just didn't work, because they were not well enough thought out or did not sufficiently leverage the "crown jewels" and thus important things got missed or left behind. Also, execution fell short of the concrete goals established, due to the managers' relative inexperience in planned strategic change (versus organic entrepreneurial change) and because the carriers of the crown jewels were holding day-to-day operations together while heavily participating in the change program. Finally, there was a relatively high degree of "brokenness" in the old way of doing things, and as we advanced forward, cracks very quickly developed into deep fractures. So, things began to look in disarray and the confidence of shareholders and the Board started to wane.

Bringing all of oneself to a task or project is easily said but rather more difficult to do, as there are so many embedded personal behaviors, operating styles, and patterns that are hard to change. I found that while I could walk the talk on a one-on-one basis, I felt paralyzed in doing so with teams and larger groups.

With the numbers running against me and my behavior not reflecting my ideals, I began to lose self-confidence and sensed that key people were losing faith in our ability to deliver. However, I felt unable to let go of my objectives to realize the strategy, deliver the short-term numbers, and stay true to myself. Something radical needed to change. But when would the numbers start to come good again, the strategy take hold, and confidence be regained? As is often the case, the tipping point wouldn't be reached until we had nothing left to lose and very little left to give.

I felt the weight of the world on my shoulders as the 7:35 train pulled out of Connolly station, Dublin. We were heading into another quarter of tough targets, and the change program was crippling us. I was scheduled to introduce our first coaching program in Belfast, and I sighed heavily, hunched over the delegate list, searching for inspiration. I needed the audience, a group of northern and southern managers to fully engage in a personal development contract that I felt was important—for them and for the business. I was blank, floored by complete and utter exhaustion. In that empty space inside me was a space for possibility that felt easeful, yet unconventional and scary.

Three hours later, I was sitting quietly among the group, combing the words in my head and feeling tense, as I do before I speak. The program facilitator finished her introduction and suddenly it was time. I stood up, and in that moment I found the strength and grace to drop my mask of invulnerability in front of peers and colleagues.

"I titled this program, Leadership Starts with Me," I said. "And I guess as you sit there you're thinking, 'well she's the Managing Director, so leadership must start with her!' I can tell you, our shareholders and Board think so, too. But it's not true. Leadership starts with you. Leadership of this business, just like leadership of your life, starts with you."

I took a deep breath and continued. "Ten years ago this week I came home from a family holiday to a telephone message that stopped me in my tracks. Three days later I was recovering from surgery brought on by a cancerous tumor. I was devastated, afraid, and grateful that it had been caught in time. In the weeks and months ahead, I felt I was in a time warp.

"I was full of fear, afraid that I might not see out my four daughters' childhoods. And gnawing away at me was an insight I found deeply disturbing: If I die now, there isn't a headstone large enough to engrave all the things not yet done, all the people not yet met, and all the experiences not yet lived. Included on that long list was taking responsibility for fully developing my own potential as a person and as a business leader. And from that point on, I did."

I looked into their eyes and said, "*Life is short, live it well; be your best because you're worth it.* This program is as much about you as it is about Grafton ESP. And if you don't make it yours, it won't be ours. Come join me in leading this business."

As group after group of managers went through the coaching

program, the penny began to drop. They got that leadership started with them and that an important part of their job was to coach for success in others. They got the importance of cross-organizational teamwork in delivering our short-term numbers and in becoming a best practice-quality business. They grasped that longer-term, superior performance was grounded in many things including living the brand values of integrity, collaboration, resourcefulness and responsiveness. And finally, they began to more fully embrace and take ownership of the changes that were happening on the ground.

By building our capability from the inside out, we were able to reposition Grafton ESP in the market. Our promise to clients and candidates is "We're here to put you first." We do this in the knowledge that there is much yet to do. But we trust in our investments and in our people to deliver.

For the company, the program provided a bridge across tomorrow. It respected the heritage and the strengths that made us who we were today, while recognizing what needed to change in order to *draw in,* and not just *drive toward,* the vision.

There were a small number of people who, in the eyes of our shareholders, embodied the heritage of Grafton ESP. And I have chosen an extract from one of their accounts to explain the impact of the coaching program and vulnerable leadership.

*The coaching program inspired me to take responsibility for my own destiny and stop placing invisible limits on myself. It helped me to make some very difficult decisions in my work and personal life. I still find it incredibly difficult to reveal my soul and seek support when I need it, but I am making progress. I realized I was spending insufficient time thinking about the future of the business, the people I was responsible for, myself, and my home life. It started to dawn on me that it had been easier and quicker to give my team the answers than to help them find their own. Using my new coaching skills, I encouraged my managers to take more responsibility for their performance and their destiny. "Leadership starts with me" is a mantra I will use for the rest of my life.*

I believe that inside ourselves are all the answers we need for this lifetime. When we empathize with another human being as they struggle with their personal process of choice making, we give a priceless gift. This is every bit as true in the workplace as in the rest of life. The coaching program gave Grafton ESP the framework within which to make supportive presence an integral part of how we do business. It provided a simple tool kit that managers could use to become coaches to each other and to their teams.

Vulnerable leadership is centered in the natural balance between the feminine (potentiality, creativity, nurturing, and vulnerability) and masculine (formulae, strategies, weaponry, and strength) within each of us. It requires that we be prepared to reveal our truths in a balanced and disciplined way in order to authentically engage with employees, colleagues, and other stakeholders.

In stepping into vulnerable leadership, we recognize that all change starts with self, and that at the core of business, as with life, are our human relationships. When we truly live from this knowledge as business leaders, we commit to developing ourselves to our full potential as human beings, not just as masters of business and entrepreneurship. And we take on the responsibility to encourage our employees to do the same, and to invest in that development.

Our leaders need to find this balance not just for the sake of business, but more importantly, because of the power and influence that business and business leaders exert in the world today. If we are in business then we are as much part of the problem as the solution. If we accept that all change starts with the self, then we have a choice: ignore that right and responsibility or do something about it.

I chose the path of vulnerable leadership, trusting in the face of adversity that the management team had its own answers, that they would find those answers, and that they might listen to and believe in their Managing Director when she had hit rock bottom and felt and looked her worst. This is what vulnerable leadership is, fully embracing the feminine as well as the masculine in the hard-nosed realm of business.

As Grafton ESP Ireland stands today, we will do our numbers this financial year and have turned the corner with our southern business. The change program is well past its midpoint and holding ground. The vision is becoming reality. Outside of Ireland, the Grafton ESP international businesses are looking to us and to what we have learned.

So, job well done? For me, this is a work in progress, a model that illustrates the fact that if we are to bring about ethical and sustainable change, we need to find new ways of leading our businesses. The leadership and cultural contract we build with our workforce is central to our success. Contracts such as the one we have made must both address the raw realities of business and put "being human" back into the business vocabulary. This requires a willingness to trust in vulnerability and potentiality, within ourselves as well as within the roles we play in the workforce.

Frankly, I don't think this paradigm shift will be an easy one. Today's business world is very tough—it's full of self-interest and suffers from attention deficit disorder. A trusted associate said to me recently, "Be careful Áine Maria, or they will think the corporate conscience has arrived in the boardroom." I hope she has.

I want a better world for my children. That means I choose to be my best and to accept that change starts with me. So, despite the many, many times I ditched it, ignored it, and pretended it wasn't there, at 45 years of age I have found the wisdom and grace to embrace what I knew when I came into the world.

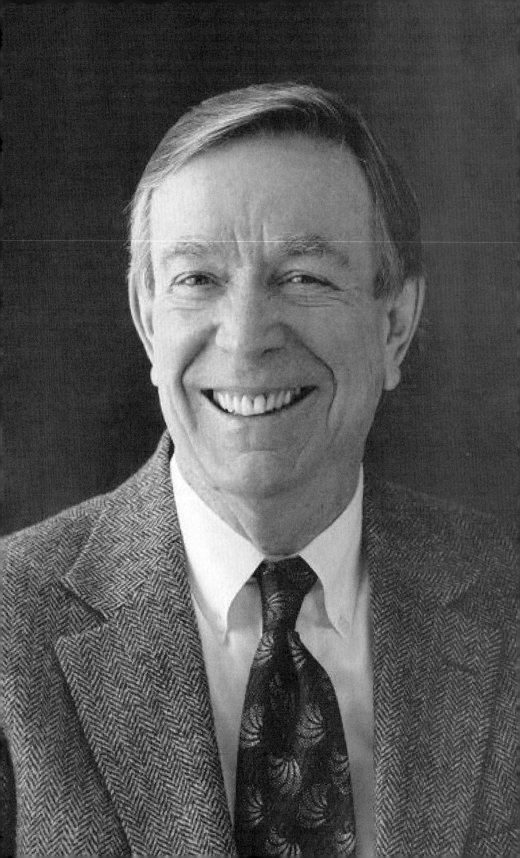

# RAY ANDERSON:

# Doing Well by Doing Good

In the summer of 1994, customers began to ask a question that we had never heard in 21 years of business: What is your company doing for the environment? The salespeople were stymied and couldn't respond. Eventually, the question made its way to my office in Atlanta.

As the world leader in the design, production, and sales of modular carpet and commercial fabrics, as well as a leading producer of broadloom carpet, Interface has manufacturing facilities on four continents and we sell our products in more than a hundred countries. Our company impacts not only global commerce but the earth's ecology as well—nearly every product we produce is petroleum-derived, and the energy used to manufacture and transport our products depends on petroleum, which contributes to greenhouse gases. In addition, many of the processes used in carpet making are water- and chemical-intensive. Our industry offers many opportunities to pollute.

However, since we had always followed all the necessary laws and regulations, including those regarding environmental protection, I assumed we were doing enough. As our customers' questions continued, however, we knew we had to find some answers and so created a task force composed of people from our businesses around the world. The leaders of this task force asked me to kick off the first meeting with a speech outlining my environmental vision. There was

Ray Anderson, founder and chairman of Interface Inc. interior furnishing company, is recognized as one of the world's most environmentally progressive leaders in sustainable commerce. He served as co-chairman of the President's Council on Sustainable Development during the Clinton administration and has been recognized by Mikhail Gorbachev with a Millennium Award from Global Green in 1996. Ray Anderson serves on the boards of The Georgia Conservancy, the Rocky Mountain Institute, and the University of Texas Center for Sustainable Development. He holds honorary doctorates from North Carolina State University and the University of Southern Maine. Visit www.interfaceinc.com.

a problem, though: I didn't have an environmental vision. I tried to write that speech, but could never get beyond, "We obey the law. We comply." Even I knew that "comply" was not a vision. I kept dragging my feet, but finally relented.

As if by pure serendipity, a book landed on my desk at that propitious moment. It was Paul Hawken's *The Ecology of Commerce.* I picked it up, not knowing what it was about or who Paul Hawken was. As I thumbed through it, a chapter heading caught my eye: "The Death of Birth." Startled and a bit mystified, I began reading to find out what that meant. "The death of birth" is a phrase coined by Harvard biologist Edward Wilson to add poignancy to the idea of species extinction—species, disappearing in great numbers, never again to experience the miracle of birth. I continued reading.

My wife and I read the book together at home, and we often wept as we read. Hawken's central point is that all the life support systems of the earth are in decline, putting the biosphere itself—which supports and nurtures every living thing on earth, including us—into decline, and there is not much time left to repair the damage and restore the biosphere. The biggest culprit in this scenario, he wrote, was the linear, take-make-waste industrial system, of which my company was an integral part.

I got it. It was an epiphanic experience—a spear in my chest, as I've often called it since. Compliance with the existing law was not nearly enough. I was convicted then and there as a plunderer of the earth.

Fortunately, Hawken did not end his book with the condemnation of industry. He left us with hope. He said the system doing the most damage—the institution of business and industry—is also the only one that is large, powerful, pervasive, wealthy, and influential enough to really make a difference and lead humankind out of the mess it is making of the biosphere.

I wrote that speech and delivered it to the small task force of about 16 people, telling them what I had learned. They were as stunned as I had been, and we wept together as I spoke. I challenged them to lead our company not only to sustainability but beyond, to being a restorative company that would put back more than it took and do good, not merely no harm. Not only would we eventually never have to take another drop of oil from the earth, we could even help restore some of the damage that had already been done.

And I let them set the deadline to accomplish this feat. They initially chose the year 2000, but later, as the people of Interface became more and more engaged and the magnitude of the challenge became clear, the deadline was re-established as 2020. It would take at least that long to accomplish this monumental transformation.

The task force met for two days, and then I came to meet with them again. They explained that they had, perhaps, found a glimpse of what sustainability might mean for Interface. But what did restorative mean? "That sounds like perpetual motion," they said. After some discussion, we decided that if we could gain a clear understanding of what sustainability meant to us and then move in that direction in a demonstrable, measurable way, we might also influence someone else, such as competitors or another businesses, to move in that direction, too. It would be this influence on others that would make Interface a restorative company.

Still later, we created a formal statement to keep us on track through the long transformation ahead. We call it Mission Zero: Our promise to eliminate any negative impact our company has on the environment by the year 2020.

## The Interface Plan

The real plan began to emerge after about two years of intensive work by many people. It flowed from such questions as, How do we do this? What does it truly mean to be sustainable and restorative? What technologies will be necessary — do they even exist? If not, how do we create them? How will we pay for all of it? I wrote about the plan in *Mid-Course Correction: Toward a Sustainable Enterprise: The Interface Model*, which came out in 1998. The Interface plan is the heart of the book. I think it applies to all of industry. Since 1996, we've been executing that plan and making amazing progress in becoming part of the solution and an example for others.

We created a metaphor to describe our process: climbing Mt. Sustainability. This mountain has a very large footprint, which is Interface's negative impact on the earth. Our goal is to meet at the top one day, at the summit, symbolizing no footprint at all. To do so, we need to conquer all seven faces of Mt. Sustainability:

1. **Eliminate Waste:** Eliminating all forms of waste in every area of business

2. **Benign Emissions:** Eliminating toxic substances from products, vehicles, and facilities

3. **Renewable Energy:** Operating facilities with renewable energy sources — solar, wind, landfill gas, biomass, geothermal, tidal, and low impact/small scale hydroelectric or non-petroleum-based hydrogen

4. **Closing the Loop:** Redesigning processes and products to close both the technical loop and the natural cycle, using recovered petrochemical products and bio-based materials

5. **Resource-Efficient Transportation:** Transporting people and products efficiently to reduce waste and emissions and offset the irreducible

6. **Sensitizing Stakeholders:** Creating a culture that integrates sustainability principles, engages all stakeholders, and improves people's lives and livelihoods

7. **Redesign Commerce:** Creating a new business model that demonstrates and supports the value of sustainability-based commerce—selling more service and less stuff

We have made significant progress since that small beginning in 1994, moving about 40 percent of the way to the top of Mt. Sustainability. Here is only one example of that progress. Traditionally, when old carpet is removed, it is thrown into a landfill, and it may remain there for thousands of years as the earth tries to digest it. Waste fiber from our carpet and textile mills used to experience the same fate. Now, under our program of eliminating waste and closing the technical loop, we have diverted more than 85 million pounds of material from landfills since 1995, with much of it being recycled. All told, we have so far saved $300 million simply by eliminating waste of all kinds from our operation, bringing us more than halfway to zero waste. This alone has more than paid for the rest of our sustainability programs—for research and development, for capital investments, and for process changes.

As a result of this broadly focused effort to eliminate our footprint, we've been the recipients of so much goodwill in the marketplace that we couldn't have bought it with all the advertising in the world. Along with our costs going down because of those waste savings, our products are better than they've ever been, inspired by sustainable design. Our customers are embracing what we're doing, and our profits have increased. We are doing well by doing good.

Sustainable characteristics of a product or a service add to the value proposition. We've taken an oath to never knowingly foist an inferior product on our customers in the name of sustainability, but we do believe that sustainability characteristics are part of the value equation, and we don't hesitate to reflect that in the prices that we quote. Our customers are willing to pay because they, too, accept the value proposition.

To those people who say becoming sustainable costs too much, I would say we have proof that the opposite can be true. The marketplace is supporting us, our products are better than ever, our costs are down, and our employees' motivation is up. We've proven there's a better way to make a bigger profit. As other companies buy into the model, that's the way the whole system moves.

Even so, we still have a very long way up to the top of the mountain. Technology has been our biggest challenge in this transformation. Some of the technologies we're now using didn't exist when we began. Some are in development but are not yet commercial, and it may take a long while for them to become commercial.

I've been asked if laws or regulations have been a roadblock to all the changes we're making, and the answer is not in the least. For a sustainable company, there's no regulatory process on earth that's going to affect it. The regulatory process is made not for the early movers, like Interface, but for the never-movers. In any paradigm shift, there are the early movers, then the fast followers, the vast middle ground of the mainstream, and finally the never-movers. We're an early mover, and the regulatory process is irrelevant to us.

## Biomimicry

Along with the image of Mt. Sustainability, we came upon another metaphor to keep us focused on our ultimate goal of becoming a restorative operation. Have you ever wondered how a forest works? The answer is so complicated that no one knows. Yet, a forest, like all natural systems, is composed of myriad symbiotic systems working together to create true sustainability; given the right conditions, it is infinitely restorative. If we can figure out how a forest works and mimic that in our industrial processes, we will have the model for the next Industrial Revolution.

This concept is called biomimicry, and Janine Benyus described it in *Biomimicry: Innovation Inspired by Nature*. She wrote, "Biomimicry is the process of learning from and then emulating life's genius. After 3.8 billion years, life knows what works and what lasts here on Earth. Mimicking these designs and strategies, 'recipes,' could change the way we grow food, harvest solar energy, run our businesses, even the way we make materials."

She described the nine operating principles in nature that we are working to emulate in Interface operations:

1. Nature runs on sunlight.
2. Nature uses only the energy it needs.
3. Nature fits form to function.
4. Nature recycles everything.

5. Nature rewards cooperation.

6. Nature banks on diversity.

7. Nature demands local expertise.

8. Nature curbs excesses from within.

9. Nature taps the power of limits.

Look at a single tree, for instance. Its root system not only takes from the earth, it gives back to the earth. A tree also transmits nourishment to other trees via its roots and receives nourishment back. Using sunlight, the ultimate energy source, the tree produces chlorophyll, which makes the leaves green in the spring and summer. But when the leaves turn red and gold in the autumn and then fall from the tree, the chlorophyll doesn't disappear. The tree husbands this valuable resource throughout the year. A tree also produces shelter and food. The tree understands the power of limits — it doesn't grow to the sky. Rather, it lives in mutual dependence and cooperation with its neighbors — flora and fauna.

In the current industrial system, we disregard most, if not all, of these natural principles in our linear, take-make-waste systems. We are depleting the earth's resources and allowing waste to accumulate in the biosphere, thus destroying natural, cyclical, living systems. At Interface, we are redesigning our processes and products into cyclical material flows where waste becomes food. For example, we're working to use petroleum-derived materials over and over and over again, to give them life after life after life. This means using technologies to close the loop on material flows so that the product is retrieved at the end of its first life to give it new life, then another and another. Another example is using the waste products from other industries as our raw material. We invested in a huge range of processing machinery to recycle a variety of raw materials to make carpet-tile backing, and we are scavenging in other industries to find their waste products to feed this machine. Like nature, we are using waste — even if it comes from a company that has nothing to do with carpet making — as raw material. We are also working to keep natural organic materials uncontaminated so they can safely be returned to their natural systems.

## Other Successes

Fossil fuels have always been Interface's most important raw material, and they play a huge role in transporting our products. When we first began implementing our plan in 1996, oil was $15 a barrel, so many people thought we were foolish. But since the price of oil has skyrocketed, the improvements we've made have given us a huge competitive advantage that plays well even with Wall Street—we're more efficient than our competitors because we're using less fossil fuel to generate a dollar of business. Additionally, even as our business has grown, we've reduced our net greenhouse emissions by 56 percent in absolute tons. (The Kyoto Protocol, which the U.S. has thus far refused to ratify into treaty, calls for only a seven percent reduction by 2012.)

Other products are coming to the market to replace petroleum in carpets and textiles, and we are taking advantage of that. Some of our textiles include a new kind of fiber, made from corn dextrose and bioengineered by Cargill to produce a polyester-like material. This is one instance of the dawn of the carbohydrate economy, which eventually will stand beside if not replace the hydrocarbon economy.

Many Interface employees fly frequently for business, and air travel is a large contributor to global warming. So we created an internal program called Trees for Travel whereby we sponsor the planting of trees to offset the $CO_2$ emissions resulting from our business air travel. Since 1997, we have sponsored the planting of more than 62,000 trees, enabling Interface to positively effect benign emissions and resource-efficient transportation.

We have already influenced other companies by our example, thus beginning our restorative mission. Every one of our competitors has had to create some kind of green initiative. Without someone setting the example, they might never have done so. Ten years ago, one of our competitors looked me in the eye and called me a dreamer. Today, he's scrambling to catch up.

Our own employees have also benefited from our new goals. Many of them have found new purpose in their work. If you were to walk the factory floor in an Interface plant and ask one of the employees, "What is your job?" he or she very likely would tell you, "To save the earth," as opposed to "Run this machine." They realize they are a part of something good and different—a higher purpose. There's a pride that comes with that.

Finally, we can't forget the power our customers wield. They were the ones in 1994 who pushed us to make these changes. They were the ones who inspired us. The demand side moved the supply side—since then an entire industry has been co-evolving to a better place.

When we enjoy a favored position with our customer, our competitors wonder why they lost that business. If they ask our customer for a reason, the reply might well be, "Interface is for real, they're sincere, and you're not." Our competitor will have to consider that and maybe even change. The power is with the people in the marketplace. They can make change happen by demanding the ethical, sustainable production of products.

For many companies considering this journey to sustainability, the easiest place to begin may be with their buildings. Because the United States Green Building Council (USGBC) has established its consensus-based LEED (Leadership in Energy and Environmental Design) rating system, green building characteristics have been effectively codified. The good news for the earth is that LEED is rapidly moving to mainstream.

The sustainability movement, of which green building is a part, is gaining momentum throughout America — not just because it is the right thing to do, but also because it is the smart thing. The reason is as old as the story of the goose that laid the golden eggs. The earth is the goose. We must not squeeze it to death.

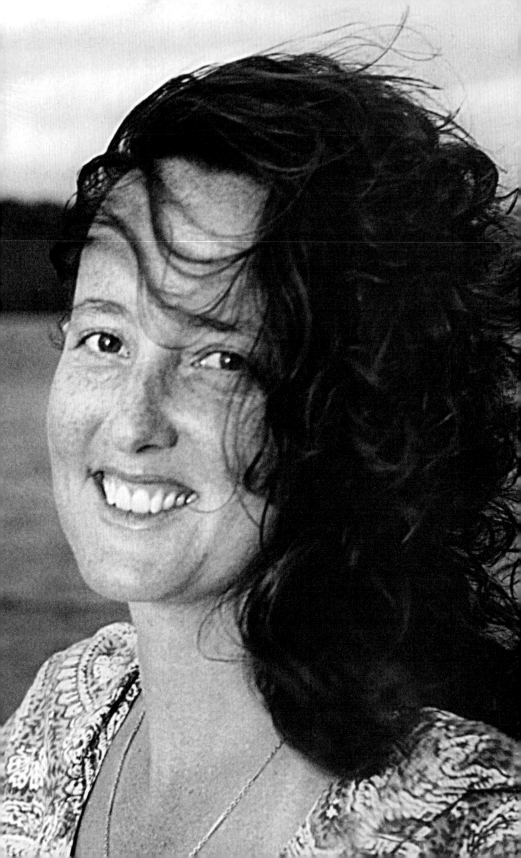

# JULIE GERLAND:

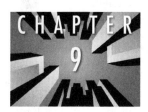

CHAPTER
9

# The Voice of Conscience

T he man's face changed suddenly, a frown replacing his smile. "Are you telling me," he asked solemnly, "that if I go home and kick my cat and beat my wife, that has something to do with peace in the world?"

"Yes," I beamed, delighted to be sharing my innermost convictions with someone so "important."

"Julie," he concluded, shaking his head, "I thought you were an intelligent young woman. Now I know we have nothing to say to each other."

If the world is run by people who think like he does, I thought, it is definitely not going to improve.

In 1980 I was an idealistic 21-year-old working at the United Nations in New York issuing planetary passports for a nongovernmental organization called Planetary Citizens. It was there that I met with this elderly member of the U.N. Disarmament Campaign, who had worked with the organization since soon after the League of Nations was founded. I had spoken of inner peace and of how if individuals were peaceful, we wouldn't have wars. I told him that if we didn't plan for wars, we could feed and provide clean drinking water for the whole human family.

Over a quarter of a century after the first planetary passports, however, the concept that we are all citizens of this beautiful planet

Julie Gerland has, for more than 30 years, inspired and helped countless numbers of people to heal and transform their lives from soul to cell. She is co-founder of Association Suryoma and director of The Holistic Parenting Programme: Preconception to Birth & Beyond, which empowers parents and training professionals to participate in the regeneration of humanity. Julie and her husband François are co-founders of Providence, a holistic community in the French Pyrenees, where they live and receive people from around the world for individual stays, sessions, workshops and professional trainings. She travels and teaches internationally. Visit www.suryoma.com, or contact julie@suryoma.com.

seems far from the general consciousness. Many people still perceive nature and one another as threats and prepare for war against *the enemy*. We project our inner realities onto the greater global life. Today wars and fighting seem ever more prevalent. Domestic violence, beginning from the moment of conception, is on the increase. So are the wars on the larger world stage. We have the "War on Terror," disease, famine, and innumerable commercial and trade wars. We are still preparing for war instead of peace.

## Fight, Flight, or Freeze

Everyone is familiar with the hormone adrenaline and its response of fight, flight, or freeze to a perceived danger. When we *perceive* a threat, our reptilian hindbrain takes over to ensure our survival. Most of the body's energy rushes to the arms and legs, making them up to 10 times stronger. This reaction is known to have saved lives: Years ago, a flight attendant jumped over a huge airport fence to escape the flames of the burning aircraft. No one could understand how she had done it, but she did! Such is the power of a sudden rush of adrenaline. When used in the context of a real danger this reaction is nature's blessing. But when we see others as a threat and live under the constant influence of these stress hormones they become harmful to us. This vision feeds fear, stimulates greed, and leads to the need to dominate and control. The result is the capitalistic global control dynamic that provokes the extreme imbalances humanity is witnessing today. This vicious cycle then causes even higher stress and adrenaline levels, leading to greater frustration, disease, and uncontrolled violence. The French unions have recently been calling for stress to be accepted as a named disease with all that that entails. It is crippling economies, yet the systems and behaviors that provoke and sustain it remain intact.

It is time for us to take a good look at what is causing this stress and come up with some *soul*-utions! When we are in stress there is no energy left for growth, repair, healing, or creative thinking. Ironically, in this nuclear age, the actual survival of humanity no longer depends on primitive, fear-based instincts but rather on creating and implementing these new solutions. The fight or flight response is now inappropriate in facing our global challenges. We need to let go of the chronic stress levels that plague humanity and start creating the world we wish to live in.

In the world of busi-ness it is important to maintain integrity and be responsible for where we invest our time and energy, making quality of life the goal. When companies work against the best interest of individuals, for example, training an "aggressive" sales staff, customers and clients can feel threatened and enter into the stress cycle. We don't have to look far to find examples of the countries, corporations, and individuals who are poisoning the Earth and enslaving humanity with fear and stress to feed their greed. Playing God and alienating people from Nature's intelligence is a symptom of very serious social illness. If we don't take these people to the crimes against humanity courts, then Nature surely will.

The late-20th century luminary Omraam Mikhael Aivanhov wrote in *Aquarius: Herald of the Golden Age:*

> Man as conceived by Cosmic Intelligence is such that if he is to be fulfilled, he must connect himself with the light and power of the Higher World. If not, if he puts all his trust in his own limited faculties, he will be unable to see ahead and in his blindness and he will make drastic errors in all domains. If he puts his faith in technology, trade and material development, sooner or later he will fail...

It is essential for us to question where and to what end we expend our energy. On a recent flight, I found myself seated next to a chemist who works for the pharmaceutical industry. Our conversation only deepened my convictions about the craziness of our current commercial terrorism. He quite overtly told me that most of the pharmaceutical drugs that are being manufactured are "blah blah blah," as he put it. They have nothing to do with helping people to heal, but merely serve commercial gain. Innocent people are being abused — as employees and as guinea pigs — to line the pockets of greedy and over-zealous apprentice sorcerers. This chemist also admitted that when not in a state of adrenaline, the body heals itself.

"We know that," he said. "I wouldn't take any of these drugs. We have better results with placebos. Madame, don't be naive. This world is about profit," he shrugged.

"Isn't this a crime against humanity?" I challenged.

And he whispered, turning inward, "There is nothing we can do."

But he was wrong, there is.

## Love: A Change of Heart

What would it be like if we began caring for our planet and each other? If all our energies went toward healing rather than toward fighting, defending, or inertia? Powerful love hormones could then replace the old, prehistoric patterning opening doors to greater awareness, creative intelligence, intuition, and bliss. Our partners, work associates, and global family members could then become co-creators in a world of living intelligence and abundance.

95

The good news is that, like new skin growing under an old, crusty scab, a silent revolution *is* generating. This new way of thinking *is* emerging. Increasing numbers of people are choosing to perceive the world and one another with love and confidence, connecting heart to heart, soul to soul. Fear and love are mutually exclusive, and people are consciously choosing the love hormone response. Once our stress is managed and we are bathed in powerful endorphins and oxytocin, doors do open. We come face to face with intelligence, intuition, healing, discoveries, creativity, and the untold treasures of the human brain and cosmic intelligence. This is the "higher world" referred to by Omraam. People from all cultures and ages are reaching this state of awareness.

## The Inner Voice

We each quiet ourselves and turn our attention inward by being still and listening to the small voice within. Feeling the bliss of being an integral part of the intelligence of life, my colleagues and I begin to make the decisions that will affect our lives, our activities, and the quality of the services we have to offer. Our objective is to be led by this voice. Our work or business is then guided and fueled from inside ourselves. The feeling that I am in love with life gives me an energy greater than anything I've known before, facilitating creative intelligence and opening vistas of previously unimaginable frontiers.

People laugh when, faced with a question, I say, "Let me close my eyes and see." But it works. Try it. When we look within, our "problems" become challenges, the solutions flow, and our faces light up as we begin to witness the synchronicities that show us we are not alone.

Though they may not realize it, corporations stand to gain substantially from offering stress management programs to their employees. Quiet meditation rooms would become the inner eye of the workplace. How about a relaxing body massage or a few minutes of meditation to calming music just before the next board meeting? An increasing number of businesses are already reaping the rewards of these practices as they align their activities with the new paradigm.

## Making the Paradigm Shift

In his bestseller, *Confessions of an Economic Hit Man*, John Perkins writes that the voice of his conscience saved him. He clearly reveals the sordid details of how he was lured into acting as an economic hit man and cheating countries out of trillions of dollars. Because he made sure that they couldn't repay their debts to the United States, these countries were forced to hand over their natural resources.

There are people who prey on our weaknesses by promising material success, while intending to trap us in unethical jobs and commercial crimes, be they overt or covert. But, we do have a choice. Perkins allowed the quiet inner voice that had haunted him to finally triumph—he resigned from hurting people and began working for their well-being. In so doing he found his own, and he now inspires others to follow in his footsteps. Perkins concludes:

These are the times that try men's souls. We will be faced with increasing acts of desperation by those who feel cheated and oppressed by the corporatocracy. Whether terrorism occurs in Manhattan, Madrid, London, Riyadh, or La Paz, it is essential that we understand that in the long term these horrible acts will not be stopped by military or by security guards in airports and along our borders. They will only be stopped when enough of us demand that our corporations, banks, and governments cease to exploit the majority of the world's population and resources and when we insist on dealing with the world from a plane of compassion—the very place envisioned by our Founding Fathers...

I learned this lesson in Hong Kong when, at the age of 19, I spent a year selling international real estate. The company sent me to Europe to visit developments and villas for sale. But upon my return I was horrified to discover that my boss had advertised one of our popular developments in Spain as having a swimming pool. Knowing that it didn't, I went to question him. Brushing me off as naive he said, "Julie, you're not going to make a fuss about that!" But I was already well set on my tracks and refused to be dishonest. I didn't need to cheat. I put myself in my clients' shoes and thought about how I would like to be treated.

I enjoyed serving people and helping them to find the property or investment that suited their real needs. As a result, I had very satisfied clients. I actually had more than all the other consultants put together. When I met them socially I felt a healthy pride for having given a good service. Many became friends and I started to sell more properties through their recommendations. However, this was not my boss *Ron-the-Con's* way of doing business. Unable to continue investing my soul in that job, I chose to resign. This experience had confirmed my belief that it is indeed possible to succeed in business with integrity. Like Perkins, I knew that when enough people refused to work out of greed and fear, our societies would blossom and flourish in love and mutual respect. Many of my friends told me that I was crazy to give up the income and prospects the job offered, but I knew that no amount of money could buy such a feeling.

Having faced emotional despair as well as a life-threatening disease, I have learned to put my trust in life and its innate intelligence. Life knows exactly what to do when we give it the right conditions. How often do we hear our inner voice warning us, showing us, guiding us? In my experience we usually get three warnings and then it goes quiet. Sometimes it is not easy to follow its advice. It takes courage. But things always work for the best when we do. It isn't the voice that screams or insists; it's the quiet one. The one that you've heard often, didn't listen to, and found yourself later saying, "Something inside me told me what was going to happen," or "I knew I should have done that."

This same inner voice led a whole tribe on an Indonesian Island during the recent devastating tsunami. They made for high ground along with the animals. Not one member of the tribe was killed or injured. You, too, can choose to listen to this voice. It will lead you, your family, and your business out of darkness into light, out of disease into health, out of sadness and isolation into happiness and prosperity.

When people visit Providence, our beautiful holistic living center in the south of France, they often exclaim that it is paradise. I smile. Many people predicted that I would not get anywhere. My home is more than a house; it's a place were people are inspired and empowered to make the life changes necessary to make their own dreams come true.

Just as stress is contagious, so is well-being. This is reflected in the dynamic increase of the natural health and wellness industry. Yet when people leave Providence saying that they want to set up the same type of center, I find myself cautioning them. A very healthy vigilance is required in order not to fall into the usual trap of becoming a business shark in order to provide a well-being product or service. As we move forward into the new paradigm, the success of a company will be measured by the degree of health and happiness of its members and employees. It is not a place or a service that makes it—it's love.

Why is it that we generally don't accept that a woman would have sex for money? According to the dictionary, the definition of a prostitute is: *A person who willingly uses his or her talent or ability in a base and unworthy way, usually for money.* Isn't this what so many people are doing with their energy and intelligence? When I question my unhappy friends and clients as to why they stay in jobs they dislike that are making them ill, the reply I often hear is, "Well, I have to earn my living." It is crucial to be able to put your heart and soul into whatever you are doing. Then you will no longer be "working for a living," but living and loving, instead. When love and mutual respect are present in our relationships and our work, everything changes. We reap the rewards of happiness, health, and financial gain.

# Global Family in Harmony with Mother Nature

Let's dare to see and side with the innate intelligence in all things. We are all a part of this web of life, held together by that amazing stuff called *love*. We now live in a global village, and it is certain that everything we do affects the whole planet.

I was reminded of this recently, in a very pertinent way, when I visited the beautiful plains of the Masai Mara in Kenya. I stood with a newfound friend, enjoying the pure warm feelings passing between us as we looked out over his homeland. This handsome Masai asked me if I would return to help his tribe with stress management. I was shocked.

"Surely you don't need that out here," I gasped.

"We are very stressed," he replied with deep sadness. His eyes fixed mine with a look that pierced my heart. He asked, "What are they doing to our planet?"

My mind's eye showed me all those sprawling cities, the consumption, the waste, obesity, starvation, disease, pollution, children committing suicide at the age of five...murder—the planet is being raped! How could I begin to answer?

What will it take for us to feel that we are citizens of the same world, brothers and sisters in a global family? It really is up to us to make it a happy family, in harmony with cosmic intelligence. Although the situation looks bleak, I know, as others do, that we can do it. That means you and me. When we choose to perceive the innate loving intelligence behind all life and create the love hormone response, we actually move our sick, unbalanced world toward health, happiness, peace, and plenitude.

Just as our body is made up of cells, our world is made up of human beings. Our personal health is determined by how we treat our cells, how they are nourished and how they feel, communicate, and grow. In the same way, our global health depends on how individuals are nourished, how they feel about themselves and the world, and how they communicate and co-create. In the global body, countries represent the various organs. Each country has a unique participation in the whole. Corporations are also organs within our societies. They employ people who fulfill certain functions. The health of the company—and its long-term wealth—therefore relies on the health and happiness of its employees. As we progress into a future shaped by love, unethical companies will be doomed to collapse, making the Enron disaster look like a little incident. Those that are grounded in integrity are co-creating a positive future in harmony with the laws of nature and the heart.

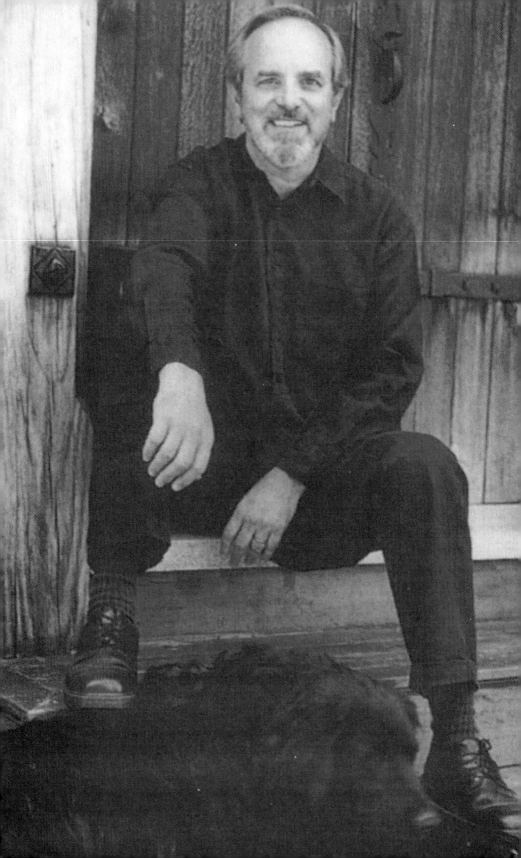

# THOMAS MOORE:

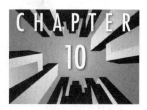

# Joyful Ethics

In light of the immense power that corporations wield today, it's been said that no significant positive changes can happen in the world until corporations decide to transform the way they operate—be more humane to their workers, protect the environment, stop demanding political handouts at the expense of the less powerful, or look beyond the next quarter to the long term, for instance. In my opinion, while it would be very useful and important for corporations to make this kind of radical about-face, I don't know what might persuade them to do so. Although certain progressive companies have begun acting in more mature ways, many businesses today are still strikingly immature, as shown by their cynicism, greed, and self-destructive policies. So, if we are interested in fostering positive change in the business world, we must remember that business does not exist in a vacuum, unaffected by or not affecting the rest of society. We ordinary citizens can create the changes we want to see in business by making decisions with our purchases and our jobs, thus casting our votes for the status quo or for change.

When people decide quite literally not to buy into the negative values around them, even in small ways, they are creating positive change in society. For instance, a growing number of people are rejecting gas-guzzling SUVs and buying hybrid vehicles. In doing so, they are casting their vote for protecting the environment and reducing their dependence on petroleum. As more people are

Thomas Moore, Ph.D., is a leading figure in the field of contemporary depth theology whose works focus on the soul and emerging ideas about spirituality. He taught at Southern Methodist University, The Dallas Institute for Humanities and Culture, and Lesley College before authoring the *New York Times* bestseller, *Care of the Soul* (HarperCollins, 1992). Since that time, he has published many books, tapes, CDs, and videos, including *Soul Mates* (HarperCollins, 1994), *The Re-Enchantment of Everyday Life* (HarperCollins, 1996), *The Soul of Sex* (HarperCollins, 1998), and *Dark Nights of the Soul* (Gotham Books, 2004). For more information, visit www.careofthesoul.net.

demanding hybrid vehicles, the auto companies are producing more of them. As people demand more "green" products or more organic foods or a home that's energy efficient, the producers take notice, and society begins to evolve in positive ways.

More people today are seeking jobs that not only pay well but also satisfy their deep hunger to be creative and productive. They want work that enables them to feel their lives are worthwhile and also allows them to have a strong family life and adequate time for themselves. So when employers do what they can to respond to these needs, as a small but growing number are doing, their employees vote their approval by often producing better quality work and improving the bottom line.

Another major way we might encourage positive change in business is to transform our notion of ethics. We need to get away from the idea that ethics is a matter of principle and what we should and should not do. America is a very moralistic nation in many ways, so our sense of ethics has become very moralistic. We label people "good" if they do the right things and "bad" if they do the wrong things. We even have a list of "evil" nations that we threaten with punishment if they don't live up to our rules. Our idea of ethics has become very simplistic, no more than a list of negative and minimal standards. This kind of ethical system does nothing to inspire and encourage people to be ethical.

One reason why people sometimes act unethically is because they feel an anger that has no particular identifiable source and which they don't know how to handle. In our society, we generally don't deal with anger very well, and it comes out as road rage or assaulting someone or just generally being mean-spirited and uncivil. I'd go so far as to say that trashing the environment is also a sign of a deep, unconscious anger that is expressed by lashing out. In our moralistic society, this anger can be expressed as a kind of judgment, where we turn our anger against someone we believe is doing something bad — and since it looks like we're being ethical, we can feel good about being angry. That feeling of being virtuous or better than someone else is more about narcissism than about ethics.

I believe that ethics could have a different base. Instead of providing a list of how to be virtuous and teaching us how to do the "right" things, ethics could be more about coming to feel like part of a community and not wanting to hurt that community, not wanting to harm your neighbors for your own gain, and not wanting to be somebody by dominating someone else. The soul of ethics, I believe, is being able to reach out beyond yourself and your own self-interest to act freely on the desire to do the most good for your community, which can encompass everything from your family and circle of friends to the entire planet, without harming anyone else.

When I wrote my book *The Soul's Religion*, which includes a section on ethics, I discovered that "ethos," from which the word ethics is derived, originally meant a place frequented by groups of animals, such as a watering hole. So in that light, we have to ask, when we gather together, how do we act? What behaviors do we allow? Do we take care of one another and the place where we gather, the common resources we all share? Do we welcome others or exclude them? With this definition of ethics, we don't have to abide by some tiresome list of good and bad, right and wrong, which is often too limited in scope to deal with many of the larger questions we face in our lives. Instead, finding out how we answer these basic questions of human existence allows us to discover our ethics.

We don't just grow up being ethical. We learn it from parents and teachers, from the culture. We learn ethics step by step as we wrestle with situations in our lives. We must find a way of teaching this community-related ethics to our children; but it's difficult because we need a certain level of intelligence and maturity to distinguish between simply laying our values on others and being able to educate them about the process of learning how to discover their own. It's much more than just telling them what they should believe and what they should do. If we can learn how to always add to the immense flow of life around us rather than obstruct it, we will have learned to be ethical.

A key point in this education process should be that ethics does not mean acting on principle alone, which can be a grim, tedious task. Instead, it is acting from the sheer joy of life and being creative instead of being destructive. We should be ethical because, in this way, we become more of who we are and because, in this kind of act, we will find the deepest joy and sense of fulfillment. Ethics is not something to keep us from enjoying life. Just the opposite. Working ethically allows us to feel our mature innocence, to be loved by our community, to feel that we are making a genuine contribution and that our lives have meaning. These are the ultimate joys and rewards. As I wrote in *The Soul's Religion*, "Ethics is a way of recognizing that although we are each alone in this universe, we are all alone together. We can make a good life not only by protecting each other but by being creative together and taking our pleasures from one another." We often forget that business can be a way of advancing the life of the community as well as the lives of individuals. By doing both, as some progressive companies are already doing, everyone benefits and we all are lifted up.

Ethics is really about a radical sense of community, a profound awareness that every other person is just like me, and we are all together in this mysterious business of life. No matter if I'm a teacher, a CEO, or a champion cyclist, I am just like you and like everyone else within our shared humanity. We all become a community with the realization of our fundamental identity as the human race. Once I profoundly feel that I am a member of this group, this community gathered together, then I will care for it. Then I will be an ethical person.

Transforming our workplaces into spiritual places would also help transform the business community. I don't mean spiritual as religious, but in the sense of transcending our small worlds in some way — transcending our egos, our selves, our families, our nations, and our own corporate groups enough so that we see the overall view of the whole of being. When we work, we're participating in the culture and in that whole of being on many levels. We're assisting in the evolution of the natural world and of culture. But at some level, we have to be creative to keep that evolution going. That is a spiritual enterprise because we're reaching beyond ourselves. Ultimately, we have to have a very broad vision to keep evolving so we're not doing things just for ourselves or for our own group, but instead for whatever it is that's beyond us.

If we don't have this spiritual, transcendent viewpoint, what is left to us? Nothing but narcissism, where we say, I'd better get what I need and forget about everyone else. If we are all out for ourselves in this way, and if we don't possess this larger spiritual sense of things, I don't see how we can survive. Instead of expanding and evolving, our culture will shrink and collapse.

In making this transition from a work culture based on competition and mistrust to one focused on collaboration and respect, we must be careful that we don't fall into a sentimental approach. We often use idealistic language about these changes: We say our aim is to create a culture of love and togetherness and community. People look at that and say, that's very nice but it will never happen. This is because people in business believe they have to be tough and practical — and in many ways they're right. So drifting off into clouds of airy idealism will only maintain the split between ethics and the hard reality of the business world. We have to find ways to appreciate the practicalities of business while moving towards the ideals.

I would even say that it's very important to assert the value of competition, the game of business with its dark side, its shadow aspect. We're never going to get rid of these darker elements, and we shouldn't try. They are part of the pleasure of the darkness of business. It's only when that pleasure of the dark aspects overtakes our sense of values that it all falls apart and we see corporate scandals like those that happened several years ago.

Those of us who want to foster change in the business world

should not be too shiny, too much like the white knight full of ideals. It would be much better if we could respect the people in business for the sharpness they exhibit and the knowledge and intelligence they have, and then bring a piece of our own vision to them so we can meld the two sides together. Trying to implant a new vision on to them while denigrating their established ways of doing things will never work.

Because business is concerned with making and sustaining community, it is by definition a transcendent endeavor, ideally always pushing beyond individual and local interests. A corporation is a spiritual entity, no matter how secular it looks. But just as secularity — the joyful participation in everyday material life — sometimes is corrupted into secularism — the loss of any sense of the spiritual — business, too, can become merely local and self-serving. Both companies and workers could benefit greatly by reclaiming the spirituality inherent in their work, and the world would be a better place.

# PART THREE

❧

# Leading Us Astray

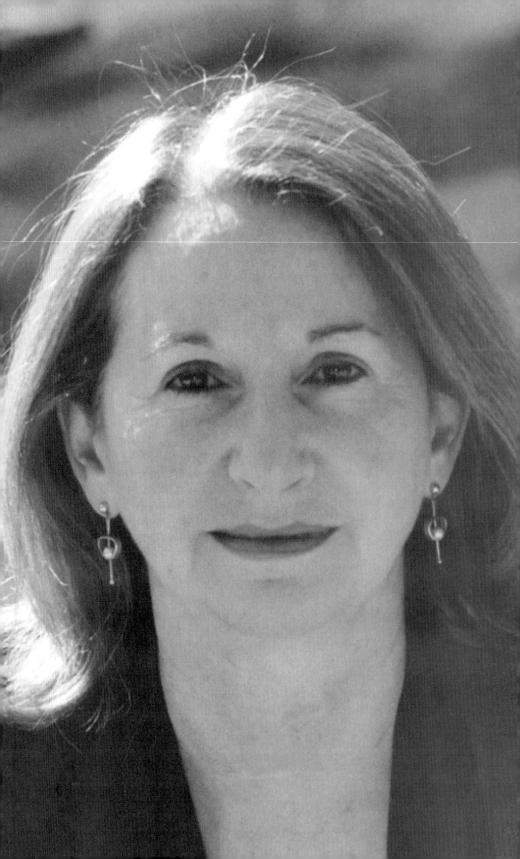

# BARBARA KELLERMAN:

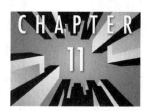

# Bad Leadership

There's something odd about the idea that somehow leadership can be distinguished from coercion, as if leadership and power were unrelated. In the real world, in everyday life, we come into constant contact not only with good leaders and good followers doing good things but also with bad leaders and bad followers doing bad things. In fact, anyone not dwelling in a cave is regularly exposed, if only through the media, to people who exercise power, use authority, and exert influence in ways that are not good. Still, even after all the evidence is in — after the recent corporate scandals, after the recent revelations of wrongdoing by leaders of the Roman Catholic Church, and before, during, and after political leadership all over the world that is so abhorrent it makes us ill — the idea that some leaders and some followers are bad, and that they might have something in common with good leaders and followers, has not fully penetrated the conversation or the curriculum.

The positive slant is recent. Historically, political theorists have been far more interested in the question of how to control the proclivities of bad leaders than in the question of how to promote the virtues of good ones. Influenced by religious traditions that focused on good and evil, and often personally scarred by war and disorder, the best political thinkers have had rather a jaundiced view of human nature.

Machiavelli provides perhaps the best example. He did not

Barbara Kellerman is Research Director of the Center for Public Leadership at the Kennedy School of Government, Harvard University. She is also a lecturer at Harvard and has held professorships at Fordham, Tufts, Fairleigh Dickinson, George Washington, and Uppsala Universities. She served as dean of graduate studies at Fairleigh Dickinson, and as director of the Center for Advanced Study of Leadership at the University of Maryland's Academy of Leadership. She is the author of *Reinventing Leadership: Making the Connection Between Politics and Business* (State University of New York Press, 1999) and *Bad Leadership* (Harvard Business School Press, 2004), among other books.

wrestle with the idea of bad — as in coercive — leadership. He simply presumed it. He took it for granted that people do harm as well as good, and so his advice to princes, to leaders, was to be ruthless. Consider this morsel about how leaders should, if need be, keep followers in line: "Cruelties can be called well used (if it is permissible to speak well of evil) that are done at a stroke, out of the necessity to secure oneself, and then are not persisted in but are turned to as much utility for the subjects as one can. Those cruelties are badly used which, though few in the beginning, rather grow with time."[1]

Today leaders who use coercion are generally judged to be bad. But to Machiavelli, the only kind of bad leader is the weak leader. Machiavelli was a pragmatist above all, familiar with the ways of the world and with a keen eye for the human condition. And so, to him, the judicious use of cruelty was an important arrow in the leader's quiver.

Although it seems counterintuitive, America's founders thought like Machiavelli, at least insofar as they also believed that people required restraint. They were products of the European Enlightenment, but as they saw it, their main task was to form a government that was for and by the people but that would simultaneously set limits on the body politic and on those who would lead it.

To be sure, the emphasis was different. Whereas Machiavelli was concerned primarily with the question of how to contain followers, the framers of the U.S. Constitution were concerned primarily with the question of how to contain leaders. Alexander Hamilton, for example, was, in comparison with his peers, a proponent of a strong executive. But even he considered it ideologically important as well as politically expedient to focus not on the possibilities of presidential power but on its limits.

In *The Federalist Papers,* Hamilton acknowledged America's "aversion to monarchy" — to leaders who inherit great power. He dedicated an entire essay to distinguishing between the proposed president, on the one hand, and the distant, detested British monarchy, on the other, an essay that made one main point: The U.S. Constitution would absolutely preclude the possibility that bad leadership could become entrenched. The very idea of checks and balances grew out of the framers' presumption that unless there was a balance of power, power was certain to be abused. Put another way, the American political system is the product of revolutionaries familiar with, and therefore wary of, bad leadership.

But as sociologist Talcott Parsons observed, on matters that relate to the importance of power and authority in human affairs, American social thought has tended toward utopianism.[2] For whatever reasons, most students of politics shy away from the subject of bad leadership and especially from really bad leaders, such as Stalin and Pol Pot. In other words, no matter how great and obvious its impact on the course of human affairs, "tyranny as such is simply not an issue or a recognized term of analysis."[3]

The question is, why do we tend toward utopianism on matters relating to the importance of power and authority in human affairs?[4] Why do we avoid the subject of tyranny in our leadership curricula, thereby presuming that tyrannical leadership is less relevant to the course of human affairs than democratic leadership? Why does the leadership industry generally assume that a bad leader such as Saddam Hussein has nearly nothing in common with a good leader such as Tony Blair, or that the Nazis were one species and the Americans another? Is Bernard Ebbers really so very different from Louis Gerstner Jr.? How did *leadership* come to be synonymous with *good* leadership?[5] Why are we afraid to acknowledge, much less admit to, the dark side? These are the questions to which I now turn.

## The Light Side

We want to read books about good leaders such as John Adams, Jack Welch, and Nelson Mandela. We don't want to read books about bad leaders such as Warren Harding, David Koresh, and Robert Mugabe.

This preference is natural. We go through life accentuating the positive and eliminating the negative in order to be as healthy and happy as possible. As Daniel Goleman put it, "[O]ur emotional and physical well-being is based in part on artful denial and illusion." In other words, for us to cultivate an "unfounded sense of optimism" serves a purpose. It is in our self-interest.[6]

In the leadership industry, this disposition has now moved from the level of the individual to the level of the collective. Those of us engaged in leadership work seem almost to collude to avoid the elephant in the room—bad leadership.[7] We resist even considering the possibility that the dynamic between Franklin Delano Roosevelt and his most ardent followers had anything in common with the dynamic between Adolph Hitler and his most ardent followers; or that John Biggs, the admired former CEO of TIAA/CREF, has skills and capacities similar in some ways to those of Richard Scrushy, the disgraced former CEO of HealthSouth.

# The Dark Side

But the leadership industry has a problem that years ago I named Hitler's ghost.[8] Here is my concern. If we pretend that there is no elephant and that bad leadership is unrelated to good leadership, if we pretend to know the one without knowing the other, we will in the end distort the enterprise. We cannot distance ourselves from even the most extreme example — Hitler — by bestowing on him another name, such as "power wielder." Not only was his impact on twentieth-century history arguably greater than anyone else's, but also he was brilliantly skilled at inspiring, mobilizing, and directing followers. His use of coercion notwithstanding, if this is not leadership, what is?

Similarly, it makes no sense to think of corporate lawbreakers as one breed, and corporate gods as another. Why would we preclude people at the top of the Enron hierarchy — chairman Kenneth Lay, CEO Jeffrey Skilling, and CFO Andrew Fastow — from being labeled leaders just because they did not "realize goals mutually held by leaders and followers"? The fact is that Lay, Skilling, and Fastow were agents of change. What they did affected the lives and pocketbooks of tens of thousands of Americans, many of whom were not Enron employees. Let's be clear here. These men were not just a few rotten apples. Rather, they created, indeed encouraged, an organizational culture that allowed many apples to spoil and, in turn, ruin others.

## Why Do Leaders Behave Badly?

Leaders are like everyone else. They — we — behave badly for different reasons, and they — we — behave badly in different ways.

Sometimes the context fosters bad behavior. A city in which corruption has long been tolerated is more likely to be defrauded by its elected officials than one that has a long and strong tradition of good government.

Sometimes followers entice leaders to go astray. People in positions of authority are not immune to the influence of others, especially close advisers who, although perhaps misguided, are nevertheless determined and single-tracked. But, in the main, leaders behave badly because of who they are and what they want.

## Why Do Followers Behave Badly?

It's one thing for followers to follow bad leaders merely by going along. It's quite another for them to lend bad leaders strong personal support. What I am arguing is this: Followers who knowingly, deliberately commit themselves to bad leaders are themselves bad.

Followers' dedication to bad leaders is often strongest when their leaders are very bad, as opposed to only somewhat bad. Again, it's a matter of self-interest. Followers usually have no particular incentive to lend strong support to a leader who is merely ineffective. Going along is good enough. On the other hand, intimates of frankly unethical leaders often stand to benefit financially or politically from the relationship.

The corruption that took place in companies such as WorldCom and HealthSouth by no means involved only the CEOs. Both Bernard Ebbers and Richard Scrushy were surrounded by small groups of followers who knew what the score was, participated actively in the wrongdoing, and stood to profit substantially from the company's fraudulent practices. These members of the two men's respective inner circles were separate and distinct from the larger group of followers, who were out of the loop and who, whatever suspicions they might have had, were not directly involved in the corruption.

The most extensive study of bad followers has been the case of Nazi Germany. At the risk of oversimplifying but in the interest of distinguishing among the kinds of followers, I will divide Germans during the Nazi period into three groups: bystanders, evildoers, and acolytes. (Only a handful of Germans actively opposed Hitler, and they often paid with their lives.)

Bystanders went along with Hitler and the Nazi regime, but they were not fervent Nazis. Bystanders' motivations ranged from self-interest (on matters relating to stability and security) to being part of a national group (Germany was, after all, their *Heimat*, their homeland) that was cohesive and provided a sense of identity.

Evildoers were members of units such as the SS-Einsatzgruppen. One of this unit's first goals during the Second World War was to massacre as many Soviet Jews as possible. The 1941 slaughter at Babi Yar, a ravine in Kiev, was testimony to its efficiency: In only two days members of this unit shot to death 33,771 Jews. Why did members of the German SS become, in the words of Richard Rhodes, "masters of death"?[9] The reasons varied. Some were genuine sadists. Others had been persuaded that they were killing "vermin." Still others turned brutal because they themselves were being brutalized by violence or the threat of violence. Finally, however weak in retrospect this line of argument, German soldiers were like soldiers everywhere. They were told what to do and they did it.

CHAPTER ELEVEN ❧

# Brief Examples
## Sumner Redstone

Viacom is one of the few mega-media companies to have survived the era of mega-mergers in good shape. But Sumner Redstone, its octogenarian CEO, had long been in denial concerning his own eventual demise. His rigid refusal even to address the issue of who would succeed him left Viacom vulnerable.

The widely reported tensions between Redstone and the company's president, Mel Karmazin, further contributed to the sense of unease. Redstone's need to dominate everything and everyone, and his reluctance to quit center stage, made the situation unnecessarily tense and even precarious.

Put bluntly, the chairman and controlling shareholder of Viacom long refused to consider himself mortal, and so he continued to resist planning for an orderly transition in the event he became disabled or dead. "Viacom is me. I am Viacom," Redstone said. "That marriage is eternal, forever."[10]

## Vladimir Putin

In 2000 the Russian submarine *Kursk* sank to the bottom of the Barents Sea, with 118 men on board. President Vladimir Putin's response was curious. Unwilling to cancel his Black Sea vacation to visit the site and commiserate with the families of the victims, he remained at a remove for more than a week.

More critically, he refused to immediately request the kinds of assistance—especially from the United States—that might have saved lives. After a week, Norwegian divers were finally permitted to come in and do in one day what the Russians had been unable to do in seven. They pried open the sunken submarine's emergency escape hatch, but by then to no avail.

"Why did Mr. Putin and his generals resist asking for foreign help until it was too late?" asked *New York Times* foreign affairs columnist Thomas Friedman. "Because they feared it would sully the honor of Mother Russia's army and puncture Russia's pretense to still being a super power."[11]

# Mary Meeker: Queen of the Net
## The Prologue

Mary Meeker was one of the legendary leaders of the frenzied boom in online stocks that characterized the equities markets during the mid- to late 1990s. A friend of Amazon.com's Jeff Bezos, AOL's

Steve Case, and eBay's Meg Whitman, Meeker was not a leader in the conventional sense. That is, she had no direct power or formal authority over her followers. Rather, she was an opinion leader. From her prominent perch as a financial analyst at the Wall Street firm of Morgan Stanley Dean Witter & Co., Meeker wielded great influence. When she spoke, people listened. More to the point, when she told them to do something, they did it. Tens of thousands bought stocks solely on the basis of Meeker's personal recommendations.

As long as the Internet bubble remained intact, everything was fine. Alan Greenspan's faint caution about "irrational exuberance" notwithstanding, Meeker gave her followers what they wanted: hot tips on hot stocks. But when the market turned bearish, she remained bullish. Long after she should have warned that owning stocks, especially the technology stocks in which she specialized, had become risky, Meeker refused to give the signal to sell. Moreover, her inability or unwillingness to adapt to new information and changing markets was not confined to a single incident or brief period. Rather, it came to define the nature of her leadership, just as it came to cost those who hung on her every word.

## The Context

In January 1995, the Dow Jones Industrial Average stood at 3,800. In March 1999 it hit 10,000, and by May it had climbed another 1,000 points. The rise in the tech-heavy NASDAQ exchange was even more dramatic. In March 2000 the NASDAQ hit 5,000—an increase of 571 percent in six years.

What happened? What accounted for this upsurge, which only a few years later was widely viewed as merely a speculative bubble?

In the summer of 1994, *Time* ran the first of several cover stories on the Internet, describing it as "the nearest thing to a working prototype of the information superhighway."[12] In other words, by the mid-1990s the media establishment had concluded that the Internet was of signal importance and that it was here to stay. Moreover, fledgling businesses were starting to capitalize on what was soon being described as a "revolution" in information technology.

Although several companies could claim the title, if you had to pick one to represent the so-called New Economy, America Online (AOL) would be as good a candidate as any. In July 1993, AOL had two hundred fifty thousand subscribers. One year later it had a million. By early 1996, five million people were accessing the Internet through AOL.

Predictably, AOL's rapid growth was reflected in the price of the company's stock, which climbed steadily. Between 1992 and 1996,

AOL's market value rose from $70 million to $6.5 billion. Moreover, strong backing by Wall Street insiders enabled CEO Steven Case to finance his plans for aggressive expansion. Mary Meeker, who by the mid-nineties was one of Morgan Stanley's star stock analysts, was one of Case's strongest and most visible supporters. As John Cassidy reported in his book *Dot.con,* which smartly and succinctly tells the story of the New Economy, Meeker had made a buy recommendation on AOL stock beginning in 1993.[13]

The rise of stocks in companies such as America Online, Netscape, and Yahoo! was part of a broader phenomenon. In the first four months of 1996 alone, Americans deposited about $100 billion in stock mutual funds. As recently as 1990, that figure had been a mere $12 billion for the entire year.[14] With all that money pouring into the equities market, prices climbed sharply. Between the beginning of 1995 and the end of May 1996, the Dow went up 45 percent, and the NASDAQ 65 percent.

For all the optimism, however, not everyone was an optimist. For example, well-known equities analysts Barton Biggs and Byron Wien—both older than most of their bullish colleagues and both also, like Meeker, based at Morgan Stanley—warned that because the markets had risen nearly without pause, they were vulnerable. Meeker, though, was undeterred. Her buy signals for stocks such as Netscape and America Online remained in place.[15]

On Friday, December 29,1999, Muhammad Ali rang the opening bell of the New York Stock Exchange. By the end of the day, the Dow was at an all-time high of 11,497. For the year, it was up more than 25 percent. The NASDAQ, in turn, stood at 4,069. During the previous two years it had climbed more than 85 percent—the best performance ever by a major American stock index.

But then the worm turned. By the middle of 2000, interest rates had started to climb, many stocks outside the tech sector had lost value, and the equities market had generally become more volatile. By October 2000, the Dow Jones Composite Internet Index was down 54 percent from its high of only seven months earlier. Whether or not the collapse of the NASDAQ was, as Cassidy labeled it, a "turning point in American history," only time will tell.[16] What can be said for certain is that it wasthe end of one era in which all things seemed possible and the beginning of another considerably more somber.

But despite the changing economic climate and dramatic declines in the markets, Mary Meeker held her ground. It was the ground beneath her that gave way. And so, with her buy recommendations for stocks such as Amazon.com, Priceline.com, and Yahoo! remaining in place, she became a scapegoat. Meeker was on the cover of the May

14, 2001, issue of *Fortune,* along with a headline that read, "Can We Ever Trust Wall Street Again?"

Still, Meeker held fast. While almost all signs were pointing downward, Meeker predicted that sometime during the next two or three years, the "nuclear winter" would give way to a "spring bloom." Soon, she proclaimed, the market value of leading stocks would make the market value just passed "look like chump change."[17]

### The Leader

Meeker was not alone in assuming two roles that would seem to be in conflict. During this same period, Jack Grubman worked for Salomon Smith Barney, supposedly as an independent analyst specializing in telecommunications stocks. What was not known then but is known now is that Grubman also advised the very companies whose stocks he was trying to sell. Grubman helped Salomon Smith Barney earn almost $1 billion in fees during the late 1990s, but by 2002 investors and lenders who had put money into the firms he recommended had lost an estimated $2 trillion.[18]

By 2000 the bloom was off the Meeker rose. Ranked by *Institutional Investor* in 1999 as the number one Internet analyst, in October 2000 she was charged with "pushing fool's gold." An article in the *New York Post* titled "Queen of the Internet Dethroned" pointed out that the stocks Meeker followed and recommended had not in fact outperformed the market, her "outperform" ratings notwithstanding.[19] The piece went on to charge that Meeker was caught in the catch-22 referred to earlier: To bring in business, she was hobnobbing with the rich and famous rather than providing the objective investment advice ordinary investors were looking for. In any case Meeker's rigidity made her unable carefully to watch and listen—and to tack accordingly.

By 2001 it was also an expensive indulgence. The investment community was calculating sums lost as a consequence of her bad calls, and the media that had built her up was cutting her down. In April, *Business Week* concluded that as a stock picker Meeker had a "mixed" record. For example, Meeker had downgraded the search engine Ask Jeeves, but only after the company warned of disappointing earnings. And she was plain wrong on Priceline.com, conceding too late that she had misjudged the size of the market.[20]

But it was *Fortune* that finally struck the fatal blow to Mary Meeker's reputation. In that May 2001 issue that had her on the cover, the magazine charged that Meeker had become "the single most powerful symbol of how Wall Street can lead investors astray." Meeker had maintained strong "buy" or "outperform" ratings on all except two of the fifteen stocks she was covering, *Fortune* reminded its readers, even in a market in which "Internet stocks have crumbled and entire companies have vaporized."[21]

## The Followers

Americans are spoiled. In one generation the average American home grew from fifteen hundred square feet to about twenty-two hundred square feet, and nearly three-quarters of new American cars have cruise control and power door locks. We spend $40 billion a year on our lawns alone—an amount roughly equal to the entire federal tax revenue of India.[22] In fact, those among us who are members of college-graduate households are richer than 99.9 percent of all human beings who have ever lived. But still we want more.

Moreover, because Americans are optimists who trust the system, we are willing to place bets on getting rich quick. This explains at least in part why, during the 1990s, many of us speculated in markets that had already gone way up. As David Brooks has put it, "The lure of plenty, pervading the [American] landscape, encourages risk and adventure."[23] An article in the *Journal of International Business Studies* confirms that Americans are more comfortable with the idea of taking risks, including financial risks, than citizens of any of the other nine nations studied.[24]

Mary Meeker could not have been a leader in the financial services industry without legions of followers willing to put their money where her mouth was. She was the expert who told us what to believe and how to behave, and we freely went along. Because many of us continued to buy after the market had by every historical measure climbed too far too fast, it can fairly be claimed that the Internet boom and subsequent bust were as much our fault as they were the fault of Wall Street professionals who misled us. In other words, even though Meeker stayed stuck, her bad leadership depended absolutely on those of us who were so eager to make a killing that we fell in line.

Meeker's bid to add to the ranks of investors in her thrall was strongly supported by, among others, the media. As Cassidy observed, the overall standard of reporting during the dot-com heyday was dismal. The print media had fawned over and finally crowned Meeker "queen," and the electronic media, especially CNBC, had become a fan club for corporate America. "All across the country—in bars, banks, health clubs, airports, and doctors' waiting rooms—televisions were permanently switched to CNBC. The network's reporters didn't hype stocks directly. Rather they helped to create a populist investing culture in which adulation of the stock market was the norm."[26]

So bad leadership is not solely the fault of a few bad leaders. We are all, every one of us, in this together.

Archbishop Desmond Tutu has said that his experience of South Africa taught him "two contradictory things." On the one hand, we "have an extraordinary capacity for good." But on the other hand, we have "a remarkable capacity for evil — we have refined ways of being mean and nasty to one another [through] genocides, holocausts, slavery, racism, wars, oppression and injustice."[27]

Because leadership makes a difference, sometimes even a big difference, those of us who desire to make the world a better place must do what Tutu did. We must come to grips with leadership as two contradictory things: good and bad.

1. Niccolo Machiavelli, *The Prince* (Chicago: University of Chicago Press, 1998), 37, 38.
2. Talcott Parsons, introduction to *The Theory of Social and Economic Organization*, by Max Weber (Free Press, 1947), 36.
3. Mark Lilla, "The New Age of Tyranny," *The New York Review of Books*, 24 October 2002, 29.
4. There are some exceptions to this general rule. See, for example, Christine Clements and John B. Washbush, "The Two Faces of Leadership: Considering the Dark Side of Leader-Follower Dynamics," *Journal of Workplace Learning: Employee Counseling Today* 11, no. 5 (1999); M.F.R. Kets de Vries, *Prisoners of Leadership* (New York: John Wiley & Sons, 1989); *Leaders, Fools and Imposters: Essays on the Psychology of Leadership* (San Francisco: Jossey-Bass, 1993); *The Leadership Mystique: An Owner's Manual* (London: Pearson, 2001), especially chapters 4 and 7; Jean Lipman-Bluman, "Why Do We Tolerate Bad Leaders: Magnificent Interlude, Anxiety and Meaning" in *The Future of Leadership: Today's Top Leadership Thinkers Speak to Tomorrow's Leaders*, eds. Warren Bennis, Gretchen M. Spreitzer, and Thomas G. Cummings (San Francisco: Jossey-Bass, 2001), 125-138; and Craig E. Johnson, *Meeting the Ethical Challenges of Leadership: Casting Light or Shadow* (Thousand Oaks, CA: Sage, 2001).
5. Edward Rothstein, "Defining Evil in the Wake of 9/11," *New York Times*, 5 October 2002, B7.
6. Daniel J. Goldman, "What Is Negative About Positive Illusions? When Benefits of the Individual Harm the Collective," *Journal of Social and Clinical Psychology* 8 (1989): 191.
7. Eviatar Zerubavel, "The Elephant in the Room," in *Culture in Mind*, ed. Karen A. Cerulo (New York: Routledge, 2002), 21.
8. Barbara Kellerman, "Hitler's Ghost: A Manifesto," in *Cutting Edge: Leadership 2000*, eds. Barbara Kellerman and Larraine Matusak (College Park, MD: Burns Academy of Leadership, 1999), 65-68.
9. Richard Rhodes, *Masters of Death: The SS-Einsatzgruppen and the Invention of the Holocaust* (New York: Knopf, 2002).
10. Michael Wolff, "Summer Squall," *New York*, 18 February 2002, 38.
11. Thomas Friedman, "A Russian Dinosaur," *New York Times*, 5 September 2002, A27.
12. Quoted in John Cassidy, *Dot.con: The Greatest Story Ever Sold* (New York: HarperCollins, 2002) 63. This section draws heavily from Cassidy's book.
13. Ibid., 111.
14. Ibid., 118.
15. Ibid., 120.
16. Ibid., 295.
17. Quoted in ibid., 309.
18. *New York Times*, 16 August 2002, A1.
19. Emily Lambert, "Queen of the Internet Dethroned," *New York Post*, 23 October 2000, 50.
20. Steve Hamm, "Tech's Cheerleader Won't Say Die," *Business Week*, 30 October 2001, 90.
21. Peter Elkind, "Where Mary Meeker Went Wrong," *Fortune*, 14 April 2001, 68-82. All the quotations in this section are taken from Elkind's article.
22. David Brooks, "Why the U.S. Will Always Be Rich," *New York Times Magazine*, 9 June 2002, 90.
23. Ibid., 91.
24. Ibid., 124.
25. Cassidy, "The Woman in the Bubble."
26. Cassidy, *Dot.con*, 168.
27. Desmond Tutu, "Let South Africa Show the World How to Forgive," *Knowledge of Reality* 19 (2000).

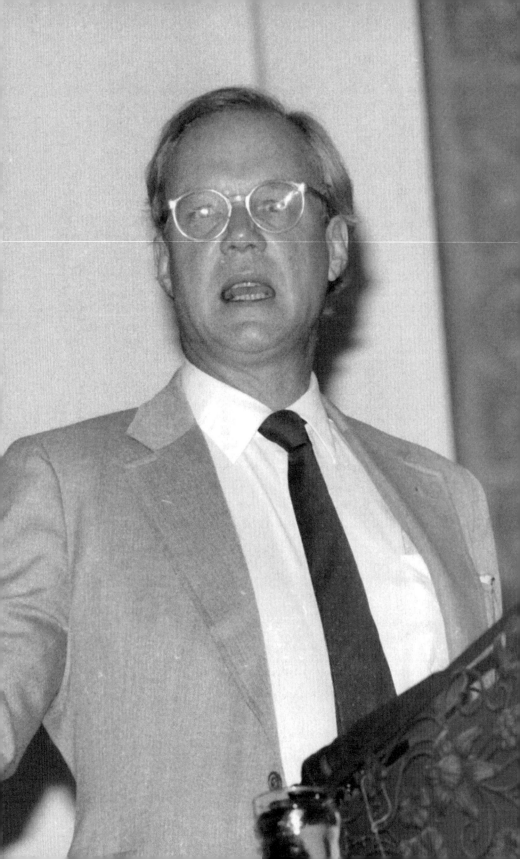

# Scott Peck:

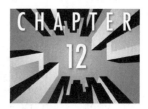

CHAPTER 12

# The Evil of Compartmentalization

In one of his letters, the Apostle Paul wrote that this human society was ruled by "principalities and powers," his phrase for "the demonic." Whether we interpret the demonic as some external force or simply our human nature and "original sin," the notion that the devil is the ruler of this world has an enormous amount of truth to it. Given the prevalence of war, genocide, poverty, starvation, gross inequality in the distribution of wealth, racism and sexism, despair and hopelessness, drug abuse, white-collar crime in our institutions, violent crime on our streets, and child and spousal abuse in our homes, evil seems to be the order of the day.

It certainly looks that way most of the time — for the forces of evil are real and varied. Some religions claim that the factors perpetuating evil originate in human sin. Psychological explanations often point to the lack of individual and group consciousness. Many social commentators view the chaos in our culture, including a breakdown in family values and the emphasis on materialism and comfort at all costs, as the primary determinants of evil. The media are often blamed for their wicked influence. Let's look at each of these factors briefly to flesh out the paradoxical reality of good and evil that has a significant impact on our choices about society.

The word "Satan" originally meant adversary. In Christian theology, Satan is also called the devil. We are being adversarial when we speak of "playing devil's advocate." Satan or the devil,

M. Scott Peck, M.D., was a nationally recognized authority on the relationship between religion and science. He authored the epoch-making book *The Road Less Traveled* (Simon & Schuster, 1978), as well as *The Different Drum: Community Making and Peace* (Simon &Schuster, 1987), *Meditations from the Road* (Simon & Schuster, 1993), *Denial of the Soul* (Harmony Books, 1997), and many others. As a result of his pioneering community work, Peck received the 1994 Temple International Peace Prize, and the 1996 Learning, Faith, and Freedom Medal from Georgetown University. He died at his home in Connecticut in September, 2005.

mythologically, was originally a "good" angel who was cast out of heaven for disobedience and pride, and became the personification of evil and the adversary of man. A certain amount of adversarialism is good for our thinking and growth. Its flippant practice, however, may hide a hint of the sinister. Any adversarial position which is persistently contrary and opposed to human growth—and directly opposite to that which is godly—contains the harsh ingredients for the perpetuation of evil.

Among those ingredients may be human nature itself. I have little idea what role the devil plays in this world, but as I made quite clear in *People of the Lie*, given the dynamics of original sin, most people don't need the devil to recruit them to evil; they are quite capable of recruiting themselves. In *The Road Less Traveled*, I suggested that laziness might be the essence of what theologians call original sin. By laziness I do not so much mean physical lethargy as mental, emotional, or spiritual inertia. Original sin also includes our tendencies toward narcissism, fear, and pride. In combination, these human weaknesses not only contribute to evil but prevent people from acknowledging their Shadow. Out of touch with their own sins, those who lack the humility to see their weaknesses are the most capable of contributing to evil either knowingly or unknowingly. Wars tend to be started by individuals or groups lacking consciousness and devoid of integrity and wholeness. I wrote of this in *People of the Lie*. Using My Lai as a case study, I demonstrated how evil at an institutional and group level occurs when there is a fragmentation of consciousness—and conscience.

In *Further Along the Road Less Traveled* and *The Different Drum*, I wrote of the evil of compartmentalization. I described the time when I was working in Washington in 1970-72 and used to wander the halls of the Pentagon talking to people about the Vietnam War. They would say, "Well, Dr. Peck, we understand your concerns. Yes, we do. But you see, we're the ordinance branch here and we are only responsible for seeing to it that the napalm is manufactured and sent to Vietnam on time. We really don't have anything to do with the war. The war is the responsibility of the policy branch. Go down the hall and talk to the people in policy."

So I would go down the hall and talk to the people in policy, and they would say, "Well, Dr. Peck, we understand your concerns. Yes, we do. But here in the policy branch, we simply execute policy, we don't really make policy. Policy is made at the White House." Thus, it appeared that the entire Pentagon had absolutely nothing to do with the Vietnam War.

This same kind of compartmentalization can happen in any large organization. It can happen in businesses and in other areas of government; it can happen in hospitals and universities; it can happen in churches. When any institution becomes large and compartmentalized, the conscience of that institution will often become so fragmented and diluted as to be virtually nonexistent, and the organization has the potential to become inherently evil.

The word "diabolic" is derived from the Greek *diaballein*, meaning to throw apart, fragment, or compartmentalize. Among the most diabolic aspects of the fragmentation of our collective consciousness are those things so common that they have become institutionalized. Where institutionalized evils such as racism, sexism, ageism, and homophobia exist, for example, we find the dual mechanisms of oppression and dehumanization. When certain segments of humanity are systemically regarded as disposable or irrelevant or are treated with derision, dire consequences for the integrity of the entire society are inevitable.

To do battle with institutionalized societal evils, we need remember that what we call good must be good for most people, most of the time, and not merely a matter of "Is it good for me?" This variant of the Golden Rule means that when we employ double standards condoning our own behavior but judging others harshly for the same breach or something lesser, we are in danger. For example, those who live in the nation's inner cities receive substantially longer prison terms than others for relatively minor crimes, like possession of small amounts of crack cocaine, according to statistics from the National Sentencing Project based in Washington, D.C. Suburban powder-cocaine users and middle to upper-class users are rarely sentenced to prison for first offenses. They are more likely to get probation and be encouraged to receive treatment for their drug problems.

Often, the forces of evil are more subtle than blatant. Almost as horrific as evil itself is the denial of it, as in the case of those who go through life wearing rose-colored glasses. Indeed, the denial of evil can in some ways perpetuate evil itself. In *In Search of Stones*, I wrote about this tendency among a number of financially well-off people whose money insulates them in their world of opulence. They fail to actually see the poverty that exists so close to them, and thereby they avoid accepting any responsibility they may have for the problem. Many ride a train to work every day from their suburban havens to downtown New York City, never looking up from their newspapers as they pass the most impoverished sections of Harlem. The slums are rendered invisible and so, too, are those enmeshed in them.

On the other hand, there are those who take a cynical view of the world and seem to believe that evil lurks behind everything. Their vision is gloom-and-doom, even in the midst of innocence and beauty. They look for the worst in everything, never noticing that which is positive and life-affirming. When despair and cynicism are like demons to us, we risk perpetuating evil as well. Although we can't avoid our demons, we can choose not to welcome or to ally ourselves with them. To be healthy, we must personally do battle with them.

A despairing vision of society can become even more clouded by media influences. Through their focus on the drama of evil, the media perpetuate an unbalanced view of reality. When a credit card is stolen, it becomes a statistic, and the headlines bombard us with crime reports. But we rarely hear any statistics about credit cards left behind on counters and quietly returned (as is almost always the case). The media's general exclusion of good news leaves the public with the impression that evil truly rules the day. If "no news is good news," it would also appear that "good news is no news." We do not hear or read about the goodness that occurs routinely—on a daily basis—in the world.

It is easy to despair, to simply throw one's hands up and believe that, since the world is so evil, nothing and no one can make a difference. But if we are to look at our society realistically, we will recognize the powerful influences of both good and evil forces. The world is not all beautiful. Neither is it all bad. Thus, the most critical challenge we face is developing the ability to gain and maintain a balanced perspective. And from this perspective, there is cause for optimism, not despair.

A story told to me by my late father helps make the point. It is the story of an Oriental sage who, back in the 1950s, was interviewed by a reporter and asked whether he was an optimist or a pessimist.

"I'm an optimist, of course," the sage replied.

"But how can you be an optimist with all the problems in the world—overpopulation, cultural breakdown, war, crime, and corruption?" the reporter asked.

"Oh, I'm not an optimist about this century," the sage explained. "But I am profoundly optimistic about the next century."

Given the reality of the world today, my response would be along the same lines.

Just as it is necessary to develop one's consciousness in order to acknowledge the reality of evil and our own potential for sin and for contributing to evil, we also need to become increasingly conscious to identify and relish what is good and beautiful in this life. If we see the world as inherently evil, there is no reason to believe it can improve. But if we see that the forces for good in the world are, at the very least, on an equal footing with the forces for ill, there is great hope for the future.

In many ways, the world is changing for the better. As I wrote in *The Road Less Traveled*, over one hundred years ago child abuse was not only rampant in the United States but blandly overlooked. Back then, a parent could beat a child severely and commit no crime. Some two hundred years ago, many children, even those as young as seven, were forced to work in factories and mines practically all day. Some four hundred years ago, children weren't generally considered worthy of attention and respect as individuals with their own needs and rights in our society. But child protection efforts have improved tremendously in our century. We have established hotlines for reporting cases of child exploitation; investigations are routine and sometimes extensive in cases of suspected child abuse and neglect. Unless you can't see the forest for the trees, there's no denying that society has made vast improvements in protecting the interests and well-being of its youngest and most vulnerable citizens.

There is also profound proof of change for the better on a world level. Consider the issue of human rights. Governments are regularly monitored to determine how they treat their citizens, and some have suffered economic sanctions in response to major human rights violations, as was the case with the apartheid system in South Africa. In previous centuries, the notion of war crimes was nonexistent. Captured women and children were routinely raped and enslaved while the disembowelment of male prisoners of war was ritualistic behavior. Wars and war crimes persist, but recently we have begun to raise the issue of why humans so frequently go to great lengths to kill one another when a most decent peace would be quite feasible if we simply worked at it a little bit. We have established tribunals to try to punish those guilty of war crimes. We also now debate whether a war should be considered just or unjust and unnecessary. That we even raise these issues is an indication of how much positive change is emerging in this society and throughout the world.

It can be argued that one reason many view evil as more prevalent than ever is a result of the fact that our standards have improved. In any case, the evidence suggests that society is evolving for the better over the long haul. That would be impossible if society were wholly evil. The truth is that both good and evil coexist as forces in this world; they always have and always will. I recognized that fact long ago. But I find it actually easier to pinpoint with greater clarity why evil exists and whence it comes than to ascertain the origins of goodness in this world without reference to God. What St. Paul called "the mystery of iniquity" is ultimately less mysterious than the mystery of human goodness.

While the prevailing Judeo-Christian view is that this is a good world somehow contaminated by evil, as a mostly middle-of-the-road Christian I prefer the view that this is a naturally evil world somehow contaminated by goodness. We can look at children, for example, and rejoice in their innocence and spontaneity. But the fact is that we are all born liars, cheats, thieves, and manipulators. So it's hardly remarkable that many of us grow up to be adult liars, cheats, thieves, and manipulators. What's harder to explain is why so many people grow up to be good and honest. While capable of evil, in reality human beings overall are often better than might be expected.

In my experience with community-building workshops, I've been immensely impressed by what I've come to call "the routine heroism of human beings." It is also common to discover how people in tragic circumstances such as the Oklahoma City bombing, or in other crisis situations, rise to the occasion. There is abundant evidence of how people can be incredibly good when they are pulling together. Still, many tend to take goodness for granted. There is a lesson for us all in these words of wisdom, uttered by some anonymous soul: "A life of all ease and comfort may not be as wonderful as we think it would be. Only through sickness do we gain greater appreciation for good health. Through hunger we are taught to value food. And knowing evil helps us to appreciate what is good."

If the coexistence of good and evil is paradoxical, we must embrace that paradox so that we can learn to live our lives with integrity. The crux of integrity is wholeness. And through wholeness as human beings we can practice the paradox of liberation and celebration. Liberation theology proclaims that Christians are called to play an active role in doing battle with the systemic sins and evils of society—called to take responsibility for liberating people from the burdens of poverty and oppression. Celebration theology has historically encouraged a focus on and celebration of the goodness and beauty found in the world.

In his book *Christian Wholeness*, Tom Langford probes the many paradoxes that Christians must embrace in order to be realistic and whole people, among which the paradox of celebration and liberation is but one. As Langford points out, people who focus exclusively on liberation become fanatic and glum, while those who focus only on celebration will be frothy, superficial, and glib. Once again, we are called to integration. Striving for wholeness makes it necessary for us to continually acknowledge and do battle with the forces of evil. At the same time, we must remain conscious of and deeply grateful for the forces of good.

In the battle between good and evil, we must be open to struggling throughout our lives. While there is reason to be pessimistic, there also is strong reason to believe that each of us can have some impact, however minuscule it may seem, on whether the world tilts toward change for good or ill. In a remark attributed to Edmund Burke, we have the basis for determining which of the two forces will ultimately win the day: "The only thing necessary for the triumph of evil is for good men [and women, I must add] to do nothing."

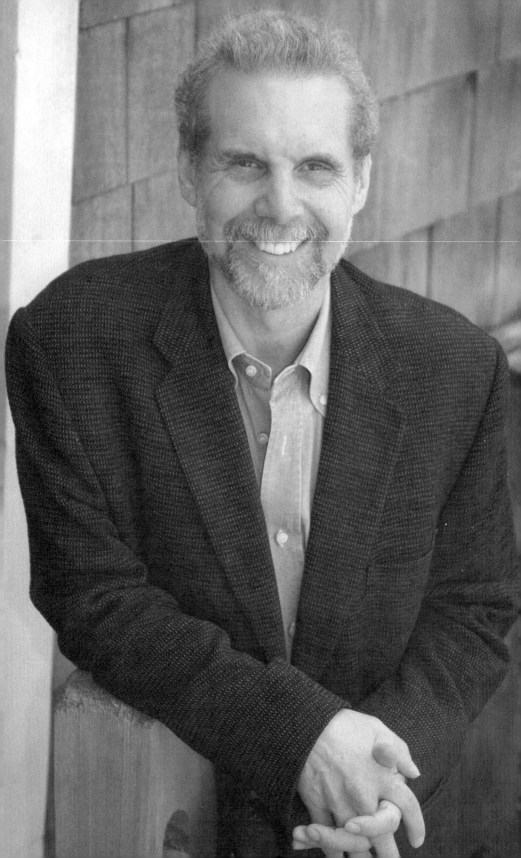

# DANIEL GOLEMAN:

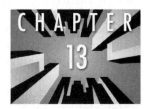

# The Discordant Leader

D issonance, in its original musical sense, describes an unpleasant, harsh sound; in both musical and human terms, dissonance refers to a lack of harmony. Dissonant leadership
produces groups that feel emotionally discordant, in which people
have a sense of being continually off-key.[1]

Just as laughter offers a ready barometer of resonance at work,
so rampant anger, fear, apathy, or even sullen silence signals the
opposite. Such dissonance, research finds, is all too common in the
workplace. In a survey of more than a thousand U.S. workers, for
example, 42 percent reported incidences of yelling and other kinds of
verbal abuse in their workplaces, and almost 30 percent admitted to
having yelled at a co-worker themselves.[2]

Consider the biological costs of such dissonance. Although
surfacing genuine complaints can clear the air — and build resonance —
when the person complaining does so with anger, the encounter can
easily spiral into emotional toxicity. For example, rather than saying
calmly, "When you're late for our meetings, it wastes our time — we'd
all be more effective if you showed up on time," the complainer
launches into a character attack.

He snarls, "I see His Highness has deigned to join us. I'm glad to
see you could fit us into your busy schedule. We'll try not to waste
too much of your time."

Daniel Goleman is a psychologist, lecturer, and author of the bestselling
books *Emotional Intelligence* (Bantam, 2005) and *Working with Emotional
Intelligence* (Bantam, 2000). He is co-chair of the Consortium for Social
and Emotional Learning in the Workplace at the School of Professional
and Applied Psychology, Rutgers University, which seeks to identify
best practices for developing emotional competence. A Fellow of the
American Association for the Advancement of Science and visiting faculty member at Harvard University, Goleman was twice nominated for a
Pulitzer Prize for contributions to *The New York Times* reporting on brain
and behavioral science. Photo by Frank Ward.

Such disturbing encounters wreak havoc emotionally, as demonstrated in studies in which physiological responses were monitored during arguments.[3] Such attacks—which send the painful emotional messages of disgust or contempt—emotionally hijack the person targeted, particularly when the attacker is a spouse or boss, whose opinions carry much weight.

John Gottman, a psychologist at the University of Washington, uses the term "flooding" to describe the intensity of the fight-or-flight reaction that such an extreme message of contempt can trigger: Heart rate can leap 20 to 30 beats per minute in a single heartbeat, accompanied by an overwhelming feeling of distress. When flooded, a person can neither hear what is said without distortion, nor respond with clarity; thinking becomes muddled and the most ready responses are primitive ones—anything that will end the encounter quickly. As a result, people will often tune out (or "stonewall") the other person by putting either an emotional or physical distance between them.

Although these studies were done with married couples, a dissonant encounter between boss and employee takes much the same emotional toll. In one study, employees were asked to recall times managers had lost their tempers at them and launched into a personal attack. Typically the employee became defensive, evaded responsibility, or stonewalled, avoiding contact with the manager. And when 108 managers and white-collar workers reported on the causes of conflict in their jobs, the number one reason was inept criticism by a boss.[4]

In short, dissonance dispirits people, burns them out, or sends them packing. There's another personal cost to dissonance: People who work in toxic environments take the toxicity home. Stress hormones released during a toxic workday continue to swirl through the body many hours later.[5]

## The Varieties of Dissonance

There are countless kinds of dissonant leaders, who not only lack empathy (and so are out of synch with the group) but also transmit emotional tones that resound most often in a negative register. Most of those leaders, we find, don't mean to be so discordant; they simply lack the critical emotional intelligence abilities that would help them lead with resonance.

In the extreme, dissonant leaders can range from the abusive tyrant, who bawls out and humiliates people, to the manipulative sociopath. Such leaders have an emotional impact a bit like the "dementors" in the Harry Potter series, who "drain peace, hope and happiness out of the air around them."[6] They create wretched workplaces, but have no idea how destructive they are—or they simply don't care.

Some dissonant leaders, however, are more subtle, using a surface charm or social polish, even charisma, to mislead and manipulate. Those leaders don't truly hold their professed values, or they lack empathy, caring about little other than their own advancement. When followers sense that kind of insincerity—when a manipulative leader feigns friendliness, for instance—the relationship dissolves into cynicism and distrust.

Dissonant leaders sometimes may seem effective in the short run—they may get a coveted promotion, for instance, by focusing on pleasing their boss—but the toxicity they leave behind belies their apparent success. Wherever they go in an organization, the legacy of their tenure marks a telltale trail of demotivation and apathy, anger and resentment. In short, dissonant leaders are the bosses that people dread working for.

When we see someone leading an organization by stirring such negative resonance, we know that trouble lies ahead. Despite any short-term rise in performance, if a leader resonates exclusively in the negative emotional range, the effect will be to eventually burn people out. Such leaders transmit their own—often corrosive—emotions but don't receive; they neither listen to nor care about other people. Emotionally intelligent leaders, in contrast, follow the more lasting path to motivation by evoking positive resonance: rallying people around a worthy goal.

## The Demagogue

Given that adept leaders move followers to their emotional rhythm, we face the disturbing fact that, throughout history, demagogues and dictators have used this same ability for deplorable ends. The Hitlers and Pol Pots of the world have all rallied angry mobs around a moving—but destructive— message. And therein lies the crucial difference between resonance and demagoguery

Compared with resonant leaders, demagogues spread very different emotional messages, ones that elicit negative emotions, particularly a mix of fear and anger: the threat to "us" from "them," and the dread that "they" will take what "we" have. Their message polarizes people rather than uniting them in a common cause. Such leaders build their platform for action on a negative resonance—on the disturbing fight-or-flight survival emotions that stream through the brain when people feel threatened or enraged. The Serbian leader Slobodan Milosevic, for example, was a master at fanning the flames of ethnic hatred, uniting his followers behind a banner of resentments, fears, and rage—to both his own and his nation's detriment.

Demagoguery casts its spell via destructive emotions, a range that squelches hope and optimism as well as true innovation and creative imagination (as opposed to cruel cunning). By contrast, resonant leadership grounded in a shared set of constructive values keeps emotions resounding in the positive register. It invites people to take a leap of faith through a word picture of what's possible, creating a collective aspiration.

Luckily, the demagogue is a rare type in business; politics seems the demagogue's more natural ecological niche. Still, some business leaders do resort to nefarious tactics. Workplace leadership built on negative resonance—for instance, cultivating fear or hatred of some "enemy"—amounts to a cheap trick, a quick and dirty way to mobilize a group toward a common goal. It may be relatively easy to get people to hate or fear something together; these emotions come readily, given the right threat. But from a biological perspective, these emotions were designed for short, intense bursts meant to prepare us to fight or run. If they last too long or are continually primed, they exhaust us or slowly burn us out. Anger or fear, then, may get a leader through the crisis of the day, but they are short-lived motivators.

There are also the leaders we call "clueless," who try to resonate in a positive tone but are out of touch with the unpleasant fact that their subordinates are stuck in a negative emotional register. In other words, the organizational reality makes people angry or anxious or otherwise unhappy, but the leader remains oblivious and so sends an upbeat message that resonates with no one.

One executive we know describes his organizational vision this way: "We are nimbly moving into a complex future, leading our industry as we reach for new heights. Our leaders look for opportunities at every turn and our managers are blasting the competition. We delight in our customers' satisfaction."

At first glance it may sound pretty good—but on second thought, it's a string of empty platitudes. We don't know what he really meant (do you?), but when we began to look at the culture and the leadership practices, we couldn't find much flexibility; tolerance for ambiguity, risk taking, or innovation; or attunement to customers. We found groups of people focused on the same old routine and cynical about the vision their leader described. The sad fact is that business jargon can be a smokescreen, so that a leader never has a real conversation about what people are actually doing in the organization — and never has to change.

Self-absorbed leaders can often be clueless. For instance, a group of managers at a consumer goods company requested a meeting with their CEO because they were deeply troubled by what they saw happening at their company. Though the company was still ranked in the top ten compared with others in their industry, the trend lines pointed downward. These managers, so close to the work, wanted to help their CEO move things in the right direction.

But when the CEO met with the managers, he didn't seem to hear them. His reply to their concerns: "People want a hero — they need one — and that's what I am to the employees. I'm like a movie star — people want to see me and look up to me. That's why I thought it was a good idea for you to come here, so you can hear what I have to say and tell everyone what I'm really like."

There was a stunned silence in the room as he spoke — a silence that the CEO no doubt took as agreement. For him, this was not about "us" but about "me." The dark side of ambition is that it can focus a leader's attention on himself, leading him to ignore the worries of the people who he needs to make him successful — and breeding dissonance.[7]

By contrast, emotionally intelligent leaders build resonance by tuning into people's feelings — their own and others' — and guiding them in the right direction. To understand the mechanisms that drive emotionally intelligent leadership, and so create resonance, we look to new findings in brain research.

## Leadership and the Brain's Design

No creature can fly with just one wing. Gifted leadership occurs where heart and head — feeling and thought — meet. These are the two wings that allow a leader to soar.

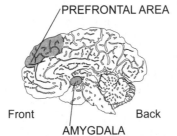

The crucial emotional regulatory circuitry runs from the prefrontal area to the amygdala, located on either side of the mid-brain as part of the limbic system.

All leaders need enough intellect to grasp the specifics of the tasks and challenges at hand. Of course, leaders gifted in the decisive clarity that analytic and conceptual thinking allow certainly add value. We see intellect and clear thinking largely as the characteristics that get someone in the leadership door. Without those fundamental abilities, no entry is allowed. However, intellect alone will not make a leader; leaders execute a vision by motivating, guiding, inspiring, listening, persuading—and, most crucially, through creating resonance. As Albert Einstein cautioned, "We should take care not to make the intellect our god. It has, of course, powerful muscles, but no personality. It cannot lead, it can only serve."

The neural systems responsible for the intellect and for the emotions are separate, but they have intimately interwoven connections.[8] This brain circuitry that interweaves thought and feeling provides the neural basis of primal leadership. And, despite the great value that business culture often places on an intellect devoid of emotion, our emotions are, in a very real sense, more powerful than our intellect. In moments of emergency, our emotional centers—the limbic brain—commandeer the rest of the brain.

There's good reason for this special potency of emotions. They're crucial for survival, being the brain's way of alerting us to something urgent and offering an immediate plan for action: fight, flee, freeze. The thinking brain evolved from the limbic brain and continues to take orders from it when we perceive a threat or are under stress. The trigger point for these compelling emotions is the amygdala, a limbic brain structure that scans what happens to us from moment to moment, ever on the alert for an emergency.[9] As our radar for emotional emergencies, the amygdala can commandeer other parts of the brain, including rational centers in the neocortex, for immediate action if it perceives a threat.

This arrangement worked well during the last 100 million or so years of evolution. Fear guided early mammals through the real dangers of predators; anger mobilized a mother to fight to protect her young. And social emotions such as jealousy, pride, contempt, and affection all played a role in the family politics of primate groups—just as they do in the underworld of organizational life today.

While emotions have guided human survival through evolution, a neural dilemma for leadership has emerged in the last 10,000 years or so. In today's advanced civilization, we face complex social realities (say, the sense someone isn't treating us fairly) with a brain designed for surviving physical emergencies. And so we can find ourselves hijacked—swept away by anxiety or anger better suited for handling bodily threats than the subtleties of office politics. (*Just who the hell does this guy think he is! I'm so mad I could punch him!*)

Fortunately, such emotional impulses follow extensive circuitry that goes from the amygdala to the prefrontal area, just behind the forehead, which is the brain's executive center. The prefrontal area receives and analyzes information from all parts of the brain and then makes a decision about what to do. The prefrontal area can veto an emotional impulse—and so ensure that our response will be more effective. (*Remember, he's giving your annual review—just relax and see what else he says before you do something you might regret.*) Without that veto, the result would be an emotional hijack, where the amygdala's impulse is acted upon. This happens when the prefrontal zone circuitry fails in its task of keeping these emotional impulses in check.

The dialogue between neurons in the emotional centers and the prefrontal areas operates through what amounts to a neurological superhighway that helps to orchestrate thought and feeling. The emotional intelligence competencies, so crucial for leadership, hinge on the smooth operation of this prefrontal-limbic circuitry. Studies of neurological patients with damaged prefrontal-limbic circuitry confirm that their cognitive capacities may remain intact, while their emotional intelligence abilities are impaired.[10] This neurological fact clearly separates these competencies from purely cognitive abilities like intelligence, technical knowledge, or business expertise, which reside in the neocortex alone.

Biologically speaking, then, the art of resonant leadership interweaves our intellect and our emotions. Of course, leaders need the prerequisite business acumen and thinking skills to be decisive. But if they try to lead solely from intellect, they'll miss a crucial piece of the equation.

Take, for example, the new CEO of a global company who tried to change strategic directions. He failed, and was fired after just one year on the job. "He thought he could change the company through intellect alone, without moving people emotionally," a senior vice president at the company told us. "He made radical strategic changes without bothering to get buy-in from the people who would execute those changes. A storm of e-mails from employees to the board complained of his tuned-out leadership, and the CEO was finally ousted."

## How the Four Core Emotional Intelligence Domains Interact

We are by no means the first to suggest that the main tasks of a leader are to generate excitement, optimism, and passion for the job ahead, as well as to cultivate an atmosphere of cooperation and trust.[11] But we wish to take that wisdom one step further and demonstrate how emotional intelligence enables leaders to accomplish those fundamental tasks. Each of the four domains of emotional intelligence—self-awareness, self-management, social awareness, and relationship management—adds a crucial set of skills for resonant leadership.

These domains are, of course, closely intertwined, with a dynamic relationship among them. For instance, a leader can't manage his emotions well if he has little or no awareness of them. And if his emotions are out of control, then his ability to handle relationships will suffer. Our research has found a system underlying this dynamic.[12] In short, self-awareness facilitates both empathy and self-management, and these two, in combination, allow effective relationship management. Emotionally intelligent leadership, then, builds up from a foundation of self-awareness.

Self-awareness—often overlooked in business settings—is the foundation for the rest: Without recognizing our own emotions, we will be poor at managing them, and less able to understand them in others. Self-aware leaders are attuned to their inner signals. They recognize, for instance, how their feelings affect themselves and their job performance. Instead of letting anger build into an outburst, they spot it as it crescendos and can see both what's causing it and how to do something constructive about it. Leaders who lack this emotional self-awareness, on the other hand, might lose their temper but have no understanding of why their emotions push them around. Self-awareness also plays a crucial role in empathy, or sensing how someone else sees a situation: If a person is perpetually oblivious to his own feelings, he will also be tuned out to how others feel.

Social awareness—particularly empathy—supports the next step in the leader's primal task: driving resonance. By being attuned to how others feel in the moment, a leader can say and do what's appropriate, whether that means calming fears, assuaging anger, or joining in good spirits. This attunement also lets a leader sense the shared values and priorities that can guide the group.

By the same token, a leader who lacks empathy will unwittingly be off-key, and so speak and act in ways that set off negative reactions. Empathy, which includes listening and taking other people's perspectives, allows leaders to tune in to the emotional channels between people that create resonance. And staying attuned lets leaders fine-tune their message to keep it in synch.

Finally, once leaders understand their own vision and values and can perceive the emotions of the group, their relationship management skills can catalyze resonance. To guide the emotional tone of a group, however, leaders must first have a sure sense of their own direction and priorities—which brings us back again to the importance of self-awareness.

These dynamic relations among the four emotional intelligence domains are of practical, not just theoretical, importance. They're the basic ingredients of effective primal leadership—of resonance.

1   We see resonance and dissonance as the two major poles of emotionally intelligent leadership. These dimensions can be thought of in terms of two dimensions: emotional tone and empathic synchrony. One dimension tracks the emotional tone and the impact of a leader's actions, positive or negative. The other dimension reflects empathy: whether or not people are in synchrony with the leader's emotional tonality, and the leader with theirs.

2   Yelling at work: Survey results reported in Vivian Marino, "It's All the Rage at Work, Too," *The New York Times*, 12 November 2000, Money & Business section, 3.

3   The physiology of arguments: The research, by John Gottman of the University of Washington, was done with married couples, but the physiology of response should apply whenever the two people involved have close and emotionally important relationships with each other, such as a boss and employee. For details, see John Gottman, *What Predicts Divorce: The Relationship between Marital Process and Marital Outcomes* (Hillsdale, NJ: Lawrence Earlbaum Associates, 1993)

4   Inept criticism: Robert Baron, "Countering the Effects of Destructive Criticism," *Journal of Applied Psychology* 75, no. 3 (1990): 235-246.

5   Stress hormones circulate for hours: See, for example, Dolf Zillman, "Mental Control of Angry Aggression," in *Handbook of Mental Control*, eds. Daniel Wegner and James S. Pennebaker (Englewood Cliffs, NJ: Prentice Hall, 1993).

6   Dementors: J.K. Rowling, *Harry Potter and the Prisoner of Azbakan* (London: Bloomsbury, 1999), 187.

7   The dark side of ambiton: See, for example, Michael Maccoby, "Narcissistic Leaders: The Incredible Pros, the Inevitable Cons," *Harvard Business Review*, January-February 2000, 69-75

8   The specifics of the neurology described throughout this chapter are far more complex than indicated here. In the interests of clarity, we have simplified the picture, focusing on key structures within the intricate web of circuitry always involved in any complex behavior.

9   When we use the term amygdala, we refer to the structure itself along with the web of circuitry that integrates the amygdala with other parts of the brain. See Joseph LeDoux, *The Emotional Brain* (New York: Simon & Schuster, 1996)

10  Cognitive abilities intact, but emotional intelligence impaired in patients with prefrontal-amygdala lesions: Neurological patients with damage to the bilateral areas of the amygdala, the ventral-medial area of the prefrontal lobe, and the right somatosensory and insular cortices show deficits on tests of emotional intelligence, whereas patients with damage to other brain areas, such as those in other areas of the neocortex, do not. These areas appear critical for being aware of our own emotions, for regulating and expressing them, and for being aware of the emotions of others. Antonio Damasio, University of Iowa College of Medicine, personal communication; Reuven Bar-On, personal communication on preliminary date collected with Antoine Bechara and Daniel Tranel, associates of Dr. Damasio.

11  The main task of a leader: See, for example, Gary Yukl, Leadership in Organizations (Upper Saddle River, NJ: Prentice Hall, 1998)

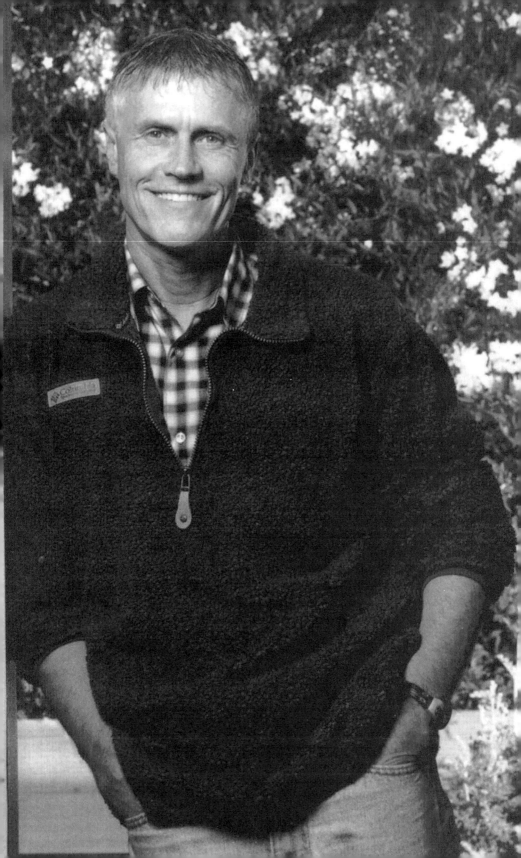

# PAUL HAWKEN:

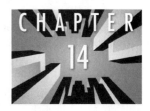

# Kicking the Consumption Habit

W e have elevated the ideology and mores of corporate life into a belief system before which we pay homage, and we have allowed it to take over the political system. We may spend an hour in church or temple every week, but we spend 40 or 50 or 60 hours at the workplace, in a job that demands and receives the greatest devotion we bestow on anyone or anything outside of (and sometimes including) our families. Work or some form of collective labor has always been a defining element of society, but never before has the output of work become the dominant organizing principle of the world's peoples.

Corporations are portrayed in the media as models of efficiency producing a stream of goods and services. But compelling evidence suggests that the behavior of many individuals in the modern corporation is remarkably similar to that of addicts. The parallels between the way addicts organize their lives and the lives business encourages suggest that there are many aspects to addiction we may not have recognized before—and many ways to define it.

At the core, an addiction is a way to keep ourselves from feeling.

Thus, anything we do that keeps us from knowing ourselves and fully experiencing the world around us can become an addiction. Work, television, food, money, sex, sports, and other activities can all be addictive when we rely on them to avoid dealing with inner

Paul Hawken is an environmentalist, entrepreneur, journalist, and best-selling author who has dedicated his life to changing the relationship between business and the environment. His practice has included starting and running ecological businesses, writing, teaching, and consulting with governments and corporations on economic development, industrial ecology, and environmental policy. His books, including *Natural Capitalism* (Little, Brown, 1999) and *The Ecology of Commerce* (HarperCollins, 1993), have sold more than two million copies in over 50 countries. He has written for the *Harvard Business Review, Resurgence, New Statesman, Inc, Boston Globe*, and *Utne Reader*. Visit www.paulhawken.com.

problems or deeper emotions. For every addiction there is a fix, an experience that we repeat over and over again, giving us the illusion that we are alive, while in fact numbing us to the real world and our real self, until it damages or destroys us.

The extension to corporate behavior is clear. We can become addicted to the deal, the power, the action, the excitement, the conflict, the aggression, the victories, the defeats, addicted even to the chaos and the stress, addicted to the point at which we feel empowered to do anything as long as it is legal (and perhaps not even legal), oblivious to many if not all of the effects of our actions on the environment, on society, or on ourselves. But like any habit, corporate addictiveness leads to chaos. Pursuing productivity and efficiency, American corporations have found anxiety. The demand to perform has become so overwhelming that, according to a recent poll, 20 to 30 percent of middle managers in the largest corporations confess that they have written memos or progress reports to their superiors that were dishonest. According to Michael Josephson, an ethics consultant for large companies, "We are swimming in enough lies to keep the lawyers busy for the next 10 years."[1] Kirk Hanson, Professor of Business Management at Stanford, says that managers feel they must be top achievers, or risk being fired.[2] A recent profile in a business magazine of a prototypical "successful executive" described his *modus operandi* as taking no prisoners, having the hands-on quality of Attila the Hun, and as not suffering fools gladly but shooting them on sight. That was all meant as a compliment. Jack Welch,[3] the Chairman of General Electric, nicknamed "Neutron Jack" because of his brutal and sudden firings, has eliminated 170,000 jobs during his reign and is considered one of the most admired CEOs in America by his peers. Some top executives have been summarily sent home from GE without warning, their personal effects shipped home by UPS. It should come as no surprise that another business magazine cover story featured a discussion of a "hot new skill" in the executive ranks, the ability to manage cultural, structural, and emotional chaos.

Business is faced with seemingly irreconcilable forces that sunder old assumptions and play havoc with employee morale. As the job base in Fortune 500 companies continues to decline (four million jobs lost in the past 12 years), as health and pension benefits are curtailed, as real wages continue to fall, and with job security becoming a nostalgic relic, workers can hardly be expected to be their most creative and productive. At the same time, decades of insulating prosperity in America have left our corporations slow in responding to global threats and competitors. Fear of the future has never been an effective human motivator, yet today the loss of jobs and benefits is never far from people's concerns, affecting their willingness to take risks, to speak up, to address critical issues of safety or long-term value.

The victims of an organized addictive system are not only those who lose their jobs, but also those who keep them. You cannot pick up a magazine that does not, at one time or another, praise, envy, or profile a woman or man who "has it all," who regularly puts in 60-hour work weeks, sits on several boards, volunteers for charity, heads the local Chamber of Commerce, works out at the health club, sails a boat, raises three children, and may even run for public office. This "successful" person is rapidly approaching burn-out, of course—you cannot "save the world" if you're destroying yourself on the altar of workaholism, wolfing food, gulping coffee, taking "red-eye" flights in the middle of the night, trying to do the work of three people—but she or he nevertheless was consistently portrayed as living a dazzling life. Many of us who feel inadequate about our own lives will redouble our efforts to climb the corporate ladder through a similar life of constant activity.

A friend tells a story about his business, a regional publishing house that began to build. With the expansion came a feeling of exhilaration and excitement. "Growth was just like being at a party," he recounted. "I could hear the buzzing of the conversation, the tinkling of the champagne glasses, the electricity in the air. I was having a good time but when I looked over at the doorway, there was this goofy, awkward guy standing there, not having fun, feeling like things had passed him by. And I realized it was me. My business was growing, but a part of me had been left behind, the me that is shy, quiet, and reflective." I suspect many people who get involved with business have a modest self that resists being adrenalized and overworked by incessant growth. In most cases, we see this subdued side of ourselves as something to overcome, a limit, a reluctant and unassuming persona that needs motivation tapes and seminars to mold it into the obsessive, success-driven, capable person the late-night cable programs assure us is hiding within.

Nothing in the modern workplace, and very little in society at large, encourages us to take our time, or be satisfied with what we have. We're being presented instead with a future where we will have to work harder, but have even less leisure time than we do today, if we are going to maintain our way of life. If that sounds like a positive feedback loop, it is. We are speeding up our lives and working harder in a futile attempt to buy the time to slow down and enjoy it.

Our economic insecurity, drifting and corrupt politics, suffocating debt, and environmental degradation cannot help but be reflected in the workplace where we spend most of our waking lives. The connections may be more obvious than we are willing to grant. For example, federal debt reduces the supply of capital for investment, and thus diminishes innovation, jobs, and productivity. High deficits were an attempt to re-create with paper the industrial growth of the past, a type of growth that depended on a unique set of circumstances in relation to the environment and resources. We have reached a point where the value we do add to our economy is now being outweighed by the value we are removing, not only from future generations in terms of diminished resources, but from ourselves in terms of unlivable cities, deadening jobs, deteriorating health, and rising crime. In biological terms, we have become a parasite and are devouring our host.

For a long time in American society, a large number of people thought they were advancing under the guidance and direction of commerce. As long as we could identify the improvements in the quality of our existence with the continuing growth and influence of big business, criticism of and dissatisfaction with the system were generally discounted or ignored. But during the past 20 years our standard of living has not increased, real wages have not risen, and, for the very first time since the Industrial Revolution, our work week is getting longer, not shorter[4] — a literally epochal development, barely remarked upon in the press. Worldwide, workplace stress has increased to the extent that the U.N. has issued a warning report calling it "one of the most serious health issues of the 20th century." Of the seven top-selling drugs in the United States, three are for hypertension, two are for angina and cholesterol respectively, and two treat ulcers — including Zantac, the top-selling drug in the world.[5] It is estimated that in the United States alone stress-related diseases such as ulcers, high blood pressure, and heart disease cost $200 billion a year in lost workdays, medical claims, and lost compensation.[6]

The question arises as to how long a company can prevail if its employees, consciously or unconsciously, perceive their products, processes, or corporate goals as harmful to humankind. We must consider whether on some deep or primordial level, we sense and embody within ourselves the strains and demands we place upon the environment. What does it mean to work at a company that produces copious amounts of $CO_2$, thousands of tons of toxins, dangerous and controversial products? A company that has a legal staff larger than its personnel department? Where gag orders are commonplace? Where lawsuits abound? And where safety is sometimes compromised? If such a company was full of depraved people, we would easily understand our dilemma and walk. But instead, it is run and operated by decent people who are friends, neighbors, and associates, people who, like ourselves, are not the least bit interested in harming the environment. Virtually no company exists or has been created to intentionally harm, society, so we can assume that destructive acts of commerce are generally well intended, or based on knowledge that was available at the time of inception. But our understanding of the environment and humankind's impact upon it has accelerated and exploded in the past decades, and with that has come a great unease.

One source of the discomfort is apparent: An economy oblivious to the environment may be equally insensitive to its workers and managers. Employees will be used in wasteful ways, leading to workplace stress, overwork, ill health or low morale. That the American workforce lives in a persistent state of anxiety further enlarges the power and control exerted over workers' lives by management. This relationship holds true in both successful and less successful companies, and it is made more acute when rank-and-file sees that a handful of executives and managers are lavishly compensated, in some cases with no apparent correlation to the performance of the company as a whole.

In sum, many employees sense that they are still caught in a fundamental inequality that they feel powerless to change. It should come as no surprise that every time a corporation offers a generous early-retirement program as a way to cut costs, it is usually oversubscribed.

It would be one problem — a serious one, granted — if our behavior within the corporate belief system hurt only ourselves, but the damage done is greater than that. It is axiomatic that people will do things in concert that they would not dream of doing as individuals. The actions required in warfare are the standard example, but business offers plenty of its own. The infamous Pinto gas tank was not designed to explode. Rather, an elaborate skein of rationalization, denial, and suppression of information was wrapped around the facts when the safety of the Pinto was questioned within the organization, even when the car was still in the design stage. When a disaster like this strikes and the corporate belief system finds itself at risk in the public eye, public relations is called in to deal with the crisis.

Denial will always prevent us from coming to terms with our actions as they affect the natural world but denial is an understandable reaction in the face of the great gulf between commercial reality and ecological reality. The fact is, if you work for a business — or even more so, if you own a business — it is highly inconvenient to fully acknowledge what is happening in the greater environment. That awareness runs counter to what we have been taught, and what we expect and want from our lives. America was founded on the "Go West, young man" principle of exploiting new lands and resources. Since World War II, we have expanded that principle, and now seek to grow more rapidly, drill deeper, speed up the economy, take more and do it faster. Today, we seem to be entering another phase, which is to deny the downside of present natural resource practices while pretending to be environmentally responsible. Our insatiable appetite for resources and the attendant waste caused by their consumption are being masked in meaningless eco-speak.

The message is much the same whatever the context: Don't worry about too much packaging, too much plastic, or too much waste. We are going to solve the problem with recycling and clean-up. You don't need to change your behavior, and we certainly don't need to change ours in any fundamental way. Recognizing that the greatest threat to their reputations and long-term fiscal health rested with children, their future customers, a number of corporations have entered the classroom, providing teaching kits to schools, many of which have been impoverished by tax-cutting programs supported by business. These teaching materials are, above all, cute: *Planet Patrol* by Procter & Gamble, *The Energy Cube* by Exxon, *Recyclasaurus and Recycle* by Dow Chemicals and Plastics, *Understanding the Waste Cycle* by Browning-Ferris Industries, and *Waste! A Hidden Resource* by Keep America Beautiful, a public relations extension of the packaging industry.[7] In the same vein, Champion International put out advertisements entitled: "Save the Wheatfields. Recycle Toast." The ad goes on to say that environmental issues are "becoming clouded by misconception and confused by a myriad of concerns... Sure, trees are a vital natural resource, but they are a renewable resource—and one that is protected by sound forest management... The critical issue is garbage dumps." The company would like us to believe that ancient forests are comparable to wheatfields: crops you can grow year after year.[8]

While social issues such as homelessness and poverty are rarely touched by corporations or TV programming because they represent no opportunities to create or maintain illusion, the environment is redolent with benign, endearing imagery. Soft-focus shots of deer in virgin forests are used as totemic proof of a paper company's commitment to the future even as they continue to clear-cut and fight congressional renewal of the Endangered Species Act. Native Americans look approvingly over a littered wildflower meadow being cleaned up by children using plastic bags advertised as biodegradable which in fact are not. (Mobil Oil was sued and chastised by attorney generals in several states for this ad.) Simpson Paper introduces a line of "recycled" paper with fractional amounts of post-consumer waste under the names of Thoreau, Whitman, and Leopold. British nuclear power companies announce that nuclear energy is green energy since it does not pollute the air.

Within the forest products industry, one of the leaders in

imaginative public relations is Louisiana-Pacific, whose chairman, Harry Merlo, was quoted as saying, "We need everything that's out there...We log to infinity. Because we need it all, now!" But in a *Fortune* magazine advertisement Merlo was wordsmithed to meet the needs of the 1990s: "Respect for the environment is nothing new to me. From the time I was a small boy in a poor family of Italian immigrants, I've understood how precious our God-given resources are, and how important it is never to waste them. The lessons I learned from my mother, Clotilde Merlo—lessons of thrift, common sense, hard work, and strength of purpose—I have not forgotten for a single day."

It was Simpson Paper Co. and Harry Merlo's Louisiana-Pacific that discharged 40 million gallons per day of toxin-containing effluents into the Pacific Ocean near Eureka, California. After documenting over 40,000 violations of the Clean Water Act, surfers who were getting skin rashes and other ailments from the ocean sued both companies and won, forcing payments of fines totaling $5.6 million. The presiding judge wrote that Louisiana-Pacific "essentially exempted themselves from all environmental protection requirements and therefore [felt] free to discharge potentially chronically toxic effluent into the waters of the Pacific Ocean with impunity. The position is disingenuous and flies in the face of the Clean Water Act."[9]

It is easy to become cynical about corporate PR and promotion, especially in the area of ecology, but cynicism may turn us away from the deeper truth, which is that environmental ad campaigns represent the limit and extent to which corporations are presently willing to accept ecological truths. Corporations do not perceive that present methods of production will deprive future generations, that there is a difference between supporting humankind with goods and services indefinitely and providing for them by relying upon environmental degradation as a means to overcome the carrying capacity of natural systems. What corporations do believe is that genuine environmentalism poses an enormous threat to their well-being. If you define well-being as their ability to continue to grow as they have in the past, they are correct.

Before the Industrial Revolution, commerce and culture were powerfully regulated by natural energy flows—mainly, the solar energy captured by food, wood, and wind. Scholars may debate the exact inflection point at which society turned to *stored* energy and, through it, harnessed the power of steam, railroads, and machinery, but once the process of industrialization commenced, the economic life of culture shifted from working with natural forces to working to overcome them. With the wholesale extraction and exploitation of stored solar energy, human beings are no longer living in synchronization with natural cycles and have accepted, however reluctantly, industrialism's shadow — waste, degradation, and dehumanization.

We have created, in essence, an artificial life, and in so doing, have lost some part of our human nature. Corporations extract resources and manufacture them into saleable products, leaving 11.4 billion tons of hazardous waste behind every year. On one level it appears that we are the customer for these goods, but on another level it is we who are being sold, offered up, and delivered to the corporations. It is we who are being extracted, mined, impoverished, and exploited. It is we who are fungible. Common wisdom holds that ecologists worry about nature while economists are concerned about human beings. But economists are in fact taking care of economics, and human beings are abandoned to the marketplace. What is for sale in America[10] is our welfare.

Author Joanna Macy writes of a type of despair that people feel when they experience the gulf between the grotesqueness of the world and the business-as-usual tenor surrounding it. At the level of the family, the gap between what a child feels and knows is right and reasonable, and what Mom and/or Dad *tells* the child is right, can lead to schizophrenia. A similar dysfunctionality can affect an entire society that knows the state of the world is one way, yet is told over and over again that the world is something else. That disparity finds its most powerful and pervasive form in advertisements.

By the time he or she graduates from high school, an American teenager will have seen 350,000 commercials. Children watch commercials at school thanks to Whittle Communication's Channel One, which beams two minutes of advertising for every 10 minutes of video "news" piped into thousands of classrooms. The average adult sees 21,000 commercials per year. Of these, 75 percent are paid for by the 100 largest corporations in America. In fact, corporations spend more money trying to get us to buy their products than we spend on all of secondary education in this country. Besides breathing, what do you do more than 3,000 times a day? What you do — or, more specifically, what is done to you — is receive several thousand messages to buy something. Not all of these are TV hard-sells. Many are marketing messages on T-shirts, shopping bags, license plates, or even stenciled on your oranges and lemons. The others are billboards, radio spots, signs, movies, newspaper ads, labels on the outside of clothing, or sponsorships at operas and sporting events. When you arrive home in the evening, one of the first things you do is collect the flyers, junk mail, catalogs, envelopes from nonprofit groups containing "personalized" letters, and free samples of shampoo hanging on your doorknob. Then the computer-generated junk phone calls start during dinner.[11]

Few of the 3,000 daily marketing messages you receive are by invitation. The fact that we are free to ignore any one particular ad doesn't diminish the fact that the commercial environment as a whole is coercive. We cannot ignore it for it is where we live. There is no other place. With newspaper readership trailing off, and book reading likewise, TV has become America's intellectual environment. Our minds are being addressed by addictive media serving corporate sponsors whose purpose is to rearrange "reality" so that viewers forget the world around them.

Advertising *is* needed to inform, direct, and educate, but in its present form, it is an invasive expression of commerce. Advertising creates envy and a sense of inadequacy; it is responsible for mediocre TV programming because the lower denominators of taste produce the highest ratings; it deceives young and old alike into purchases that are inappropriate, unnecessary, or wasteful, feeding the frenzy of consumption that is responsible for civilization's overshooting present carrying capacity. It is a type of "disvalue," the *removal* of value from a product by transferring the monies that should go into quality to promotion and hyperbole instead. Mass-market advertising reinforces economic centralization because of the high costs required; it is anti-democratic because it is not designed to allow dissenting voices that challenge the product's value or merits, and serves no social needs. Advertising permeates our souls, and denigrates women, the intellect, and spirituality.

The relentlessness of corporate promotion is matched by the passivity of consumers. Both parties are implicated, but both exonerate themselves gracelessly and easily by pointing a finger at the other. Businesses say they are responding to market forces and will change when the consumer changes. Consumers feel economically trapped by corporations and see only the narrowest of options afforded in their daily acts; consciously or not, we feel abused, objectified, taken for granted. American consumers may continually astonish even themselves by their base behavior and wants, but they have also tried to express themselves to business in thousands of other ways, from MADD's campaign against the promotion of beer and liquor to youth and citizens' clearinghouses on toxic waste issues, to local activist groups concerning open space. People are organizing to fight what they feel are the larger forces that infect their lives and values, forces that are almost invariably rooted in economic self-interest. The giant corporations are silent, immobile, and unmoved by our stirrings and longings. When they do speak, it is almost always through the disingenuous voice of "corporate communications." Fixing, restructuring, and reorganizing the corporation to serve a restorative economy will not be a solution unless businesses level with their customers. As the therapist wisely counsels: honesty does not harm, dishonesty always does. Today's deteriorating culture, environment, and economy are the fruits of decades of corporate dishonesty, a dishonesty that we have created, sanctioned, and supported.

The potency of industrial systems is overwhelming. No culture in the world has been able to resist the allure, convenience, ease, and wonder of materialism. Industrial corporations have overturned thousands of years of beliefs and practices, sometimes overnight, replacing cultural traditions that linked human welfare to deities and great natural laws with a managerial system that showed how mankind could intervene with, overturn, and even replace natural law with engineering, mechanics, technology, and systems. The growing power of corporations has not been accompanied by any comprehensive philosophy, any ethical construct, other than the accumulation of wealth as an end in itself. Very few principles guide the commercial conduct of corporations other than those randomly adduced or self-proclaimed. Everyone—managers, employees, customers—is left in limbo.

Those who would carry us to a new world of computerization, robotics, bioengineering, and nano-technology see their role as architects of a future that is controllable, and thereby made secure against the random and seemingly unpredictable patterns of nature. They would create molecular machines that would eat pollution and create ozone. They would fertilize the oceans with iron dust to reduce global warming. They would engineer our animals and plants and tailor them to human requirements: bacon with less cholesterol, tomatoes that have no genes telling them to decay, chickens without feathers or legs.

Whenever those moments arise in life when we become aware, fully and wholly, of the transiency of our experience, we seek those tasks and roles that give our hearts, minds, and hands the potential to serve truly another human being. While paying off mortgages and raising the kids can often provide all the "meaning" people can handle in their middle years, people are searching for higher values, both in what they do, as expressed in their work, and in how they interact with the world. What this world desperately needs is to have more value added to it. Too much has been taken away and destroyed. Businesses have this opportunity and challenge to create meaningful work for those who cannot find it in what they are presently doing.

# KICKING THE CONSUMPTION HABIT    Paul Hawken

When Pacific Gas & Electric, a utility in northern California, announced a new division called the Energy Efficiency Department, they expected only a trickle of internal applicants. The new division had an agenda that was the opposite of the company's as a whole: It was to institute measures that would create energy out of conservation, and to initiate programs, rebates, and incentives to generate "negawatts" — energy created through efficiency rather than new power plants. PG&E was overwhelmed with applications. People are hungry for ways in which they can integrate their need to be employed and support their families with work that improves the world in which they live. That department now has 300 employees.

People are either in denial or anxious that the disparity between what we experience in our own country and how most of the world lives is widening. Our prosperity in the North often results in the victimization of cultures and women and children in southern nations. People should be concerned about the difference between a population in the North that eats high on the food chain, and the 1.1 billion people worldwide, especially children, who are malnourished or hungry. It is tragic that America's largest export after food is weaponry, often sent to governments with repressive domestic policies, governments whose military superiority is frequently used to wrest resources away from indigenous cultures to pay the debts incurred in the first place by weapons purchases.

Literally thousands of native cultures around the world have been destroyed by economic development. Lost with those cultures have been languages, art and crafts, family structures, land claims, traditional methods of healing and nourishment, rites and oral histories. Despite all the economic growth in the Third World between 1960 and 1980, the gap in real income between the rich and poor nations increased from a factor of 20 to a factor of 46, and that gap continues to increase. Rather than uplifting the less developed nations, industrial economies have caused increased polarization of rich and poor, unleashed ethnic conflict, destroyed lands, urbanized the poor to marginalized conditions, and made the developed nations richer in the process. According to former World Bank President Robert McNamara, "Even if the growth rate of the poor countries doubled, only seven would close the gap with the rich nations in 100 years. Only another nine would reach our level in 1,000 years."[12] That is, in part, the result of the richer nations expanding their carrying capacity by exploiting resources in other countries. And while the United States may be richer, it has suffered some of the same fate as its neighbors internally: the skewing of the economic pie, a loss of traditions, the destruction of culture. The top 1 percent of the population increased its wealth 150 times faster than the bottom 99 percent during the 1980s.

Business *can* provide meaning for workers and customers but not until it understands that the trust it undertakes and the growth it assumes are part of a larger covenant. As long as nature, children, women, and workers are abused by institutions espousing free-market theories, the real deficit will continue to grow — the difference between what business has taken and what it has returned, the difference between value added and value subtracted. For most people meaning is derived from just the opposite relationship, one in which one gives more than one takes, where one's life is intricately bound to the promotion of the common good.

If adding value is what business is, or should be, all about, then it follows that you can't contribute values unless you have them. Our personal values, which have become so distant and removed from the juggernauts of commerce, must become increasingly important and, finally, integral to the healthy functioning of our economy. Business offers us rich and important ways to improve the world. Every transaction in the scheme of things is small, incremental, seemingly inconsequential, but each moment has the potential to create real change.

When Jerry Kohlberg withdrew from the Kohlberg Kravis Roberts partnership, dismayed that KKR had changed from a friend of innovative small companies to a predator, he said that "Around us there is a breakdown of...values in business and government... It is not just the overweening, overpowering greed that pervades our business life. It is the fact that we are not willing to sacrifice for the ethics and values we profess. For an ethic is not an ethic, and a value not a value, without some sacrifice for it, something given up, something not taken, something not gained. We do it in exchange for a greater good, for something worth more than just money and power and position."[13]

1. 1. Kenneth Labrich, "The New Crisis in Business Ethics," *Fortune* (April 20, 1992), p. 167.
2. Ibid.
3. John Huey, "Managing in the Midst of Chaos," *Fortune* (April 5, 1993), p. 38.
4. Juliet Schorr, *The Overworked American* (New York: Basic Books, 1991), pp. 17-41.
5. Shawn Tully, "Why Drug Prices Will Go Lower," *Fortune* (May 3, 1993), p. 56.
6. "U. N. Report Calls Job Stress Global Problem," *San Francisco Chronicle, March 23, 1992.*
7. "This Teacher Means Business," *Earth Island Journal* (Spring 1992), p. 4.
8. "Straight Talk" (Stamford, Conn: Champion International Corporation, 1991).
9. "Greenwash!" *Mother Jones* (April 1991), p. 23; "Surfrider Forces Pulp Mills to Halt Ocean Pollution—Costs Two Firms $5.6 Million," *Los Angeles Times,* September 10, 1991.
10. Jerry Mander, *In the Absence of the Sacred* (San Francisco: Sierra Books Club, 1991), pp. 78-79.
11. Kalle Lasn, Adbusters, "The Ecology of Mind," vol. 1, no. 4, p. 8.
12. Steven Gan, "The Global Poverty Crisis," *Earth Island Journal* (Fall 1992), p. 30.
13. *Fortune,* June 3, 1991, p. 172

# PART FOUR

# The Power of Mistakes

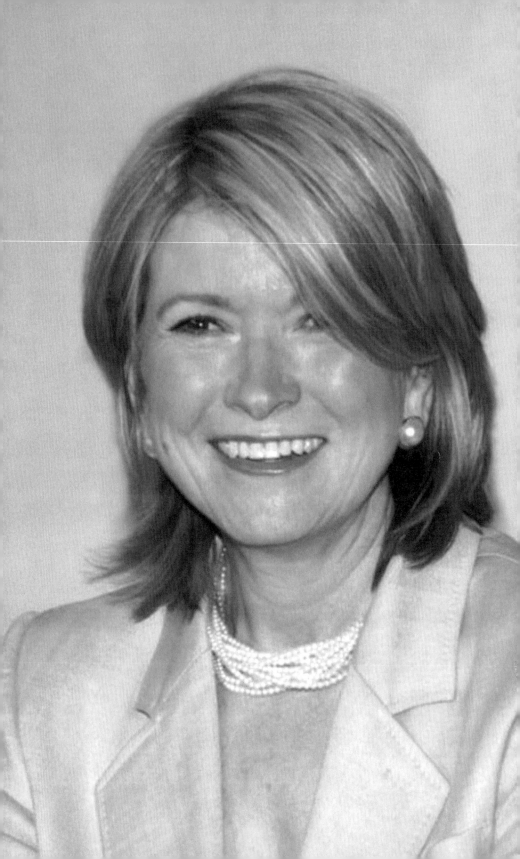

# MARTHA STEWART:

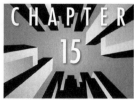

# So the Pie Isn't Perfect? Cut It Into Wedges

## Martha's Rule:

*When faced with a business challenge, evaluate or assess the situation, gather the good things in sight, abandon the bad, clear your mind, and move on. Focus on the positive. Stay in control, and never panic.*

Back in my catering days, I was fortunate to have many wonderful repeat customers, and some of my clients were well-known celebrities. When I was hired to cater a dinner for my fellow Westporters, Paul Newman and Joanne Woodward, I almost had to pinch myself. Not long before this booking, I had taken a driving tour of Morocco with my husband. Morocco was a feast for the eyes: craggy mountains, endless deserts, and miles of snow white, flowering almond orchards. Morocco was also a feast for the palate. I sampled the most incredible stews, called tagines, bursting with flavors both sweet and savory. The tagines were served over pale yellow mounds of steaming couscous. I was served a pigeon pie, called b'steeya, the savory contents encased in the flakiest pastry. Its flavors were deep and exotic. I thought this cuisine would make extraordinary party fare. At the bustling markets, I bartered for spices, canned condiments, and the necessary implements to prepare these dishes, including special copper couscous steamers and the heavy, terra-cotta-colored two-part clay tagines. We returned home with suitcases bulging and laps piled high with heavy pots.

Martha Stewart shares her creative principles and practical ideas through her magazine, *Martha Stewart Living,* her best-selling books, Emmy winning television show, syndicated newspaper column, national radio show, and product lines. Named one of the "50 Most Powerful Women" by *Fortune Magazine* (October 1998 – October 1999); she has been counted among "America's 25 Most Influential People" in *Time Magazine* (June 1996) and "New York's 100 Most Influential Women in Business" in *Crain's New York Business.* Her latest book is *The Martha Rules: 10 Essentials for Achieving Success As You Start, Build, or Manage a Business* (Rodale Books, 2005). Visit www.marthastewart.com.

When the Newmans called for a consultation, I was well prepared with a unique idea, and they were enchanted with the concept of a Moroccan buffet. I described the huge platters and colorful dishes, and they hired me to recreate many of the dishes I had sampled, including eight b'steeya, four made with chicken and the others with squab, which was more like the pigeon I had eaten in Marrakesh. Just a few hours before the party, I put the prepared b'steeya into the preheated oven. During baking, they looked just fine to me, and then I made the fatal error of getting distracted and leaving the kitchen. When I removed the b'steeya from the oven, I was horrified to see that each pie had a very badly burned crust on that portion of the pie that had been closest to the oven wall. (Now I make it a rule never to leave anything cooking without taking a timer in my pocket. When cooking shrimp, I do not even leave the stove.)

The pies, one of three main courses, were central to the buffet. My mind was full of horrifying visions. My reputation as a caterer was at stake. The pies were time-consuming to prepare, and it would be impossible to recreate them. I took a deep breath and made an assessment. I saw that although the pies were no longer perfect, the vast majority of each was fine and undamaged. I picked up a serrated knife, cut each pie into wedges, discarded the damaged portions, gathered the perfect pieces, sprinkled them with crisscrosses of powdered sugar and cinnamon, arranged them on huge brass trays, took them to the party, and served them. I acted as though nothing were amiss, and the party was a huge success. I never breathed a word of this to the Newmans or to anyone else, for that matter. I did what had to be done. The pies, now in wedges, were utterly delicious. Problem solved. Sorry, Joanne and Paul, but you may not have understood at the time.

## From Kilimanjaro to Alderson

I always smile at the memory of that day. After all, if every party, every idea, every business venture succeeded without unexpected setbacks and the occasional threat of disaster, the world would be a rather boring place. Getting over these unexpected hurdles may not be exactly enjoyable, but ultimately I believe that such challenges and the solutions we find give us more confidence. They teach us that, with common sense and determination, we can turn what looks like a disaster into a triumph.

Never in my wildest dreams did I imagine that I would draw on the basic lessons of this Moroccan party to help me endure something far more critical. From early 2002 through 2005, I was involved in a protracted and exhausting legal battle. I was encouraged by my board of directors and attorneys to resign as CEO and chairwoman of the company I had started, the company that still bears my name. This was despite the fact that the legal issues were in no way related to my activities as a corporate officer. Ultimately, I was sentenced to a five-month term in Alderson and another five months under home confinement.

During the long months of investigation and the trial and while waiting for the sentencing to occur, I awoke each day hoping that I was only having a really bad dream. I had spent my career and built my company's reputation working hard to bring Good Things to as many people as possible. And yet a personal stock trade was threatening to destroy everything: my successful television show, my much-loved magazine and book projects, a nationally syndicated radio show, a vibrant product design and merchandising business, and a highly creative staff that was never at a loss for ideas. Wall Street valued us, our growth was good, and our prospects were extremely bright.

When the press broke the story that the government was investigating me, so much changed. Media coverage became increasingly negative, horrible rumors spread, and the stock of my valued company plummeted. But one thing remained constant. From day one of this horrible nightmare, I received enormous numbers of letters and e-mails—supportive, positive messages from my viewers, readers, listeners, and customers. Partners such as Kmart stood firmly behind my company.

I remember all too well the weariness, frustration, and the surreal quality of those days. Nearly a decade before, I had experienced something akin to those feelings on a trek up Mount Kilimanjaro. On the last day of the journey, our small party departed our camp at Kibo hut a few minutes after midnight. The strategy was to make it to the summit before dawn to watch the sun rise over magnificent Africa. The climb was exhausting, and with the peak in sight, the group had split into two. One guide led my two fellow climbers, and the other paired off with me. At 19,000 feet, with the oxygen so thin that it was difficult to breathe, my guide suddenly became ill. His nose was bleeding from the effects of the high altitude, and it was imperative that he descend. I weighed the choices: to proceed alone or return with him, as he advised, and miss my chance at the summit. I could not fathom the idea of turning back without having reached the top, but I was also aware that I was on a dangerous trail, that I was physically exhausted and feeling light-headed, even giddy in the thin air. There were no guarantees that I could catch up to the lead group or even finish the climb. Plus, if something went wrong, I would have to resolve the problem myself. I trudged on, determined, eating snow to keep myself going (my guide had forgotten to bring water or food, an indication that he was indeed ill before we began our ascent) and breathing deeply and slowly in the very thin air. The apex, after all, was in sight. I climbed, step after treacherous step, but I made it just in time to witness the first rays of sunlight illuminating that part of the continent. I had followed my instincts and persevered.

Over the course of the legal investigation and the trial that followed, I felt many of the same physical sensations. I was exhausted, barely sleeping, and worried constantly about the future of my company and my employees. My executives were facing intense pressure to disassociate the company from me. They looked to me for assurance, which I tried to give, but the legal snows grew ever deeper.

## What's In a Name?

At my lowest point, just before conviction, I was pondering something that today seems utterly ridiculous. "Maybe I should change my name," I actually thought. "Maybe I can protect my company and my wonderful employees by distancing myself from the brand. If I become Martha Kostyra again, maybe then people can separate this personal matter from the value and worth of my company." This actually seemed like a real solution to me at the time.

I have already mentioned how the enormous support of my customers and fans and those hundreds of thousands of e-mails and letters helped to lift my spirits. But the verdict, when it was finally read aloud on March 4, 2004, was sad and discouraging for me, as was the judge's sentence, handed down a few months later.

Just as with my b'steeya mishap, it was time for me to fully evaluate the situation, cut the pie into wedges, gather the good parts, and move on. My lawyers were adamant that we would appeal; and, of course, I was in full agreement. However, there was simply no telling how long an appeal would take. It could very well drag on and on and on, and in the end, I might go to prison anyway. In order to save my company from irreparable harm, I knew it was time to slice my situation into wedges.

I realized that it would be in everyone's best interests for me to complete my prison term and home confinement, even as my lawyers aggressively pursued my appeal. I had built a great company, but that company had been battered — and yet I firmly believed it could weather this terrible storm. The company's good, solid core was intact—an enormous library of valuable information, a powerful brand identity, and an outstanding and creative staff. We had millions of loyal fans who were still buying our products, still reading our magazines, and still eager for us to introduce them to a myriad of useful, beautiful things. Those realizations gave me strength and courage to make the preparations that I hoped would put the crippling, toxic uncertainty far behind all of us.

I had a lot of work to do to get ready for my term of incarceration. Each piece of the pie had to be in order. Many parts of my personal life had to be attended to. When I flew off to the facility, I felt confident that many things could proceed without me because the correct wheels had been set in motion.

I must tell you that, although my stay at Alderson had none of the fun and spice of a Moroccan buffet, it was a far better experience than I had anticipated. It is no secret that I am accustomed to being in control—of my life and of my company. What became all too apparent during my confinement was how many, many women are not in control of their lives or what happens to them. They endure extraordinarily difficult situations, yet remain very strong, nonetheless, both physically and emotionally. I made it a priority to really try to understand my fellow inmates, and they did the same for me. They were so curious about my business and how and why I had accomplished so much. One group, who were followers of the Muslim faith, asked permission to have me speak at a forum about business practices, and I was allowed to do so. It was gratifying to share ideas—everything from how to develop a Big Idea to the ins and outs of Internet advertising. They were so grateful, so warm, and so excited to have answers to their questions. In fact this book began there, at Alderson, with my preparation for that business seminar.

When I was released from prison, draped in a beautifully crocheted poncho from my friend and fellow inmate, Xiomara Hernandez, I knew it was time to assess my life again. During my stay, I had been so fortunate to have a steady stream of family and friends who visited me. Believe me, many women in prison are visited by no one for years. There were many things that I had missed—my animals, my homes, fresh food, travel, and the daily challenges of managing an endlessly interesting business. But there were just as many wonderful things that I had gathered during those five months—new friendships, so many ideas, and so much information and knowledge from fascinating books that I actually had the time to read. I also gained a new appreciation for the complexity of every single person's situation. I even emerged with a funny and memorable new nickname: M. Diddy. Despite the reality of the situation, good humor prevailed at Alderson.

## Detours Are Part of the Journey

It is important to be realistic and to always remember that no matter how high you set your standards, no matter how intense your devotion to quality, no matter how detailed your business plan, stuff—I choose to use the more polite S word here—will happen. Great employees will quit; competitors will appear out of nowhere; critics will disparage you unfairly; fire will rage through your warehouse; investors will want you to go in one direction while you want to go in another. Perhaps a hurricane will ravage your state and destroy what you have built. Or perhaps your confidence will simply waiver when too many little problems mount up together.

As an entrepreneur, be prepared for these occasional dark nights and remain steadfast. However bleak things may at first appear, if you are a good person doing things for the right reason, there is always something to grasp onto to help you carry on or start over again. There is no entrepreneur, anywhere, whose journey is without setbacks and crossroads. Take a look at my very dear and funny friend, the petkeeper Marc Morrone.

## Marc Morrone: Flying Above Adversity

I first met Marc in 1997. While staying at my home on Long Island, I tuned into a local cable television channel, and there was this Dr. Doolittle type chattering pleasantly and intelligently about animals, specifically pets. A colorful parrot named Harry was perched on his shoulder, tugging on his glasses with its enormous beak. The table before him was covered with all sorts of animals—feathered, scaly, and furry—all getting along perfectly well. Marc introduced each one by name and explained its characteristics. As you know, I love animals, and I was mesmerized. Marc clearly had a real gift for communicating with his pets, and I wanted him on my show. I called Marc the next morning at eight, and he and his menagerie became regular guests. Today, he is one of our stars, with columns in two of our magazines and a weekly show called *Petkeeping with Marc Morrone*.

Marc is one of those passionate entrepreneurs to whom I always enjoy talking. He is a creative thinker; and no matter what kinds of challenges he faces, he always finds a way to prevail. He does not panic, and he does not complain. Instead, he sets out to find a solution.

# So the Pie Isn't Perfect? Cut It Into Wedges    Martha Stewart

Marc opened his pet store, called Parrots of the World, in 1978 in Rockville Center, Long Island. Specializing in exotic birds imported from tropical climates, his business was soon thriving. The animal import business has had many difficulties, including smuggling, endangered species investigations, customs problems, tariffs, and more. There have been some very unethical people involved in that world who have been notorious for abusing and neglecting the animals they have sold. Unfortunately for humane dealers like Marc, the U.S. government acted to stop the abuses by banning the import of parrots and other exotic birds, which had been the mainstay of Marc's business.

That was a huge blow to Marc. It destroyed a major portion of his business and a tremendous source of income. That was when he realized that specialization led to extinction, a principle he cites freely that is in keeping with his avocation, his attitude, and his business philosophy. Rather than closing his business, he adapted. He broadened the array of products that he sold; and he used his expertise, passion, and hard work ethic to shift his strategy. He became a breeder of magnificent, exotic birds and became so well known that he has developed a large export business selling his birds to aficionados in other countries.

You would think that his hard work and determination would pay off, and it did for many years. Marc's first store was a 15- by 40-foot space; today he and his brood share a 15,000-square-foot facility. In addition to becoming a TV personality, he started a number of related businesses, including aquarium maintenance and dog grooming.

Enter another cruel twist of fate. A duck in New York State became ill with an influenza virus much feared in the Far East, where many of his exports find a home. Because of concerns about the virus, in June 2005, Japan issued a six-month ban on the importing of birds from New York State. Although Marc's birds are well cared for and perfectly healthy, his exporting business has been shut down until the ban is lifted. Another big blow, and yet Marc is not bitter. "The world is constantly changing," he explains. "I have known that I wanted to work with animals ever since I was conscious. Bad things happen to good people all the time. You can't get angry. I have different things going on, and I can always find a way to make more money. I always look at the big picture."

Marc Morrone is an entrepreneur after my own heart. He has thrived despite his business setbacks by following the lead of some early, intrepid Arctic pioneers. Marc believes, "The most important thing in business is to make as many friends as you can. The Arctic explorers used to catch fish as they traveled, and they would bury one in the snow before they left camp. It was hard to sacrifice that fish sometimes. But on the way back, they could always count on having some food if they could make it to the next camp. That is how I look at business. You make as many friends as you can when things are going well. You do things you don't have to do in order to make friends. If you run into some difficulty and have to backtrack, they will be there, like the fish."

Marc's advice is sound. There are certain things that just cannot be taken from you: not by a change in government regulations, not by a fire in the warehouse, not by a betrayal of a trustee, not even by a federal trial and incarceration. The precious things that remain are your ideas, your determination, your work ethic, your loyal colleagues, your mentors, and all of the other friends who care about you and encourage you.

## There Is Always Value, Even Among the Ashes

Several years ago, I was honored with an invitation to take part in a book project conceived by actress and author Marlo Thomas. Marlo, a former neighbor of mine in Westport, came up with the wonderful idea of asking 100 prominent people about the most valuable advice they received during a difficult period in their lives. The list included actors, politicians, businesspeople, sports stars, and other celebrities. Marlo explained that the proceeds from the book were to go to her favorite charity, St. Jude Children's Research Hospital, founded by her father, entertainer Danny Thomas. Her book was my favorite kind of Big Idea—it offered helpful, useful, and important advice that people need and want, and it was to contribute generously to a most worthy cause.

In her book, Marlo tells her own story of when she appeared as the lead in Gigi, her first big stage production, at Los Angeles's Laguna Playhouse. Thrilled as she was, Marlo experienced unfortunate treatment from reviewers and interviewers, who compared her endlessly to her father instead of focusing on her talents. She told her father she was so frustrated that she did not "want to be a Thomas anymore." He looked her in the eye and said that he had raised her to be a thoroughbred and that thoroughbreds run with blinders so they can keep their eyes focused straight ahead, with no distractions. "Don't listen to anyone comparing you to me or to anyone else. You just run your own race." The next night, there was a knock on her dressing room door, and a stage manager delivered a box holding an old pair of horse blinders and a note from her father reading, "Run your own race, Baby."

My contribution to the project was about a predicament I found myself in during my teenage years. My ninth-grade English teacher had assigned a book report, and I chose Nathaniel Hawthorne's *The Scarlet Letter*. This proved to be a very difficult novel for a naïve 13-year-old who had no idea what the word *adultery* meant. I turned to my father for some helpful advice and encouragement. He was, after all, very well read and an excellent writer. But my dad, with his strong work ethic, said, "Martha, you can do anything if you put your mind to it. Anything!" He carefully explained the definition of adultery, and I reread the book and completed my report.

To this day, I can still hear those wise words. You can come up with a Big Idea for something that millions of people need and want. You can become a self-made billionaire. You can refuse to cave in to detractors and manipulators despite enormous pressure. You can become friends with a fellow inmate and learn all about her life over a lunch of inedible prison food. You can emerge intact even through the toughest of times. *You can do anything!*

## It Is Okay to Overreact, but Never Panic

When building a business, you will face many challenges and find yourself in some very difficult situations. I cannot emphasize strongly enough that when this occurs, you cannot panic! Panic is a debilitating thing. Your heart races, your blood pressure rises, your breathing gets shallow, you may even feel ill. You revert to a primitive survival mode as your body sends adrenaline coursing through your veins and your brain stem tells you that you have two choices: flee or fight.

When something awful and unexpected occurs and threatens your business, I believe it is acceptable to overreact. You are the entrepreneur, the creator of a business that rides on your shoulders. When something negative is thrown your way, it is fine to let your staff know that you have intense feelings regarding the development. They will expect that from you and will actually want it from you. It is your business, your creation, after all, that has come under attack, and they are involved.

Panic, however, creates irrational behavior and actions that have not been well considered. These are often short-term solutions designed to make the pain stop, rather than thoughtful, strategic approaches that will actually help to solve the problem. When you sense danger approaching, go ahead and get upset, but do not do anything that cannot be undone. If I had panicked when I burnt my Moroccan b'steeya, I might have picked up the pigeon pies and thrown them away. By remaining calm and making good decisions, I was able to serve each guest at the Newmans' party a smaller sliver of a wonderfully unique dish. Not ideal, but hardly disastrous.

## Take Time to Assess

When faced with a difficult challenge, remember the telescope, the wide-angle lens, and the microscope. Using the microscope, examine up close what exactly has occurred. By looking closely at the details, you may find the problem is far smaller and less daunting. First assess what has happened very specifically and whether the situation demands immediate action.

Here is a scenario: Suppose you are a florist, and you arrive at your shop at 6:15 a.m. with a van full of fresh flowers that you just picked up from the wholesaler. On this particular Saturday, you have an order for two dozen arrangements—centerpieces that must be delivered for a wedding reception by 4 p.m. Your best floral designer was supposed to unlock your doors at 6 a.m. and meet you, ready to get to work. It surprises you that the shop is still closed. Once inside, you find your answering machine blinking. Your arranger's husband left a message saying his wife will not be in today because she has broken her wrist and is at the hospital.

You are in a difficult situation. There were only two of you scheduled in the shop today; she would have made the arrangements while you helped and served customers at the counter. You have two immediate problems: You have an excellent employee who has suffered a painful mishap. Your first call should be to put her at ease and wish her well. Your relationship is important. But, you also have two dozen centerpieces to compose to satisfy your customer. What do you do? You could close the shop and do the work yourself; you could call other employees for either a floral designer or a counter person to fill in; you could call another florist and either divide the work or subcontract him or her to do it; or you could alert your customer that you may not be able to deliver the order—hardly an option, in my opinion.

Grab the wide-angle lens. Look at the consequences of each choice. If you decide to protect your reputation by subcontracting out the job, how will the loss of those profits impact you? Should you lose a day's walk-in business so as not to disappoint the bride? How important is this order? How important is your walk-in business?

Next, peer through the telescope. What are the long-term implications of your options for solving this problem? Should you protect your good reputation at any cost? Can you form a backup relationship with another florist that could become a valuable partnership for the future?

## Figure Out What to Cut and What to Keep

When things are not looking so bright, sometimes the most difficult decision is knowing what to keep and what to cut, what to sell, what to discard. That is why a thorough assessment is so crucial. Look meticulously at your particular problem—is the thing really ruined or is it just damaged and still reparable? There is a big difference between the two. And stay focused on the core of your business—its heart and soul.

Let us revisit the flower shop. You have to consider the impact to your reputation if you disappoint a bride on her wedding day. She and her family will be furious, and rightly so. The damage to your business from a very public failure would far outweigh the impact of not opening your retail shop for one day. This little crisis may even help you realize that you can no longer run both a special order and a retail shop successfully at this stage of your business's life. Making the right decision requires evaluation, perhaps even advice from trusted mentors.

What if MSLO, during my troubles, had decided to change its name to something generic like Good Things Incorporated? What if they had purchased other businesses having nothing to do with our core competencies—a tropical resort, perhaps, or a shoe company—in order to diversify beyond the brand I had come to represent so personally? I can guarantee you that it would have been as nonsensical as if I had changed my name back to Martha Kostyra. My image and my name are intrinsically intertwined with the brand. What we did instead was to trust that our customers could separate my personal challenges from the brand's values. We continued to work hard to maintain the strength of the name that was the heart and soul of that brand.

This lesson is evident in the Gibson guitar example. When that company was faced with competition and other distractions, rather than cherishing and supporting their esteemed reputation, the management retreated to a low-price strategy. That proved to be the wrong choice. Restoring the company's reputation as a maker of high-quality guitars was the right choice. It is rarely ever the right choice to address a business problem by abandoning the thing that a company is known for.

There are, however, examples of companies that have changed their profile and even their products while staying true to the values customers associate with the brand. Abercrombie & Fitch is one such company. In 1892, the company known as Abercrombie & Fitch produced fabulous sportswear worthy of a weekend of foxhunting or shooting at the Windsors' estate. The store was frequented by worldly adventurers and explorers, and people from high society bought their jodhpurs and trekking apparel there. Unfortunately, the brand declined during the 1960s and 1970s, and the remaining stores closed their doors in 1976. The market for very-high-end sporting goods had given way to specialty retailers and to manufacturers who use high-tech, advanced materials. A newer and more successful company, The Limited, loved how the name, Abercrombie, rolls off the tongue and knew it still meant something to high-end clientele, so they purchased the brand. They repositioned it as a young adult label with very hip clothing styles and targeted customers who aspired to something more. The company went public in 1996, and since then the new Abercrombie has been embraced by a new generation as a trusted purveyor of young, contemporary classic sportswear.

## When a Good Thing Masquerades as Trouble

I want to share with you some insights from one of America's leading entrepreneurs, Steve Jobs, the founder of Apple Computer. Steve presented the commencement address at Stanford in 2005, and a friend kindly sent me the text. During his freshman year of college, he was confused and directionless. Feeling guilty about tuition costs, he thought it best to drop out. At age 20, Steve had a passion for computers, and he and his friend Steve Wozniak became classic garage inventors. Together they built Apple Computer, which grew at an astounding pace. Within 10 years, they had $2 billion in sales and 4,000 employees. In 1985 the company was doing very well on the strength of the Macintosh computer, which was a year old and really selling to consumers. "And then I got fired," he told the Stanford graduating class. "How can you get fired from a company you started?"

He explained that they had hired a soft-drink executive to run the business side of the company. At first, the executive and Steve got along quite well, until they had a major disagreement. Siding with the executive, the board of directors determined it would be best for the company to fire Steve. So there he was, 30 years old and fired from the company that had been his life for 10 years. "I was out. And very publicly out," he told the students. "What had been the focus of my entire adult life was gone, and it was devastating." You can imagine why his speech resonated with me.

Steve described the mourning period he went through, but he also told of a reawakening that led him to start his new computer company, NeXT, and then the extraordinary animation company Pixar. He also fell in love and got married. And then an uncanny thing happened—Apple bought NeXT. Suddenly, there was Steve, running Apple again. "I didn't see it then, but it turned out that getting fired from Apple was the best thing that could ever have happened to me."

## A Martha by Any Other Name...

I would like to add Steve Jobs's name to the list of entrepreneurs who believe that overcoming challenges not only builds character but often can lead to something better than that which existed before the problem ever appeared. At MSLO, despite my brief absence, we managed to plan and execute many exciting and wonderful new things—from my new television show in front of a live audience to *The Apprentice: Martha Stewart*. Great furniture was designed; housewares created; a newly acquired magazine, *Body+Soul*, was beautifully redesigned; and we planned the content for a 24-hour-a-day, 7-day-a-week satellite radio program on the Sirius radio station. Would we have done all these things were we not forced to step back and reevaluate who we were and where we wanted to go? Possibly not.

Call me Martha Kostyra or Martha Stewart or even call me M. Diddy. I have never been prouder of my company or looked to the future with more optimism.

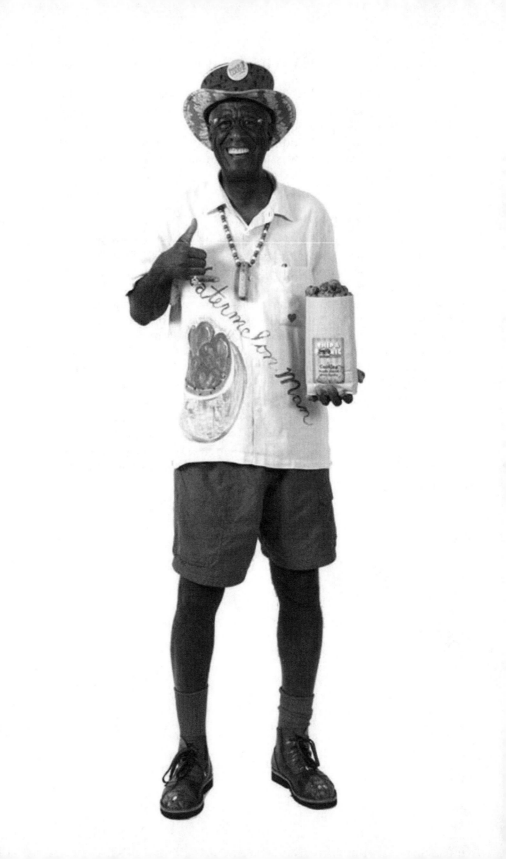

# WALLY "FAMOUS" AMOS:

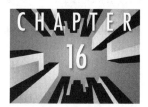

## The Grass is Greenest Right Where You Are

O nce there was a pious man whose father had just died. A geo-mancer instructed the man to bury his father at the mouth of a sea cave. Only once in a hundred years was the water low enough to permit access to this cave, and a family that utilized this window always experienced great good fortune.

Although the son had qualms about this unorthodox advice, he threw his father's casket into the sea at the mouth of the cave at the indicated time.

For weeks, the son doubted that he had done the right thing. To calm his incessant worry, he consulted a competing geomancer, who, out of jealousy, advised the son to raise the casket.

The son did so. When he opened the casket, he found that a fine layer of gold had been deposited on his father's bones, a clear indication of the auspicious transformation that had already begun. Full of regret, the son wanted to throw the casket back. But the window of time had closed, and there was no remedy for what he had done.[1]

The message in this story is that our spiritual practice must be uninterrupted. Like the slow accumulation of the gold, each day it seems that very little has happened. Yet if we are patient, in time we will see the yield of the accumulation of our efforts. Self-cultivation means steady, gradual progress.

Wally Amos is known by over 150 million Americans. His fame is grounded in quality and a positive attitude. Originator of the gourmet chocolate chip cookie industry, Wally founded the Famous Amos cookie company in 1975, and his current venture, Uncle Wally's, in 1992. Wally is active in philanthropic endeavors, and long served as national spokesperson of Literacy Volunteers of America. He is a well-known inspirational speaker and is the author of eight books. Wally is the recipient of many honors and awards including the President's Award for Entrepreneurial Excellence. He lives in Hawaii with his wife Christine. More at www.WallyAmos.com.

The grass is greenest right where you are. Many of us spend our lives chasing the next relationship, the next job, or the next opportunity. We'll have the free time *then*, we'll have the money *then*, we'll have the satisfaction *then* — any place but the present.

Yet the truth is just the opposite. Not only is the present moment the *best* moment there is, it's the *only* moment there is! You can't inhabit the past or the future, and when you learn to accept the now, right where you are, you have a sense of peace. What you plan to do next is less important than the accumulation of all the thoughts and actions you've done in all the nows behind you.

If you're in an uncomfortable job, you have to accept it — because it's where you are. You can't change it until you accept it. You have to accept whatever is going on in your life, whether you like it or whether you don't. You have to accept that it exists, because it does. Once you accept that this situation is real, than you can begin to evaluate what is you would like to change. But you must first accept and acknowledge what is going on in your life. If your job or your relationship makes you feel uncomfortable, that discomfort prods you to do something to change it. If you pretend it's not what it is, you repeat the same mistakes. They may take a different form, but you will repeat the pattern.

I began my first real career in the mailroom of the William Morris talent agency. My work seemed very limited: sorting mail and running errands. But I set targets for myself that went beyond the boundaries of the mailroom walls. I read memos that came through the mailroom to get a sense of the company's direction. I reorganized our cramped little office. I immersed myself in learning the meaning of the activity around me. I went out of my way to cooperate with the people I worked with. I took pride in my work; my life was my art, and my work was the medium. I imagined a day when I would reflect on my accomplishments as though they were paintings — and I wanted to see masterpieces. Before the end of my first year with William Morris, I had been promoted to become the agency's first-ever black talent agent. I went on to book and promote The Supremes, Simon and Garfunkel, Dionne Warwick, Helen Reddy, and Marvin Gaye, to mention a few.

In 1970 I began baking chocolate chip cookies at home regularly. I found the exercise therapeutic after a long day at work. I also used my cookies as a calling card in meetings with producers and Hollywood executives. My edible gifts became a hit, and in 1975 I opened the Famous Amos Chocolate Chip Company. My intention from the start was to build the business on sound principles and high ideals, as well as to make money. In the early 1970s, this was an alien idea to most businesspeople.

I had faith in my convictions, despite many setbacks: By the time Famous Amos cookies became a supermarket staple, I no longer owned any part of the company, and under the terms of a later non-compete agreement, I was not even allowed to use my own name in food-related ventures.

Yet I still had all the choice in the world about the shape of my life—and I'm the only one who truly has that choice. I don't have choice in anybody else's life, but I control the choices that I make in my life, every single day. In 1992, despite being broke and locked in a lawsuit with the company that bore my name, I launched a new cookie company, Uncle Noname, and was soon selling cookies to Costco by the pallet-full. Cornel West describes faith as, "stepping out onto nothing and landing on something." When we have faith, we reinforce the abilities latent in our subconscious minds to make our lives flourish.

Attitude is a determining factor in every choice. A woman woke up in the morning and saw that she had only three hairs on her head. She said to herself, "I think I'll braid my hair today." So she did, and she had a wonderful day. The next day she looked in the mirror and saw she had only two hairs on her head. "Hmm," she said, "I think I'll part my hair down the middle today." So she did, and she had a grand day. The next day she woke up, looked in the mirror, and noticed that she had only one hair on her head. "Well," she said, "today I'm going to wear my hair in a ponytail." So she did and she had a fun, fun day. The next day she woke up, looked in the mirror and noticed there wasn't a single hair on her head. "Yay!" she exclaimed, "I don't have to fix my hair today."

Regardless of the appearance of a situation, there is always good to be found there. Perhaps a vendor decides not to carry my Chip & Cookie product line. That's his choice. Then I make a choice to find another vendor. I'm not going to go around convincing vendors to carry my product. It takes too much energy. You can change their minds perhaps, but you have to expend a lot of energy. I find it much easier to find another vendor. For every door that closes, another one opens. A great salesman realizes that every "No" gets him closer to a "Yes." You waste time and money trying to convert a "No" into a "Yes." Accept that "No"—then go look for the "Yes"! We always have choice. We are always in charge.

We've all heard these principles before. Yet using them is another matter. One and one are two whether you use the information or not. If you go to school and gain knowledge, what's the point if you don't use it? You can have the most beautiful and expensive Rolls Royce in the world, but if you park it in your driveway it does you no good.

Having information and using information are two different things.

When we're challenged by our circumstances, we may cry, "I'm going through this terrible situation." Yet the answer to our dilemma lies before us: We're going *through* it. I've faced many difficult situations in my life, and I've found that it's vital to keep going.

I do this every single day; it doesn't matter what I'm going through, I just keep going through it. Last year I opened a Chip & Cookie store in Hawaii that has yet to turn a profit. My wife, Christine, and I loaned the company a considerable amount of money that we didn't even know we had. How did we come up with that money? I don't get up everyday and think, "Oh my God, what am I going to do?" I get up everyday and think, "What do I need to do today? What do I need to do in order to move through today?"

Many days I feel as though I don't have enough personal or financial support to keep going. But I still do the best I can. Focusing on what you don't have will get you nothing. Even though you have a minimal amount, you have something—so *use* the something that you have. That's what I always focus on. I can't wait for the perfect amount of money and the perfect people to show up in my life. I have to do something myself, today—otherwise I'm lost. I cannot do everything, but I can do something, and doing the something I can keeps me moving forward.

Too many people stop. Too many people wallow in their problems, feeling sorry for themselves. Looking for sympathy, they share their griefs with others around them, including people who can't even begin to help them. But that will not get them out of the situation. You must keep going. My friend J.T. O'Hara says, "When you're going through hell, don't stop to take pictures." It's one of the big ideas I've utilized in my life. No experience is bigger than I am.

Really applying these truths in my life has shown me that they work. I don't have some magic formula for success. The information I gather doesn't work until I work it. It's called a spiritual practice because you have to *practice*. Some days my best is better than other days. It's the best that I can do at any given moment.

Self-awareness is vital. You have to step outside of yourself and see what you are doing. How many times will you walk down the same road and fall into the same hole? We often think that some famous author or well-known guru is going to give us the answer. And they do give us answers. But we have to use them in our lives in order to succeed.

If you live in the moment, you will realize that you have everything you need to deal with your life. The past cannot be changed nor the future predicted, but each moment in the present is a building block to creating a happy existence. Enthusiasm creates joy. Joy creates more joy. Maintaining a joyful outlook and keeping a high level of enthusiasm can sometimes be difficult, but the more you do it, the easier it gets. The rewards reflect what you invest. And the good things are often found in the middle of life's difficult lessons.

1.   Based on a story from *Everyday Zen: Daily Readings,* by Jean Smith (HarperSanFrancisco, 1999).

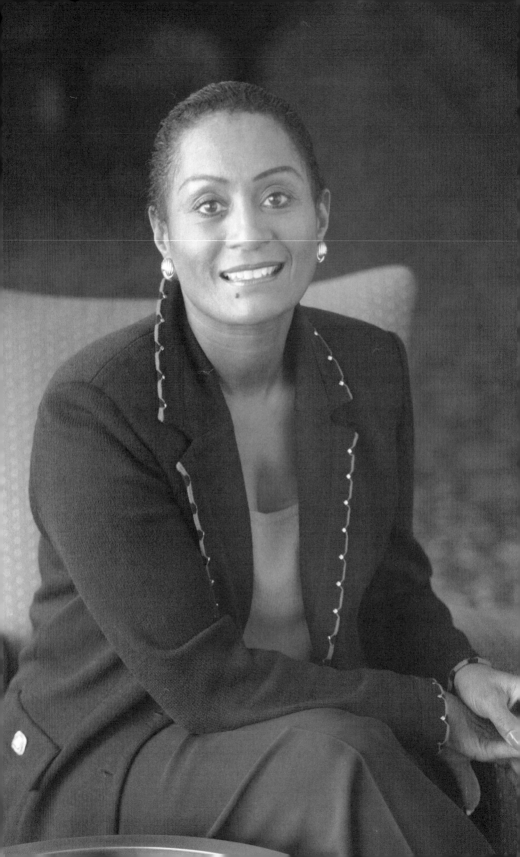

# FRANCINE WARD:

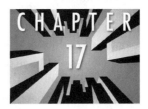

CHAPTER 17

# Essential Mistakes

One of the greatest compliments I ever received was from a woman who said she didn't believe my story. "I look at you today," she said, "and it's hard to imagine that your life was ever so bad." As we continued to talk, I realized that sometimes it's hard for even me to believe. Yet, as I look back over my life I'm reminded of the path I took and where I wound up:

§ When I was 14 years old I was strung out on heroin and alcohol. Today I am 27 years without a drink or a drug.

§ At 18 I dropped out of school and was literally living on the streets in New York. Today I am a graduate of one of the top law schools in the country, Georgetown.

§ By 21 I was a prostitute, selling my body to support my drug and alcohol habit and a lifestyle that had become more important than my life itself. Today I am a lawyer, a successful businesswoman, a twice-published author; most of the time I am a loving wife.

§ When I was 26 I was hit by a car and told that I would never walk again, and in my early forties I ran two marathons.

§ Finally, at 28, I was a poster child for selfishness. Yet today, at 53 years old, my life is about service.

How did I get from the lowest place a woman could ever find herself to where I am today? By doing what I call esteemable acts — not by thinking or feeling, but by being willing to behave differently.

Francine Ward is a life coach, inspiring author, and powerful motivator with a proven track record of achievement. From high school dropout, drug addicted, alcoholic prostitute to Georgetown educated lawyer, successful entrepreneur, and twice published author, her message is simple—take courageous, life-affirming action and the results will follow. Her mission: To encourage and support people in walking through their fear, so they can live amazing lives! She is the author of *Esteemable Acts: 10 Actions for Building Real Self-Esteem* (Broadway, 2003) and *52 Weeks of Esteemable Acts: A Guide to Right Living* (Hazelden, 2005). Visit Francine at www.esteemableacts.net.

Not surprisingly, many of the lessons I learned along the way came as a result of making mistakes…then learning from them.

One lesson I have learned is that we always know the difference between right and wrong, whether we admit it or not. Deep within our soul there is a little voice that tries to guide us in the right direction. Sometimes we listen to that voice, and sometimes we don't. Sometimes even though the red flags are waving in our face, we pretend not to notice. We live in a culture that has become lazy when it comes to living our values. We want to play, but don't want to deal with the hangover the next morning. Why? Because it's easier, because everyone is doing it, because it's often the familiar path, and because it's more fun. On any given day, we unconsciously make decisions as to how we want to live. We decide when to wake up in the morning, when to go to bed at night, who to do business with, how engaged we want to be in our own self-care, how we spend our time, and where we'll place our attention. Each choice has a price.

How do you decide what's right for you? Our choices are limited by many things, such as our emotions, other people's opinions, family commitments, lack of funds, lack of necessary skills, and fear. Fear is perhaps the greatest of these, because its impact is subtle, yet powerful. Fear of taking a risk, fear of pain, fear of making a mistake, and fear of rejection are just a few of the fears that stand between us and success. For years I was afraid to put pen to paper and write the book that was in my heart, because I was afraid that people would judge my writing. But at some point in time I made the right decision for me: to feel my fear and write my book anyway.

How do you shift the fear pattern and make the right choices, especially when you don't trust your instincts?

§ **First, as hard as it is, admit that your choices have been a little shaky.** Recognizing the need for change is the first step in altering the pattern. Twelve-step programs talk about making an admission of powerlessness as the first step in recovery; spiritual teachers talk about it, too; in the corporate arena, a "needs assessment" precedes training or coaching. We have to acknowledge that there is an issue before we can correct it.

§ **Act as if you have a choice in the matter.** The concept of acting as if is so powerful that it has the ability to turn the impossible into possibility.

§ **Consider several options in dealing with any situation.** Sometimes when we opt for the wrong choice it's because we think we have no alternatives. It is important to clearly see the possibilities.

§ **Ask yourself what the worst-case scenario would be if you did the right thing.** Thinking a problem or situation through can sometimes help you realize that it's not as bad as it seems—or, even if it is, that there are ways to deal with it.

§ **Don't go it alone.** Is there someone you can go to for help? Sharing often gives you a different perspective that you might have missed.

One of the greatest benefits of doing the right thing is that it keeps me out of the victim role and transforms me into someone who thinks about my choices before jumping into them.

Another lesson that has served me in life and in business is understanding the value of feedback. Nobody likes feedback. No one wants to be criticized. But being open to hearing the truth ultimately does wonders for us. Ken Blanchard calls feedback "the breakfast of champions." That is because if we are willing to open ourselves up to hearing what is true—even if it is painful in the moment—we benefit, our businesses benefit, and our relationships benefit.

Louise Robertson was a blessing and a terror. I loved her and I hated her—all at the same time. She was my first mentor, and loved me long before I was capable of loving myself. Some people care about your feelings to the degree that they can't or won't tell you the truth. And sometimes not knowing the truth can hinder your growth or stand in the way of your success. That was not Louise's problem. She had the courage to tell me the truth about my inappropriate behavior. It's easy to think that your behavior doesn't impact others, but in reality, our behavior does affect others—our kids, our co-workers, our spouses, our parents, our friends. And while we shouldn't tailor our lives to completely suit others, it is important that we understand how we affect the people in our lives. Louise helped me do that.

So how do you open yourself up to feedback?

§ **Imagine you are a business.** What would it take for your business to thrive and be successful? Attention to its assets and liabilities. So, perhaps making a list of your assets and liabilities, or strengths and challenges, is the place to begin. I have found that periodically taking an assessment such as the Myers-Briggs aids in the discovery process. In beginning any new coaching project, I encourage my clients to take an assessment.

§ **Get an objective pair of eyes.** I have had many objective supporters who have given me honest advice. When I repeatedly failed the New York Bar exam, a close friend sat me down one day and said, "Francine, you keep failing the Bar because you're allowing yourself to be distracted." He continued," If you are going to pass this test, you must make it your top priority — not the fifth or sixth item on your to-do list."

§ **Ask yourself, "Is it true?"** The other day after a speaking engagement, I reviewed my feedback. The evaluations were great overall, but there were about four that were less than glowing. As I read each of them, my dander immediately went up and I thought, "Who cares? It's only four people." But then, as I have trained myself to do, I reviewed their responses again and asked myself the tough question: "Could what they say be true?" And in each instance, while it was hard to admit, there was a modicum of truth to what those people said. It is not easy to receive feedback, even though I solicit it all the time. But the more we practice being open to hearing the truth, the better off we are — in business and in life.

§ **It's only their opinion.** Finally, there comes a time when we must separate the real and relevant from the false and unnecessary. Oftentimes, feedback is the result of someone else's stuff. The trick is to be open to hearing what we need to hear for our own growth, and at the same time to be able to separate it from that which is not useful for us to take on.

Another hard lesson is that failure is not the worst thing that can happen to us in life. We're taught from the time that we are infants that to fail (or to make a mistake or be rejected) is bad. Consequently, many of us find ourselves regularly making safe choices in order to avoid failure. We go to great lengths to never feel the pain or hurt attached to experiencing life. Sadly, when we don't put ourselves in a position to feel the pain, we don't experience the joy, either. No one likes to fail, but it's not the worst thing that can happen to us. Actually, the worst thing that can happen to us as human beings is staying stuck in a safe box and not going for our dreams, our goals, or our heart's desire because we are afraid to fail. It was not fun to keep failing the Bar; but had I stopped trying, I would have missed out on the wonderful lessons learned and the extraordinary feeling I felt on the day I passed.

What I've discovered is that when you fail, you get up, dust yourself off, and start all over again. Having the courage to risk failure, to risk making a mistake, to risk being rejected is critical in business, whether you're an entrepreneur, a small business owner, or a manager in a large company. This is because failure is really an opportunity to get to the next level. It's not something to be avoided, just part of the journey.

So how do you deal with failure, making a mistake, or being rejected?

§ **Acknowledge the pain you feel.** Feel the feelings. Pretending that they don't exist doesn't make them go away.

§ **Talk to a friend,** perhaps someone who has gone through a similar experience. There is a power in sharing feelings with someone else.

§ **Be honest with yourself.** Sometimes it's easier to blame someone else for what happened. But while that may feel good in the moment, if you are to get past it, you must ultimately own it!

§ **Explore ways to overcome the objection.** Most successful salespeople I know have been rejected at some time in their career. What they learn to do is acknowledge the objection to their sales pitch and then think of ways to overcome it. When I failed the Bar it wasn't because it was impossible for me to pass. I just needed to sit down and figure out how to overcome the objection or unsuccessful attempt. When I received 16 rejection letters from literary agents, I could have given up. Instead, I hired a book doctor to help me identify the problem. It worked.

§ **Break the task into small pieces.** Anything can be accomplished — one baby step at a time. After a failure, trying again often feels like an insurmountable challenge. Reducing the seemingly impossible into small action steps makes the impossible doable.

The last lesson that has served me in life and in business is that success is not contingent on me believing in myself. Many self-help authors and speakers teach the importance of self-confidence in creating positive change. They tell us that to achieve anything in life we must first be confident. We must believe that we can do what it is we want to do. Fortunately, I don't mind being a minority voice. I'm one of those people who believe that if you just take the action and keep doing what's necessary, you'll eventually get where you want to go. If I had waited to feel confident back in the day, when I was struggling with drug addiction and had no hope of having a different experience, I'd still be waiting. Instead, I took action. I behaved in a way that was contrary to the way I felt, and eventually my life changed. Confidence is nice work if you can get it. It's great to have. But for many people in need of a change of condition, starting at the level of the behavior — not the belief — is the key.

This might sound like a lot to digest, but all it takes is a beginning, a small step in the direction of your dream. You can begin today doing one thing that you've been putting off — maybe because you're afraid, maybe because you don't know how or someone told you that you couldn't, even though you really want to. All it takes is a willingness to walk through your fear and take action. That's all.

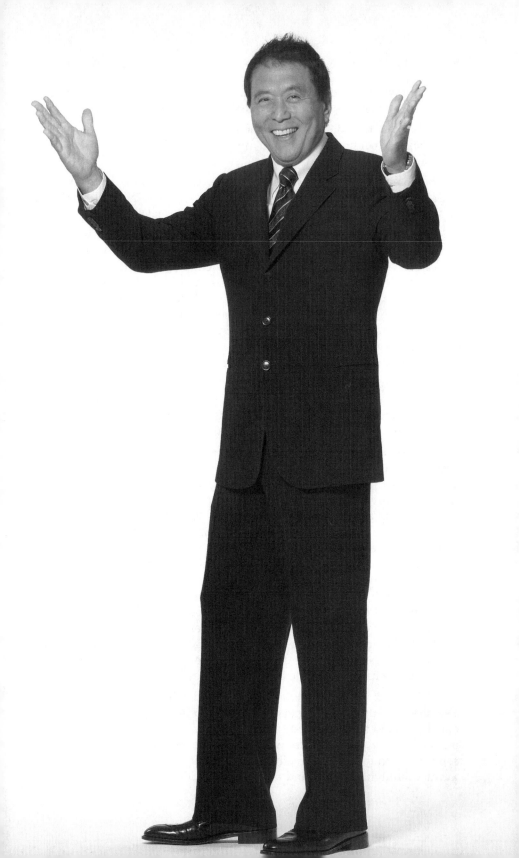

# Robert Kiyosaki:

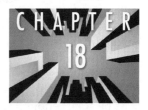

# When Being Wrong is Right

The school year had begun. Students and their teachers were still checking each other out in eighth-grade math.

"I give tough tests and I have no mercy," our teacher, Mr. Barber, began. "Either you know the answers or you fail."

I could feel the fear building inside me. I glanced around the room, seeing some of my friends rolling their eyes as if to say "not again." I sat confused. As much as I enjoyed learning mathematics, I hated the pain and pressure from the way it was taught and the stress presented by the teacher. The course was tough enough without him acting so macho. Why didn't he motivate us by making it fun instead of driving us by fear?

Despite these methods, we all passed and proceeded to high school. What we studied that year I don't really remember, but by the time I finished high school I had been through calculus, plane trigonometry, and spherical trigonometry. How much of that math do I use today? None. Today, could I solve those same problems for which I had studied so hard and had gotten the correct answers? No, I have to admit that I couldn't.

Today I don't use much of what I learned after the fifth grade. But that's not to say school didn't leave its permanent mark on me. The fact is, I left school with several behavioral traits I hadn't walked in with. Engraved in my mind was the belief that making a mistake, or

Robert Kiyosaki, author of runaway bestseller *Rich Dad, Poor Dad* (Warner Books, 2000), is an investor, entrepreneur, and educator whose perspectives on money and investing fly in the face of conventional wisdom. He has, virtually single-handedly, challenged and changed the way tens of millions of people think about money. There are currently 12 books in the *Rich Dad* series, which has been translated into 45 languages and sold over 25 million copies worldwide. Robert writes a bi-weekly column, "Why the Rich Are Getting Richer," for Yahoo! Finance and a monthly column titled "Rich Returns" for *Entrepreneur* magazine. Visit him on the web at www.RichDad.com.

"screwing up," got me ridiculed by my peers and often my teacher. School brainwashed me into believing that if a person wanted to be successful in life, he or she had to always be right. In other words, never be wrong. School taught me to avoid being wrong (making mistakes) at all costs. And if you did happen to make a mistake, at least be smart enough to cover it up.

This is where all too many people are today—not allowing themselves to make mistakes and thus blocking their own progress. The symptoms of this "disease" are feelings of boredom, failure, and dissatisfaction, although most of us never come to understand why we feel this way. After having it drilled into us for so many years, ifs hard to imagine that being "right" could cause such unhappiness.

In 1981, I had the opportunity to study with Dr. R. Buckminster Fuller. Although I can't quote him exactly, the first lesson I learned from him still sticks in my mind. He told us that humans were given a right foot and a left foot...not a right foot and a wrong foot. We make progress through our lives by advancing first with the right foot, then with the left. With each new step we both move forward and correct the prior step so that we come closer and closer to our destination. Most people, however, are still trying to walk the straight and narrow, avoiding mistakes and thus getting nowhere. What's wrong with the straight and narrow path? Perhaps nothing except the fact that straight and narrow paths simply don't exist in the real world. Not even physicists have ever found anything that is absolutely straight. Only curves have been found. Straight lines exist only in human minds.

In *The Abilene Paradox,* Jerry B. Harvey writes about the "paradox of paradoxes." He explains the universal principle that "unity is plural." Just as "up" cannot exist without "down," or "man" without "woman," a "right" cannot exist without a "wrong." Similarly, people who can only be right eventually wind up being wrong. And people who are willing to risk making mistakes in order to discover what is "wrong" eventually end up knowing what is "right."

In maturing as a businessperson, I have learned to be cautious of people who act as if they have all the right answers. At the same time, I have had to acknowledge my own over-zealous desire to be right. I had to learn that a person who stayed on his right foot too long would eventually end up on the wrong foot—or worse yet, with that foot in his mouth.

Allowing ourselves to be wrong, to make mistakes, isn't easy. Think about how you feel when you hear the words "you're wrong." If you're anything like me, you become defensive and try to think of ways to prove you are right. In my own struggles, as well as in working with thousands of other people on this issue, I continue to be amazed at how terrified we humans can become at the thought of being punished for being wrong. Our efforts to prove ourselves right are often carried to the extreme, destroying marriages, businesses, and friendships.

To finally discover that knowing the wrong answer can be the most powerful beacon we could ever hope to have, shining a brilliant light for us on the right answer, is greatly liberating. But to be able to enjoy the vast benefits of this insight we need to re-think how we handle mistakes; rather than punishing us for them, education should teach us the art of learning.

Our fear of making mistakes is so ingrained in us that we habitually react to our errors in ways that blind us to the real learning in them. Here are four of the most common and destructive "skills" that we have learned for handling those times when we make mistakes. These are the key reactions that stop the learning process:

1. **Pretending we did not make a mistake.**

The last U.S. President I recall accepting full responsibility for his actions was President John F. Kennedy for his part in the Bay of Pigs incident. Since then there have been such classic statements as "I am not a crook" (Nixon during Watergate) and "I don't remember" (Reagan during the Iran-Contra hearings). These men's avoidance of any responsibility has kept the issues alive and smoldering — as jokes, if nothing else.

It has been shown through other examples that the public demonstrates understanding and compassion for people who commit errors and then acknowledge responsibility for their actions. This seems odd in a world where we are taught to avoid making mistakes. Yet, it seems that each of us continues to be responsive to the wisdom that still lies buried deep within us that, as the poet says, "To err is human; to forgive is divine." Perhaps there is something in the act of forgiveness that makes us remember how we are meant to learn.

Comedian-actor Richard Pryor, after making the "mistake" of free-basing and badly burning his face and upper body, went on national television to come clean about drug use. TV evangelist Jimmy Swaggart admitted to visiting "women of the red-light districts." As a result, both their careers continued and their "wrongs" were put behind them. I cannot say whether they truly learned from their mistakes, but at least they didn't pretend they were not responsible.

2. **Blaming something or someone else for the "mistake."**

Immediately after the failure of my business in 1979, I blamed my two partners for the money loss. I was very stubborn, refusing to look at the role I had played in my downfall. I continued to dig in my heels and deny my own part in it for two years. I was angry, hurt and broke. It was not until I calmed down that I realized the experience was probably one of the best things that ever happened to me. I am not saying I would want to lose everything again, but I am grateful for the valuable lesson. Had I not lost my money in 1979, I am certain I would have lost it later because of my ignorance. There is the saying that "A fool and his money are soon parted." My mistake allowed me to better understand how I had been a fool, and how to avoid making similar mistakes again.

I know many people who are not successful because they are still consciously or subconsciously blaming other people for things that happened to them. I hear many horror stories about money or romance and how someone "did them wrong." The problem with that point of view is that the source of the mistake continues to lie dormant, just waiting to come to the surface again. One example of this is found with people who divorce and then marry a "different-same" person again and again, because they didn't learn the lesson from the previous marriage. They continue to blame the previous spouse for the failure of their relationship. Had I continued to blame my partners for what I did not know, I am certain I would have made the same mistake again and again, with different partners, until I either got the lesson, gave up, or died broke, frustrated, and bitter.

American society has become "blame-happy," and the term "victim" has become a part of everyday conversation. Courts are jammed up with lawsuits brought on by "victims" wanting compensation for being "wronged." No one can deny that there are legitimate claims, but we also know that the practice of suing has gone to extremes. Doctors have become fearful of delegating any of their duties to other clinicians with whom they work for fear of malpractice suits. This single factor has caused an increase in medical costs and a decrease in insurance benefits.

Similarly, the highest single cost of producing a car in North America is not steel, but insurance. Insurance of all kinds is a hidden cost of every car produced—for a commodity that benefits the consumer in no way.

We could do with fewer victims and with more people willing to learn instead of wanting to blame.

3. **Rationalizing the "mistake" instead of learning from it.** (Also known as the "Sour Grapes Syndrome.") "Oh, well, I really didn't want that anyway."

The world is filled with people who are always ready with perfect rationalizations about why they are unsuccessful. For a short time after I lost my business, I used the rationalization that I failed because I didn't have an MBA. By clinging to this rationalization I only prolonged my mental poverty and slowed down my comeback.

One of the most prevalent justifications today is, "Oh, the money doesn't matter to me." I often hear it from people who are not winning at the game of financial well-being. Does money really not matter? Let's ask the question another way: is it a mistake to put yourself and your family in the position of not having enough money? At the very least, not having enough money should be interpreted as a "tap on the shoulder," a signal to change something in our lives.

4.   **Punishing oneself.**

Possibly the most destructive behavior of all is the emotional torment people inflict on themselves as retribution for making a mistake.

When asked who is hardest on them, most people will point to themselves. They often do this with an apparent sense of pride and humility. And yet, punishment is one of the most destructive aspects of human behavior there is, whether it is self-inflicted or inflicted by a third party. One reason people are not successful is that they are consciously or subconsciously punishing themselves for something they did in the past. They cannot allow themselves to be successful because deep down inside they do not feel they deserve it. They are punishing themselves by withholding the opportunity to enjoy a successful life.

Truly successful people learn to take full responsibility for their actions; they apologize and do whatever is appropriate to correct their errors. They acknowledge the mistake, seek the lesson, make whatever corrections are required and then move on to become more successful.

Unsuccessful people harbor the emotional pain of self-blame and fail to get the valuable lessons made available to them through their mistakes. Not acknowledging mistakes makes for narrow-minded, self-righteous people who ultimately hinder their own ability to be happy and find financial success.

## Always Having to be Right

Along with denying that we've made a mistake, there are several problems associated with having to be right:

1.   **Inability to see the future.**

The person who has to be right often clings to old information, information which might have been right in the past but is no longer appropriate or true in the present. Most people confuse facts with truths. Prior to Orville and Wilbur Wright's successful flight in a heavier-than-air machine, the "fact" was that humans could not fly and never would fly. While it was a fact at that moment, it was not a "truth." Similarly, prior to the day Roger Bannister broke the four-minute mile barrier, sports physiologists presented dozens of very convincing articles "proving" that such a feat was "humanly impossible."

Most of what we call human knowledge is only information we that we have jointly agreed is "true." Another word for it is "consensual reality," meaning simply that it is knowledge that most people recognize as "true." History is filled with stories of great new ideas or inventions that were ridiculed because society adamantly refused to look beyond consensual reality. Businesses have been destroyed by failing to recognize a new reality that was staring them in the face. Today, changes are coming at a pace never experienced before, making it more hazardous than ever to cling to the notion that "what worked today will work tomorrow."

To learn from mistakes, we need to learn never to say, "That's a crazy idea. It will never work," no matter how crazy it may seem. We need to learn how to at least suspend our belief in consensual reality long enough to listen openly to new ideas and new possibilities. Rigid thinkers cannot hear new ideas as long as they cling to what they believe is "right."

2. **No increase in wealth (knowledge).**

People who have to be right rarely learn anything new because they are too busy having to be right. It is only when they are willing to be wrong that learning comes alive. Wealth only increases when people learn how to learn from their mistakes. After all, there is very little knowledge in the world that won't be obsolete tomorrow, or next year, or in the next decade. Facts change—and so must our minds.

3. **More conflicts.**

I remember, as a child, going to our family's Methodist Church. I remember asking my Sunday school teacher what the difference was between our church and the Catholic Church. She told me, "The Methodists are following the right teachings of Jesus and the Catholics are wrong." I was only ten, yet something about that statement struck me as ridiculous. But how ridiculous is it? People cause pain, grief, and bloodshed in the name of needing to prove that they are "right."

Remember the slogan that was so prevalent in the years of the Cold War between the United States and Russia? The saying was "Better dead than Red," and indeed there were many times when our two nations stood on the brink of an atomic holocaust in the name of defending their beliefs.

Again, what most people and most nations insist is "right" or "wrong" is often only their point of view or opinion. Each of us has our own hidden agenda, an opinion that we are right and that anything to the contrary is wrong. We need to learn to think more broadly and to accept that there are probably infinite numbers of answers for every question.

Change in these matters can begin with our educational system, letting go of the belief that students should strive for the ideal of always being "right." It is the need to be "right" and the subsequent neglect of any real understanding that causes conflict between individuals as well as nations. As our planet shrinks, becoming increasingly crowded, "right-wrong" thinking will need to be reevaluated or the world is going to become uncrowded very quickly through global war.

As an ex-Marine and a person who grew up fighting, I've noticed much more peace in my life since I have allowed that other people also have "right" answers. I have greatly lessened my use of the words "right" and "wrong," as well as "good" and "bad." Instead, I try to comprehend different points of view and acknowledge that people differ. I have learned the hard way that opposing points of view don't mean that someone is right and someone else is wrong.

In our schools, however, I am afraid that we are still teaching our children to be narrow-thinkers. We are planting the seeds of war, not peace.

4. **Stagnating income.**

In most businesses, people are paid for what they know. People who have to be right all the time, as we've already seen, tend to stagnate, sticking tenaciously to the "nests" of what they know instead of taking the risks that would provide them with new knowledge. Since their knowledge never changes, neither does their income. In the worst-case scenario, they are discharged from the company because it has gone on to new technologies or is making a new line of products for which this person's knowledge is no longer useful. We see this every year in the hundreds of thousands of people who are let go or offered early retirement because the knowledge they have no longer serves the company.

5. **Dimming futures.**

A person who holds onto old ideas finds that his path becomes increasingly narrow. Often frustration and justification increase and opportunities decrease. The world is changing, but the person clings to the ways of the past or waits for the "good old days" to return.

### 6. Progressive inner blindness.

Growing up in Hawaii, I learned to love diving in the ocean for fish and lobsters. I used to see other divers coming home with octopi caught in the same area. I had never seen one.

One day, I asked a seasoned diver to take me out and show me where the octopus lives. He soon had me looking into a pile of dead coral. He pointed into a hole. I looked and stared as long as I could hold my breath but saw nothing. Then I pushed my spear into the hole. Immediately, an enraged octopus leaped out, scurried along the bottom and disappeared right in front of me. I realized the octopi had always been there, right in front of me, except I could not see them.

It is the same with business and investing. I find it amusing when a person tells me there are no more opportunities out there or that all the good investments are taken. Opportunities are always out there. Over the years, I have noticed that the more calculated risks, mistakes, and corrections I made, the better my "eyesight" became. However, I would have to say too that people who are afraid of making mistakes frequently never see the opportunities, even the ones staring them in the face. The people who can't see call the people who can "sharks" because they are able to take advantage of opportunities that nobody else could see. The real problem is that the person who always needs to be right stops looking in new places.

### 7. Inability to reap the benefits of "doing poorly."

All too many people become so fixated on doing things right that they spend their entire lives doing nothing at all. This is the typical pattern of "perfectionists;" their own fears of making mistakes literally paralyze them. Progress is made by following the path with "both feet," as Bucky Fuller pointed out. We discover new paths and move forward by taking a new step, looking around to see where it has taken us, then taking another step with which we can both correct our course. Could we ever have built a 747 jet had the Wright Brothers not risked their financial resources and reputations, to say nothing of life and limb, to build and fly their crude heavier-than-air machine? What the history books often fail to tell us is the number of times they failed to get their machine off the ground and the number of times they crashed. Through this seemingly endless series of "mistakes" they made they became the brunt of journalists' jokes. Only their willingness to take these risks carried them forward to success and eventually won them a permanent place in the history books.

### 8. Personal potential turning to frustration.

I frequently meet people who have great potential but no cash or professional success. The same people seethe with envy and frustration. Much of their frustration stems from being too hard on themselves. They know they have what it takes to get ahead but they won't let themselves make the necessary mistakes and go through the learning curve which leads to personal satisfaction.

"Your son has so much potential," was the statement on the report card I took home. I remember going to school conferences with my parents and every time the teacher said the same old thing: "Robert has lots of potential, but he doesn't apply himself."

Now I understand my teachers' frustrations and my own. How could they expect me to manifest my full potential when I was always being punished for making mistakes? I went through those years knowing there were things I wanted to do and could do; however, I was living my life in the straightjacket of feeling that it was bad to make mistakes, that above all I had to be right. I didn't begin to grow and learn until I threw off that straightjacket and dared to make mistakes.

9.  **Being increasingly out of pace with the moment.**

People who fear making mistakes are slow because they are too cautious; as the world speeds up, such people tend to slow down. This doesn't mean we should be reckless. But once free of the fear of making mistakes, we are much more likely to stay in the race. Asking a person who is afraid of making mistakes to keep up in the modern world is a little like putting a Volvo driver in a high performance Indianapolis 500 race car. The car has all the speed and power necessary to win the race but the driver is conditioned to a slower, more sedate pace. He can't get past his own habits and his cautious outlook on life long enough even to test the car's full potential. Thus, it's the driver and not the car that loses the race.

Successful race car drivers are conditioned to respond with swift but very small incremental corrections, which is the only thing that works at high speed. They know what happens when they don't recognize and acknowledge their mistakes and correct their course accordingly; they end up in the pits — or worse, on the wall.

As much as we may dislike it, our fast pace is a fact of modern life. Whether he's aware of it or not, the person who fears mistakes is constantly resisting this pace. And this resistance only compounds his stress and actually increases his chances of making mistakes. Unable to acknowledge or perhaps even recognize that he is straying off course, he cannot correct his actions and so ends up crashing.

# A Major Turnaround Needed

The long-term effect of our grossly inadequate educational system is all too often the erosion of our ability to function well in the real world. All too many of us come away from the system with a lack of self-confidence, drummed into our hearts and minds by what we've failed to learn about the positive side of making mistakes.

We can no longer afford to tolerate an educational program that punishes honest mistakes and fails to design programs that make full use of our natural learning abilities. We must change the course of this antiquated behemoth that is degrading our society, eroding our children's desire for knowledge while causing pain and frustration. True learning can be frustrating enough without a system that makes it worse.

We must find a way to teach through love and kindness so that the "right/wrong" systems of education can be exposed for what they really are: filter systems for rejecting those who won't buckle under and conform to the system. We must have the courage to create new learning environments, where mistakes are applauded and seen as the invaluable source of wisdom that they are. We would prosper both in terms of tapping the full potential of our human resources and in terms of bringing greater happiness into all our lives. We must take this next step in our evolution so that we can finally see that we all benefit exponentially when we reach for the very best in ourselves and support others to do the same.

# Part Five

From the Bottom Up

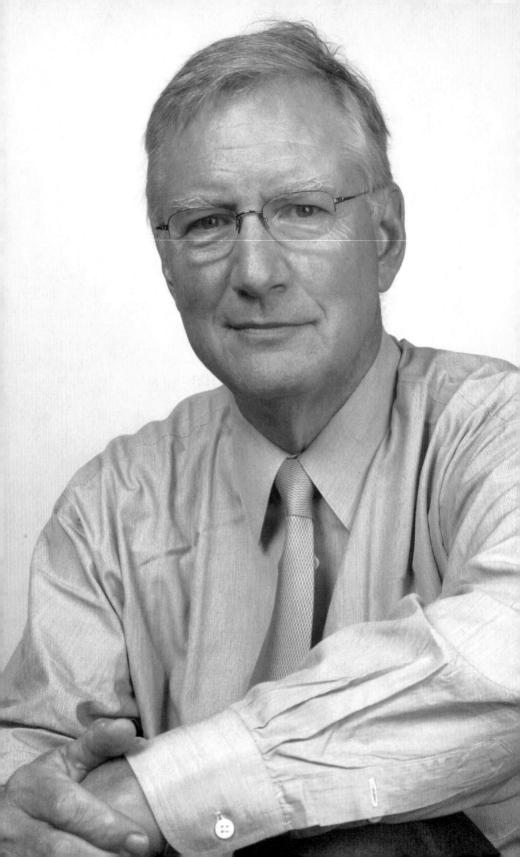

# TOM PETERS:

# The Power of Powerlessness

We labor under the delusion that we must "wait out turn"... that we must "work our way up the organizational ladder." But the decimation of hierarchies, the deconstruction of career ladders, and the re-definition of Work-of-Value make that a false—nay a dangerous—assumption. So we must Grasp the Nettle at the beginning of every job and every assignment. We must appreciate the power that comes from being "powerless"...we turn every mundane "task" into a remarkable (WOW!) project.

I imagine...a 24-year-old "independent contributor" who gets totally turned on by...Wi-Fi. She chats up some Wi-Fi experts. She leverages her growing knowledge—and her boundless enthusiasm—to cadge some bucks from vendors. (Perhaps with minimal "chain of command" approval. Perhaps not.) And she gets a beachhead Wi-Fi Project going at Enormous Enterprise Inc. Afterward, the world is never the same again at EE Inc. (or for our 24-year-old).

## Autobiography: "Powerless" Like Me

My seminar had gone on for a couple of hours. It was time for the first break. A relatively young man approached me. A fairly junior staffer in finance, it turns out. He began with flattery: "This is really great stuff." (I beamed. Naturally.)

Then it came...the phrase that mothballed a thousand ships. "But

Tom Peters has been called the "father of the post-modern corporation" by the *Los Angeles Times*. He is the author of *Re-Imagine!* (DK Adult, 2003), among many other books, and co-authored *In Search of Excellence* (Collins, 2004), which topped the bestseller list for two years. Peters presents about 80 seminars a year and serves as chairman of The Tom Peters Company. He holds two engineering degrees, two business degrees, and various honorary degrees, and served four years in the U.S. Navy, a stint on the White House staff, and eight years at McKinsey & Co. Visit www.tompeters.com.

I'm not a vice president," he said. "I can't implement any of this stuff. I don't have the power."

*"I don't have the power."*

What do I do? I flip out. Ok, not true. My mom taught me to be polite, so I'm polite.

But inside I'm flipping out.

-§-
IN THE "MEAN" TIME
Schrage cites an interview with former Sony CEO Nobuyuki Idei, who said that the key to that company's extraordinary record of new product development was this: At Sony, the "Mean Time To Prototype" (the elapsed time between the glimmer of an idea and a one-sixteenth-baked test of that idea) is a scant five days.
-§-

Can you imagine Martin Luther King, Jr. saying, "Civil Rights is Cool, but I don't have the power"? Can you imagine Gandhi saying, "The Brits stink, but I don't have the power"? Or de Gaulle in Britain following the fall of France in 1940: isolated, a longtime maverick and outcast within the French Army, recently convicted of treason by a kangaroo court in Petain's France—Can you imagine de Gaulle, at that moment, saying, "FuhgeddabouditIdon'thavethepower"?

Now, intellectually, I know that this young man was making a fair point. "I don't have the power" describes a common (indeed, ubiquitous) state of affairs. Still, talk like that does get my dander up.

I read—and think and speak and write—about many, many things. Major issues in business. And beyond. (That's how I earn my living.) But this issue is different. *It's up close and personal!* It gets right to the core of how I've lived my life ever since I was a "powerless" junior officer in the U.S. Navy in 1966...ever since I was a "powerless" new-kid-on-the-block-consultant at McKinsey & Co. in 1974.

In each case, I reveled in my powerlessness. It was precisely the challenge (and cover!) I needed. I urge you to think about your "powerless" situation in the same way.

## The Power of "Powerless" Thinking

"Getting Things Done" is not about "power" or official "rank." It is ultimately about...PASSION and IMAGINATION and PERSISTENCE.

Say you've got a Seriously Cool Idea. The very worst thing you can do—*the biggest waste of time in the world*—is to try to "sell" the idea "up the chain of command." Doing so will only remind you of how (officially) "powerless" you are. (De Gaulle didn't stick around and try to talk Petain out of executing him.)

The "chain of command": What is that, anyway? It's a bunch

of people who have been promoted for skillfully adhering to "the certified pure way we do things around here." In other words: They are the Designated and Appointed Guardians of the Yesterday. For your purposes—as a "powerless" junior type with a Seriously Cool Idea—the "chain of command" might as well be...a chain gang.

Query: What constitutes a Seriously Cool Idea? Simple. It's something that runs directly counter to..."the way we do things around here." That is, a Seriously Cool Idea is—by definition—a Direct Frontal Attack on the Holy Authority of Today's Bosses.

Oops!

Hence, as I said, the power of the "powerless" lies in what I call "Boss-Free Implementation." Or: What "they" can't see, "they" can't kill!

# What's Wrong with This Picture? Or: Reframe It!

So there you are, low person on the organizational totem pole, "powerless" to create your own WOW Project. But look around. What projects—non-WOW projects, to be sure—are you involved in? Ask yourself: Can I *reframe* one of them in a way that lets me do...under the radar...Boss-Free Implementation of a Seriously Good Idea?

My View: The answer is almost invariably "Yes!" Accordingly, I bid you to consider the following Reframers' Rules, as I call them.

**Rule #1:** *Never accept an assignment as given.*

Only idiots accept assignments as given! Those who will change the world (in the smallest of ways, even) twist any assignment until it can be turned into a...Seriously Cool/WOW Project.

**Rule #2:** *You are never so powerful as when you are "powerless."*

When are you truly hemmed in? When everybody is watching? (Welcome to VP World.) Everybody views your slightest twitch through an electron microscope. But when you are Officially Powerless...you are virtually free to dig into any assignment...and Raise Hell at Will. "They" are effectively blind to your machinations.

**Rule #3:** *Every small project contains the DNA of the entire enterprise.*

Perhaps this is the "real" secret-of-secrets. Every "small" project is a...Transparent Window"...on the Soul of the Organization. A Far better window than "official policy."

-§-

THE REAL "FAIL-SAFE": FAIL QUICK Variations on the theme of "quick loss": A high-tech executive who attended a seminar of mine shared his philosophy: Fail. Forward. Fast. IDEO founder and innovation guru David Kelley gives it another twist: Fail faster. Succeed sooner. Glib? Perhaps. Profound? Surely.

-§-

**In sum:** You don't need an *Officially* Big Project to attack a *Very Big* Real Opportunity.

# The Army of WOW Credo: Always Volunteer...

Opportunities! They are always (ALWAYS!) lying around. More often than not they're lying around in the form of...Crappy Jobs. Jobs that nobody else wants, seemingly for good reason. But think again...and follow what I call the VFCJ Strategy. That is:

# Volunteer For Crappy Jobs

Yes, *volunteer*. In the Army, there used to be a credo: Never Volunteer. Don't step out or stand out. Well, that was the Old Army. In the New Army, every soldier is...An Army of One. Likewise, in the New Economy, you must...Create our Own Army of WOW. Which means: Volunteer! Even for...Crappy Jobs. *Especially* for those... Crappy Jobs. Because...Crappy Jobs...let you take independent charge of things quickly and easily in your tenure.

The pivotal question: *Is that "unwanted" project a "throw-away task," a distraction to be "gotten out of the way?" Or is it a Seriously Cool Chance to turn a "trivial" problem into a...Stealth Opportunity...a chance to address a...Great Cultural Issue...that strategically affects the entire organization?*

Let's get down to cases:

# Voluntary Contribution #1: A Memorial Day to Remember

Which is it? The "Oh–Shit-I-Wish-It-Were-Over Memorial Day picnic"? Or the "First Annual Seriously Cool Celebration of Our Incredible Staff"?

Nobody wants the job. Yes, the job of "boss" of the Memorial Day company picnic. But you say "Aha! What an opportunity! Nobody wants this thing. Everybody hates it. But ain't it true that we do have a...Seriously Cool Staff...in our 73-person telemarketing department. Doesn't it make sense to Celebrate their Seriously Cool Greatness? And what better opportunity than the dreaded...Memorial Day Picnic?"

So you cobble together a little band of "powerless" but determined volunteers. You all throw Heart & Soul into what may be on the verge of becoming a...WOW Project. You find some entertainers on the cheap. You discover untapped skills among the staff. Friends of friends provide other resources. For two months you let your "real work" slip. The powers-that-be think you're nuts...that you're taking your eyes off The Ball. ("The Ball," meaning...Your Official Career.)

But the Dreaded Picnic becomes…an Insanely Great Event! There is Buzz. Serious Buzz. "Powerless," you are "on the map." (Your betters were watching!) Plus, you gained the Unstinting Respect of 73 folks in the previously underappreciated but vitally important telemarketing department. Plus, it was Fun! Plus, you added Members to your Network. (It's all about The Rolodex, Baby!")

## Voluntary Contribution #2: Safety First

Is it "Wrestle that damn safety manual into line with the nutty new OSHA regs?" Or: "Make an Advance in the All-Important War for Talent by figuring out how Safety Matters help make this…an Insanely Great Place to Work!"

Once more: Nobody wants the job. (To put it mildly.) But you see it as an…Incredible Opportunity…to Win a Major Battle in the Great War for Incredible Talent.

## Voluntary Contribution #3: Process Makes Perfect

Is it "Fix the bloody customer problems that have dogged the release of the new 2783B machine?" Or: "Work with a hotshot young division boss who's using Internet Speed to gather customer input — not just after, but before and during the product-design process?"

Yet again: Nobody wants the job. Except you. Okay, by now you get the idea. Opportunities are wherever you see them. Power…not official power, but the power of Initiative and Imagination…is yours for the taking.

## Plan Well with Others: The F4 Way

So success with several reframed crappy jobs has earned you Gold Stars…and a flicker of recognition. But truth be told, you're still preoccupied with your own Seriously Cool Idea — and frankly not much closer to launching it in the world. As a young engineer, your power score is still low, and your discretionary budget is zero.

Is there any hope?

There's more than that: There's a Eureka Moment awaiting you.

Find a playmate! What you need is…ONE…*sympathetic, enthusiastic, piratical, conspiratorial* friend. Yes, one. (One is plenty. For now.)

You've done some research on, say, your radical notion of Totally Transforming Project Management. And you've done some serious reading. You've chatted up some people who've tried similar ideas in other places.

Your excitement level rises. So, too, your frustration level. You desperately want to collar your boss and announce…that you have figured out a way to…Change the World.

Don't do it!

Resist the temptation!

Instead: Head to a company online chat room. Attend a company meeting. Start cold-calling to set up lunches with interesting people in the company you've gotten rumor of. In short, the time has come to take this Seriously Cool Idea...and start talking it up with some Would-Be Seriously Cool Allies.

Another name that I like for this "playtime" strategy is...the F4 Approach: Find a Freaky Friend Faraway.

## A (Play)Date with Destiny

An example of the F4 (Find a Freaky Friend Faraway) Approach:

You have a colleague—call her Nancy—who runs a medium-sized engineering unit within a subsidiary of your company. Her office is a few hours' drive from the divisional HQ where you labor away as that Junior Dude on the Engineering Staff.

You already know Nancy slightly. The grapevine says she's aggressive and energetic, and willing to try damn near anything—as long as it's interesting. You drive out to meet her, and the two of you dive into conversation. You talk up your Seriously Cool Idea.

Nancy enthuses over your pitch. Particularly since she's now working on a project that has become stalled—and for which your Seriously Cool (and Potentially Subversive) Idea might be just the thing.

Nancy says that while she's not quite "in love with" your idea (that's *your* job!) she is "very intrigued" by it. She tells you that she'll mull over your approach, sound out some of her staff about it, and look into testing some version of it in her shop.

Eureka! (Redux) You're closing in on Finding that first Freaky Friend Faraway.

Again: *One* is the critical number. One excited recruit at a time, at least in the beginning, at least until Dramatic Demos and Small Wins are in place (see below).

## Try, Try Again: The Power of Prototyping

You're junior. You're "powerless." No vice-presidential chevrons on your sleeves. But you've got that Seriously Cool Idea. And you've found Nancy—That first Freaky Friend Faraway. Now what you need is...a track record, a record of events-nuggets-stories that send the signal "something's up."

I believe there is one—and in fact only one—way of getting your

Seriously Cool Idea honed and ready for Prime Time. One and only one viable approach to creating a track record. And for that, I turn to innovation expert Michael Schrage.

Michael has spent most of that last decade on what may seem like an obscure, dry-as-dust topic: *prototyping.* That is, the process by which enterprises move from abstract concept to concrete working model, and then put that model through its paces...over and over again. Prototyping has its origins in manufacturing, but the idea goes way, way beyond that.

Schrange goes so far as to claim that excellence in Rapid Prototyping is the *chief* difference between organizations that innovate brilliantly...and those that don't. "Effective prototyping," he writes boldly, "may be the most valuable competence an innovative organization can hope to have."

Strong Language. The message: *Become a rapid prototype maniac.*

## Big "Wins" Come in Small Packages

Years (and years and years) ago, in my Ph.D. dissertation at the Stanford Business School, I coined another term for what I now call Rapid Prototyping. (Or "Serious Play," to use Schrange's language.) Namely: the "small win." That is, the wee "demo" whose success adds to your track record...and thus to your credibility.

Yes, that "small win," that "little test," that "successful prototype" shows that your Seriously Cool Idea isn't just fantasy, after all. It shows that your Seriously Cool Idea may well become...One Very Big Deal. An all-important entry on the credit side of your nascent track record. In fact, a giant and necessary leap from Gleam in Your and Your First Freak's Eye to Dirt Under Your Fingernails. A matchless tool for attracting future Freaky Friends. A catalyst for buzz that begins to ooze up the chain of command.

Nor does the "small win" even need to be a "win" in the obvious, conventional sense of the word. Sometimes a small win comes in the form of a "quick loss." That's certainly how Thomas Edison saw the matter. The Greatest Inventor of All went through some 9,000 experiments before he finally landed upon the right design for his incandescent bulb. Did he see the first 8,999 experiments as "failures"? Hardly! Each of those earlier "prototypes" was...a Brilliant and Unequivocal Demonstration of something that didn't work...in other words, a Clear Victory!

"Ouch," you shout. Save me from "those stories" management gurus love to tell. Who has the time for an 8,999-game losing streak? Fair enough, but the Edisonian "secret" is an Eternal Truth. We only win in the long run by getting out there and bloodied in the short run. As Churchill put it, "success is the ability to go from one failure to another with no loss of enthusiasm." Not so incidentally, the story of his life prior to the Ultimate Win in 1945. Another platitude? Sure. But…all of the Truly Great Ones seem to sing from the same page of the same hymnal.

## The Dance of Innovation

Rapid Prototyping turns out not to be about discreet "tests." It is…a Way of Life. Think of it as a *dance*. With a particular series of steps and a particular rhythm. Think of it as…the Dance of Innovation. It goes like this:

You get an idea. You run a (very) quick and (very) dirty test. That's great. But you've only begun. Now, after that first hair-brained test, you immediately sit down with your co-conspirators, and you ask yourself: "What happened? What can we learn from that test? What can we do differently next time?" And then you get on with that "next time"…RIGHT AWAY. And so on. Again and again.

After a while, you get good at it. You develop…a *rhythm*. And that's when innovation really starts to occur. Yes, your initial idea is Seriously Good. (Don't let anyone tell you otherwise.) But it's just that—an idea. As yet, it is only *potentially* subversive. As Schrage astutely observes, the Real Work of Innovation consists of…*the reaction to the prototype.*

True innovation is not a cool idea. True innovation is instead that we learn what we learn when we observe what goes down when we actually test a potentially cool idea. The Big-Big idea: We can't innovate until we have something tangible to…PLAY WITH.

# PLAY! INNOVATE! FAST!

Thence your goal: rapidly executed prototypes…prototypes that may succeed or may fail…but which have Charisma…and from which we reap Quick Learning, and generate Growing Excitement and Growing Credibility. And yes…Growing Power.

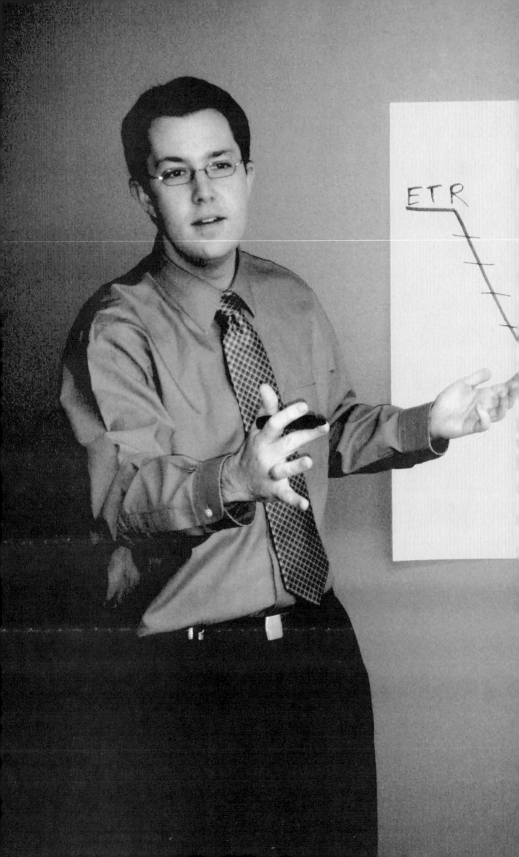

# HUNTER ARNOLD:

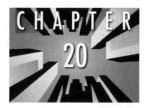

CHAPTER 20

# Paying it Forward

At some point, nearly every one of us has asked the most standard of Life's Big Questions: Why am I here? My personal moment of questioning came early in my professional career. An ugly misunderstanding between a client and an employee had left me on the phone for nearly three hours issuing mea culpas and enduring verbal abuse ad infinitum—two of my least favorite activities. As I hung up the phone I found myself wondering not only "Why am I here?" but "How on earth did I get here to begin with?"

As a kid I never sat around daydreaming about what my future might be like if I could just become a boring corporate suit. I spent my time as most of us do, imagining all of the ways I was going to change the world and the fabulous lifestyle and experiences I would have along the way. The future had seemed so full of opportunities.

Fifteen years later, however, I was making already wealthy people even wealthier while contributing absolutely nothing of lasting value to the world at large. I was a naturally talented capitalist; in fact, I was incredibly good at building up businesses and turning out profits. The problem was that being good at business wasn't what I wanted, my job wasn't what I had imagined and the idealism and energy of my childhood seemed to have been lost entirely amidst the corporate rubble.

What I wanted more than anything was to feel like I was making an impact on the world. I wanted to know that when I was no longer

Hunter C. Arnold fiercely advocates reinventing the corporate paradigm and using capitalism as a tool for global change. His unconventional approach to business focuses on creating challenge-based communication environments that push innovation and results beyond the limits of customary business practices. He consults with businesses to improve their bottom line while increasing their impact in the community, and is deeply involved in cultural outreach with Chicago public schools, international green energy initiatives, and the U.N.-supported organization Millennium Promise. He is a Vice President with Careerbuilder.com. Find out more at www.makemoreofyourjob.com.

here I would have left the world at least marginally better off than I'd found it. It didn't take a very hard look at my life to realize that I had failed at that goal. Sitting in my office that day I knew for a fact that I had become just another anonymous, grey-suited lemming headed for the proverbial cliff. I resolved that day to make some serious changes.

Then why, you may ask, am I sitting here typing these thoughts on a company computer, in a high-rise office, wearing a sport coat and tie? It isn't because I decided to swap my ideals for a Mercedes and a Brooks Brothers suit; it's because I finally figured out that the one place where I can make the deepest and most significant positive contributions to the world just happens to be behind a desk at a major corporation.

I know what you're thinking: *He's delusional, or worse a sellout.* It's ludicrous to insinuate that the capitalist machine can in fact be used as a tool for global empowerment. But I assure you it can. In fact, I challenge you to find a more productive tool for philanthropic betterment. The only problem is that it's a tool that lies too frequently unused.

You see, back on that illusion-shattering day when I decided to change my life's direction, I realized that while I could put up with the indecencies of the corporate world and the rigors and demands of my job, I couldn't stand knowing that I wasn't doing anything to make the world a better place. At the time I wanted to just give it all up, maybe become a teacher or join the Peace Corps...something, anything to become a productive member of the human race; but I had a family to think about, and such drastic decisions just weren't realistic. I'd have to find a more conservative way to bring philanthropy into my life.

I talked with friends who were deeply involved with charities and was horrified to discover that they had similar frustrations. It seemed that for those in the philanthropy sector there was never enough money or manpower to make a scaleable difference. Ninety percent of their time was spent trying to recruit the support they needed, with just a sprinkle here and there of actual progress made. It became obvious that a career in service would have many of the same frustrations I was already experiencing. I was disturbed but not defeated.

I looked into volunteering opportunities, and donated my time and money to several organizations that were near and dear to me. But I still felt that as just one person I could never make enough of a difference. I would never have enough time or money to give, and the results of my efforts felt temporary at best.

It seemed like both the corporate and philanthropic worlds lacked the full toolbox needed to create change on a large scale. The corporations had the money, skill, and scale but lacked the interest in changing the world. The philanthropic side was paved with good intentions but fell short when it came to support and organization. I felt trapped, like there was no way to balance my desire for personal success with my drive to make a difference. Neither world seemed like it could offer what I was looking for, and I found myself wondering if maybe life was just going to be less fulfilling than I thought.

At around the same time, a struggling employee approached me at work. We'll call him Dave. He was frustrated both personally and professionally, failing at his job, and on the brink of being terminated. When I looked at Dave from across the desk I saw plenty of passion and potential, but when he looked in the mirror all he saw was incompetence and failure. I gave Dave the requisite pep talk and sent him on his way, but over the next few days his situation continued to pop into my mind.

I found myself wondering if I could make a difference in Dave's life. Was it possible that with adequate support and guidance he could change his life for the better and achieve the kind of success that had eluded him thus far? The possibilities intrigued me. Perhaps, if I could focus on changing just one person's life, I would feel better about my contribution; perhaps it wouldn't seem fleeting or insignificant.

I met with Dave again and offered my support in exchange for his increased commitment to his job and his development. We immediately set out to turn his performance around.

Over the first few weeks we arrived early and worked late, because it was important to me that Dave prove his commitment and understand that change would take lots of hard work and dedication. As the weeks passed, Dave showed amazing improvement; in a matter of months he'd gone from the poorest performer in his department to the top of the heap. Each successive improvement in Dave's life brought me a greater sense of accomplishment, and at the same time, Dave's value and contributions to the company skyrocketed. The results of our little experiment were impossible to ignore, and I soon began to realize that the greatest opportunity I had to improve the world had been right in front of me all along.

I set out to change the entire scope of the way I did business. From that day forward we would shift our hiring focus from specific skills and experience to look for people with the energy, potential, and passion for personal improvement. Sure it was a risk to hire people who sometimes had no proven track record; but if it worked we would end up boosting both the company's profits and people's lives. Each new success would allow us to scale our efforts further, hiring more employees and providing more life-changing opportunities.

I envisioned a workplace where these newly successful employees would "pay it forward," helping others in the workplace and their communities on the path to self-betterment. With increased workforce productivity, our company would be more financially successful as well, giving me the leverage to request that we make donations to philanthropic organizations outside of the company. We could become a working model to prove that a focus on contributing to the world could also be wildly profitable, and we could finally begin to put our money where our mouth was.

I enlisted my management team, which soon included Dave, and we quickly began working on our model. While we didn't turn away proven, qualified candidates, we did become more lenient with our requirements. We added significant training for both job-based learning and required life learning like personal finance, cultural understanding, and so on, and it wasn't long before these new employees began to shine.

It turned out that Dave wasn't just a fluke—people really did rise to the occasion when educated and given an opportunity.

Fast forward to the present: Several years later, our current achievements have outshone our original plan in many areas. Each year dozens of our employees double—and sometimes triple—their incomes, achieving success they may have never imagined and contributing enormously to the company's bottom line. Our internal polls show that our employees today are much more involved in their communities and in philanthropic efforts, and many of them are financially able to contribute much more than before.

Dave's personal story has a happy ending, too—he's an executive in our company now, with an income 600 percent of what he made when he was first hired, less than five years ago. The changes in his professional life have been a boon to his family and his spirit, and today Dave is one of the most highly regarded mentors in our organization. I routinely hear from employees about what change he has helped them achieve in life. Like many others, Dave has embraced our model and is exponentially paying forward the help that he was given.

The company, too, is more productive than ever—some 10 times larger than seven years ago. We are blessed with the capacity to support many amazing organizations, from public school mentoring programs to efforts to spread economic stability, health programs, and education in Africa. It is now common to see a group of employees setting up a fund-raiser or heading off to work on a Habitat for Humanity home, and I'm proud to come to work each day with a group of peers who put my own contribution efforts to shame with their talents, passion, and commitment.

As it turns out, capitalism itself can be a force for change—if it is used as a tool. I no longer suffer from the feeling that I don't make a difference in the world. Today my challenges include trying to do more, finding new ways to improve, and keeping up with the boundless energy of my peers. When I look back at my company's journey to becoming a community for change, it becomes clear that we are not unique. Our path is one that anyone can follow, and you can make the decision to become a force for change in your own organization, no matter how large or small.

There were four key steps that our company took in establishing our model and mission. By using these steps you can begin to not only put your philanthropic wheels in motion, but also secure your company's future with increased commitment, productivity, and morale.

## Step 1–Identify Your Contribution

Now that you're ready to take the plunge, you'll need to decide where to begin. The task of changing the lives of others will require that you change your own as well. Like any new habit, it's going to require small, incremental steps and a large amount of commitment. Remember that the work comes before the results, so it will be important to set your expectations appropriately to avoid becoming discouraged and lapsing back to your old habits.

The first step in this process it to figure out what you have the most of to give. Our natural talents are usually the last tools we think about using when we're ready for a change. Avoid focusing on skill sets that are foreign or challenging to you, and instead use your primary assets to your benefit. By using talents that you already have at your disposal you will create an enormous amount of momentum as your project takes off.

Some of us are already conscious of where our natural talents lie, but for others it may require the guidance of our friends and families. If you have loved ones who are good at providing honest and clear feedback, don't be afraid to ask them to help you isolate your most dominant skills. Sometimes it requires the objectivity of others to give us the clarity and perspective we need.

Once you have a firm grasp of your skill set, begin to put those tools to use. If you're great at organization, fantastic, really spend some time mapping out how your strategy is going to work and understanding what other skills you'll need to acquire along the path towards change. If your greatest talent is sales, you might work aggressively to recruit the supporters you need to get your project off the ground. If you're a natural leader or mentor, you may jump right into the process of opportunity hiring or mentoring, and then figure out the long-term strategy further down the road. The possibilities are endless, but the key is sticking with your strengths early to guarantee that your efforts don't fizzle.

Many people become frustrated during this initial phase because it tends to feel very status quo. Since you're really just doing more of what you're already used to, it may not feel much like progress. Stay vigilant and remind yourself often that while not every step of the process is guaranteed to be fun, each is necessary. Before you reach your destination there will always be less exiting tasks to check off of the list.

I often use the metaphor of travel to keep myself moving forward. I love traveling to new places, meeting different people, and experiencing different cultures. Unfortunately, I absolutely hate planes. When I'm on a plane I am usually bored, uncomfortable, and irritable—but it happens to be nearly impossible for me to get to new places without them. If I were to throw in the towel and refuse to get on another plane, then I'd be missing out on a multitude of amazing new experiences. The reward is ultimately worth the cost, and getting on a plane ends up being a small price to pay.

Doing more of what you're best at might feel like being on that plane: boring and less than ideal. Just know that you can't reach your destination without it. Soon enough you'll begin to see the changes that you are effecting and the work will become less banal and more stimulating. When the people you're working with begin their metamorphosis you'll be far too exited about the destination to notice that you boarded your plane in the first place.

Once you've identified your personal strengths and begun to get the process off the ground, it's time to build up your network of support.

## Step 2–Identify Your Revolutionaries

For any worthwhile cause to gain momentum, supporters are required. Almost as soon as you have formed your strategy it becomes vital that you identify two key types of supporters: targets for change and ambassadors of change.

Your targets for change are the people you will commit yourself and your talents to. Avoid looking exclusively for workplace impact and consider your broader ability to raise people's overall quality of life. Depending on your position in the company, these targets for change may be either current or prospective employees.

If your job description doesn't involve having employees that report to you, it is unlikely that you'll be able to convince your company to change their hiring profile without proven results. This means that you'll have to pick someone that is already working at your company as your target for change.

Looking down the organizational chain, find employees who you believe have a great amount of potential that is currently untapped, either due to their direction or their position. It may be someone who would make a great supervisor, but is held back by the lack of a degree, or someone who could be a great salesperson but doesn't have the experience to qualify. The most important thing is to find targets who have energy and ambition, who with your help could build a better life for themselves.

If you're in the position of hiring employees yourself, your targets for change will likely be new hires to fill your open positions. Take some time to analyze the actual requirements of these jobs and separate them from the filters you're used to using in the selection process. For example, a sales position might require product knowledge and a certain kind of personality, but it would not, in fact, require a college degree or previous sales experience. In this example a degree and experience are filters that you may have become accustomed to using but are not necessary for the actual job duties.

Once you have separated your requirements from your filters, think through the support mechanisms that you would need if you made your hiring process more liberal. For instance, if you plan to loosen your filters on experience, it may require additional training at the beginning of the new hire's timeline. Find a way to balance these new responsibilities so your company doesn't absorb any burden up front. In our sales example you might accomplish this by reducing the salary for that role in order to pay for the training that your new candidates will require. In this example, your targets for change will still be happy to take the position, as even at the reduced salary it is an opportunity they would never have otherwise received, and your company will not have to reduce its short-term expectations for profits. I cannot emphasize enough how important it is for your program to have no negative side effect for your company; anything else will create extra roadblocks that you just don't need. The key to success in this area is opening the process to people whose lives your skill sets can change for the better, but keeping the opportunity for these people and the costs for your company balanced and in the win/win column.

Once your targets for change are in place (whether by hiring or internal search) and you have begun working with them on self-actualization, it is time to gather some "ambassadors of change." Ambassadors of change will be people like you, who want to make a difference for others, the world, and the company's bottom line. Look for people whose skill sets and passions supplement your own and will provide a long-term boon to the program. Start talking to your peers and superiors about what you're trying to accomplish and begin spreading the word about your vision.

Some people are hesitant to start this "internal marketing" because they are afraid to look as though they are seeking credit for their efforts. Remember, this part of the process is a necessary evil, because large-scale change will require that you have more than one person working for the cause. What you are likely to find is that your co-workers will be excited by the prospect of making a difference. There are very few people who don't want to make a contribution—most of us just don't know how. By discussing your vision, your enthusiasm for change will become infectious and others will join your cause freely.

At this point you have a strategy and a team. Now it's time to start generating some results.

## Step 3—Build Your Case Studies

Now that you're ready to officially launch your project, the first item of business it to get everyone together for a kick-off meeting.

The purpose of this meeting should be to provide each person with a clear set of commitments, goals, and expectations. Your ambassadors of change should commit to who, where, and how frequently they are going to contribute, and should compile a list of the impact areas they will be focusing on. Your targets for change should then receive this information as a guide to the support they will receive as they progress. Additionally, each target should agree to responsibility for certain deliverables (either inside or outside the company) to confirm their commitment. Finally, you should work as a group to set realistic timelines and expectations for the project. Try to be conservative with your goals, as nothing takes the wind out of a project's sails like the failure to achieve unrealistically set goals.

Remember that there will be roadblocks and failures along the way. Not every ambassador will deliver what you expect; life has a way of distracting us all, and you will have to focus on keeping these people engaged and committed. Similarly, not every target will be up to the challenge, so you should expect that a certain percentage of the people you are trying to help won't really want to put in the effort required to take their lives to the next level. Setting the expectations and guidelines at the first meeting will help minimize this fallout, but know that it will not prevent it entirely.

The expectation of these unavoidable setbacks will also be important when determining the size of your startup project. It is vital that you do not have so many people involved that you are unable to control the project. An enormous group of people may prevent you from being able to keep track of the vast amount of learning that takes place in the early stages. On the flip side, you also want to be cautious of placing all of your eggs in one basket. If you have only a single ambassador or a single target and they fail to live up to expectations, it can blast your entire project all the way back to step one—something you want to avoid at all costs. Balancing quantity with quality will take some trial and error, and it is something most of us never perfect; but willingness to adapt on the move and patience when facing challenges will allow to keep your end goals firmly in sight.

Once your project is off and running it is important to set regular meetings for all parties involved. Discussion of best and worst practices will be frequent and passionate in the early stages, and you must be willing to adapt in order to keep things moving at full speed. Soon enough you will begin to develop a standard for what works, and productive results will begin to pour in.

Keep a record of the performance and return changes that evolve as a living record of the project's timeline and impact. This is the data that you will ultimately need to take your idea to the next level and scale your project. As soon as your targets for change begin experiencing an increased quality of life you should begin talking about how they can contribute to others and facilitate ways they can pay forward the experiences and opportunities they have received.

As the people involved in your project start seeing results, you will begin to notice an interesting change occurring. Targets will begin mentoring others even while their personal evolution is still in its early stages. Ambassadors will begin to seek out mentors themselves, and will develop a renewed desire for self-betterment. As your program matures it will become clear that once we are focused on productively contributing to the world, most of us become both ambassadors and targets of change at the same time. The roles become less stratified and the goal more communal, since none of us is ever finished with our self-evolution. Each of us can always work towards our own next level, but in no way does that mean we cannot benefit those around us at the same time.

When your project is rolling steadily in the right direction you will notice a staggering level of commitment and passion from the people involved. Without even focusing on it, their overall productivity will improve as they commit to being the most they can become. All of a sudden you will have the data you need to prove your project's value—and that is when you'll know it's time to take things to a whole new level.

## Step 4—Refine and Scale

At this point you should begin to gather all of the anecdotal and data-based evidence you need to increase the size and impact of your program. Depending on where you began, that could mean simply recruiting more targets or ambassadors or it could mean taking the program to your corporate leaders in an attempt to make it a fully scaled company initiative.

Before you pump up the volume, however, it is important to get your participants together once again and set the stage. Discuss how you would have done things differently if you had the benefit of your current knowledge and experiences. Were there decisions that impeded your speed or effectiveness?

Spend some time streamlining the process at the individual level and then move on to considerations of scale, reorganizing your program in a way that could ultimately support an unlimited number of participants. Your goal at this point is to create a system that could continue whether you were personally involved or not. Some key questions to ask are:

§ What is the necessary ratio of ambassadors to targets?

§ Are the current expectations and timelines realistic with broader impact?

§ At what point (if any) would the project require a paid administrator, and is that a realistic request given your company? If not, could you fund-raise or open a nonprofit externally to support the company program?

Once you have addressed these issues and believe that you have a scaleable model, commit to the next round of ambassadors and targets. There is no right answer to how fast your program can grow, but try not to double the size from any one growth round to the next, as it will reduce your chance for equivalent success rates and make it difficult to keep track of the next round of learning.

It is also important, at this point, to promote reflection on the process. By now, through your hard work and commitment, you will have helped changes the lives of those around you and the future of your organization. It's amazing to look back and see how much good can come from something that started out so small, and the sense of fulfillment is overwhelming. These opportunities for reflection are often all the fuel that is required to keep the passion for change burning brightly into the future.

## Looking Ahead

As the cycle of contribution continues you will become aware of many different opportunities to make a difference. As you improve your company's productivity, you may become an advocate for organizations that you would like to see your company support monetarily. You may find ways to extend your program into the community, helping your original targets pay it forward beyond the walls of your corporation. The possibilities are truly endless, as are the rewards. Over time you will realize that there are always opportunities to be seized, and your network of supporters will increase. Someday your impact may become truly global—and all from a single decision.

Ultimately, it only takes one person to begin the change. You can make a decision that may ultimately enrich the lives of countless others. Corporate culture can be a force for progress, and you could be the catalyst that your community desperately needs. The only question is: Are you ready for the greatest ride of your life?

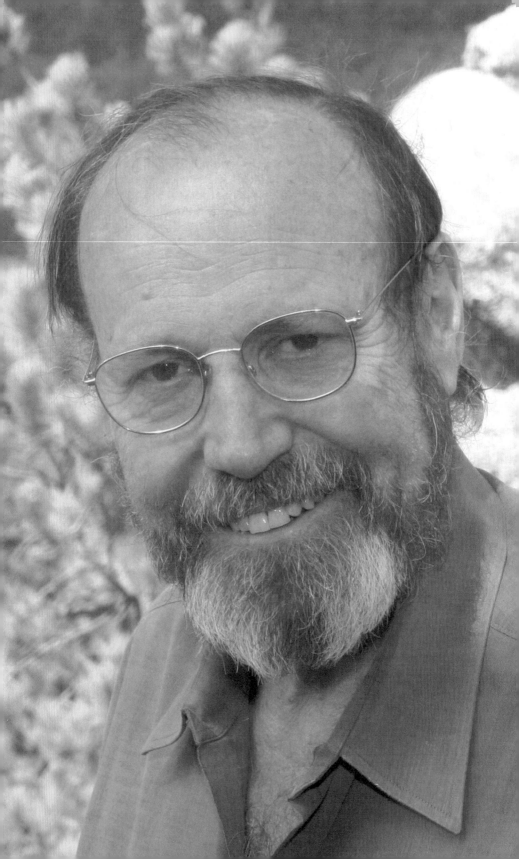

# BERNARD LIETAER:

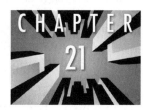

# New "Green" Currencies

W hen Jaime Lerner became mayor of the medium-sized Brazilian town of Curitiba in 1973, he had a tricky garbage collection problem. The majority of the 500,000 people of Curitiba lived in shanty towns *(favelas)*, which had been built so haphazardly that even the garbage trucks could not get into them. The accumulation of garbage attracted rodents, which in turn spread diseases at alarming rates. The classical solution would have been a welfare program to try to clean up the mess, but Lerner did not have that option because there were too few rich people in Curitiba and the necessary funds were not available.

The mayor was forced to invent another way. His solution was to pay public transport tokens to people for their garbage, under the condition that they pre-sort and deposit it in recycling bins around the favelas. For organic waste, which was composted for use by farmers as fertilizer, people received chits that could be exchanged for food. The program worked spectacularly: The favelas were clean-picked by the kids, who quickly learned to distinguish between the different types of recyclable products. People could leave the favelas by public transport and travel to the center of town where the jobs were. The additional buses and gasoline were paid for with the proceeds from the sale of the pre-sorted garbage to the glass, paper, and metal manufacturing companies. Even "normal" money was saved because fewer trucks and less gasoline were required to pick

Bernard Lietaer is one of the original architects of the convergence mechanism for the Euro, the European single currency. A former Central Banker and currency trader, he provides evidence for the validity of complementary currencies in *Of Human Wealth: New Currencies for a New World* (Citerra, 2006), *The Future of Money* (Random House, 2001), and at www.transaction.net/money. He is a Fellow at the Center for Sustainable Resources at the University of California at Berkeley, and Chairman of the ACCESS Foundation (www.accessfoundation.org). He can be reached via blietaer@earthlink.net.

up the pre-sorted garbage. And all this does not even include the savings due to reduced disease and a more efficient labor market. Today, Curitiba is clean, prosperous, self-sufficient, and the only Brazilian city I know to refuse money from the federal government. It has a state-of-the-art public transportation system and a popular mayor who has been repeatedly re-elected. Perhaps most significant, a strong sense of community and pride has arisen in a place where none was visible before.

Many cities, even entire countries around the world face a fourfold dilemma that echoes the earlier problems of Curitiba. They are experiencing unemployment, inflation, and ecological degradation, and they lack enough money for everything they want to do. There are strong indications that these same issues will remain on top of the agenda for the coming century. Emerging technologies promise to keep unemployment a major issue, even if all Western economies stay out of recession. And community breakdown is one of the most systemic, deep, and complex societal trends of the past 30 years, with no signs of any reversal. Green community currencies provide powerful social leverage to change this equation.

Money is like an iron ring we've put through our noses. We've forgotten that we designed it, and it's now leading us around. It's time to figure out where we want to go—and then design a money system that moves us toward sustainability and community.

Precisely because we will have to live with these issues for the foreseeable future, only a long-term systemic approach can successfully resolve these problems. Local community currencies could contribute to tackling all three problems and also permit us to "retrofit" economic motivation to desirable human behavior.

While economic textbooks claim that people and corporations are competing for markets and resources, in reality they are competing for money—using markets and resources to do so. So designing new money systems really amounts to redesigning the target that orients much human effort.

Greed and competition are not a result of immutable human temperament; I have come to the conclusion that greed and fear of scarcity are in fact being continuously created and amplified as a direct result of the kind of money we are using. For example, we can produce more than enough food to feed everybody, and there is definitely enough work for everybody in the world, but there is clearly not enough money to pay for it all. The scarcity is in our national currencies. In fact, the job of central banks is to create and maintain that currency scarcity. The direct consequence is that we have to fight with each other in order to financially survive.

## New "Green" Currencies — Bernard Lietaer

Money is created when banks lend it into existence. When a bank provides you with a $100,000 mortgage, it creates only the principal, which you spend and which then circulates in the economy. The bank expects you to pay back $200,000 over the next 20 years, but it doesn't create the second $100,000 — the interest. Instead, the bank sends you out into the tough world to battle against everybody else to bring back the second $100,000. When the bank verifies your "creditworthiness," it is really checking whether you are capable of competing and winning against other players — able to extract the second $100,000 that was never created. And if you fail in that game, you lose your collateral.

Complementary currencies do not suffer from this drawback, and for this reason I expect them to become a major tool for social design during this century. They won't replace national currencies; that is why I call them "complementary" currencies. For instance, in France, there are now 300 local exchange networks, called Grain de Sel, literally "Grain of Salt." These systems — which arose exactly when and where the unemployment levels reached about 12 percent — facilitate exchanges of everything from rent to organic produce, but they do something else as well. Every fortnight in the Ariège, in southwestern France, there is a big party. People come to trade not only cheeses, fruits, and cakes as in the normal market days, but also hours of plumbing, haircuts, sailing or English lessons. Only local currencies accepted!

Local currency creates work, and I make a distinction between work and jobs. A job is what you do for a living; work is what you do because you like to do it. I expect that the industrial age idea of "jobs for everybody" to increasingly become obsolete, but there is still an almost infinite amount of fascinating work to be done. For example, in France you find people offering guitar lessons and requesting lessons in German. Neither would pay in French francs. What's nice about local currency is that when people create their own money, they don't need to get currency from elsewhere in order to have a means of making an exchange with a neighbor. That does not mean there's an infinite amount of this currency, either; you cannot give me 500,000 hours — nobody has 500,000 hours to give. So there's a realistic ceiling on this creation, but there's no artificial scarcity. Instead of pitting people against each other, the system actually helps them cooperate.

Local currencies create both employment and community. For example, I would feel funny calling my neighbor in the valley and saying, "I notice you have a lot of pears on your tree. Can I have them?" I would feel I needed to offer something in return. But if I'm going to offer scarce dollars, I might just as well go to the supermarket, so we end up not using the pears. If I have local currency, there's no scarcity in the medium of exchange, so buying the pears becomes an excuse to interact. There are lots of people who love gardening, but who can't make a living from it in the competitive world. If a gardener is unemployed, and I'm unemployed, in the normal economy we might both starve. However with complementary currencies, he can grow my salads, which I pay for in local currency earned by providing another service to someone else.

Local currencies have transformed the economies of other regions in the 20th century, and done so quickly. During the depths of Germany's post-World War I depression in 1930, Herr Hebecker, owner of a small bankrupt coal mine in Schwanenkirchen, Bavaria, decided in a desperate effort to pay his workers in coal instead of Reichsmark. He issued a complementary currency — which he called "Wara" — redeemable in coal. On the back were small squares where stamps could be applied. A bill would remain valid only if the stamp for the current month had been applied. This negative interest charge was justified as a "storage cost." The workers paid for their food and local services with these Wara. For example, the baker had no real choice but to accept them, and convinced his wheat suppliers to accept them in turn.

Is such an unconventional concept as "storage charged money" a theoretically sound one? The answer is a resounding yes, and is supported by economists of no lesser stature than John Maynard Keynes. Chapter 17 of Keynes' *General Theory of Employment, Interest and Money* analyzes the implications of such money, and provides a solid theoretical backing for its merits. Keynes specifically states: "Those reformers, who look for a remedy by creating an artificial carrying cost for money through the device of requiring legal-tender currency to be periodically stamped at a prescribed cost in order to retain its quality as money, have been on the right track, and the practical value of their proposal deserves consideration."

However, the real proof is in the pudding.

Dr. Hebecker's monetary innovation was so successful that by 1931 this *Freiwirtschaft* (free economy) movement had spread through all of Germany, involving more than 2,000 corporations and a variety of commodities as backing for the Wara. But in November 1931, the German Central Bank, on the basis of its monopoly of currency creation, prohibited the entire experiment.

Similarly, in 1932, Herr Unterguggenberger, mayor of the Austrian town of Wörgl, decided to do something about the 35 percent unemployment of his constituency (typical for most of Europe at the time). He convinced the town hall to issue 14,000 Austrian shillings' worth of "stamp scrip," which were covered by exactly the same amount of ordinary shillings deposited in a local bank.

Soon Wörgl became the first Austrian city to achieve full employment. Water distribution was generalized throughout, all of the town was repaved, most houses were repaired and repainted, taxes were being paid early, and forests around the city were replanted.

It is important to recognize that the major impact of this approach did not derive from the initial project launched by the city, but instead had its origin in the numerous individual initiatives taken in the process of recirculating the local currency instead of hoarding it. On the average, the velocity of circulation of the Wörgl money was about 14 times higher than the normal Austrian shillings. In other words, on the average, the same amount of money created 14 times more jobs.

More than 200 other Austrian communities decided to copy this example, but here again the Central Bank blocked the process. A legal appeal was made all the way to the Supreme Court, where it was lost.

Today, local currencies are again mushrooming all over the world in an impressive diversity and increasing sophistication. As Hazel Henderson has pointed out, the key to the success of a community currency, just as for any currency, is trust. In this case it is trust in your neighbors, in the community as a whole, and in the community's leaders.

Today's official monetary system has almost nothing to do with the real economy. Just to give you an idea, recent statistics indicate that the volume of currency exchanged on the global level is $1.9 trillion per day. This is 30 times more than the daily gross domestic product (GDP) of all of the developed countries (OECD) together. The annual GDP of the United States is turned in the market every three days!

Of that volume, only 2 or 3 percent has to do with real trade or investment; the remainder takes place in the speculative global cyber-casino. This means that the real economy has become relegated to a mere frosting on the speculative cake, an exact reversal of how it was just three decades ago.

For one thing, power has shifted irrevocably away from governments toward the financial markets. When a government does something not to the liking of the market—like the British in 1991, the French, in 1994 or the Mexicans in 1995—nobody sits down at the table and says, "You shouldn't do this." A monetary crisis simply manifests in that currency. So a few hundred people—who are not elected by anybody and have no collective responsibility whatsoever—decide what your pension fund is worth, among other things.

In a community currency system, people would only use money as a medium of exchange, but not as a store for value. That would create work, because it would encourage circulation.

This has been tried on a large scale during three historical periods: classical Egypt, about three centuries in the European Middle Ages, and a few years in the 1930s. In ancient Egypt, when you stored grain, you would receive a token, which was exchangeable and became a type of currency. If you returned a year later with 10 tokens, you would only get nine tokens worth of grain, because rats and spoilage would have reduced the quantities, and because the guards at the storage facility had to be paid. So that amounted to a demurrage charge.

Egypt was the breadbasket for the ancient world, the gift of the Nile. Why? Because instead of keeping value in money, everybody invested in productive assets that would last forever—things like land improvements and irrigation systems.

Proof that the monetary system had something to do with this wealth is that it all ended abruptly as soon as the Romans replaced the Egyptian "grain standard" currency with their own money system, with positive interest rates. After that, Egypt ceased being the grain-basket and became and remained a "developing country," as it is called today.

In Europe during the Middle Ages—the 10th to 13th centuries— local currencies were issued by local lords, abbeys, or bishops and then periodically recalled and reissued with a tax collected in the process. Again, this was a form of demurrage that made money undesirable as a store of value. The result was the blossoming of culture and widespread well-being, corresponding exactly to the time period when these local currencies were used.

Practically all the cathedrals were built during this time period. If you think about what is required as investment for a small town to build a cathedral, it's extraordinary. Besides the obvious spiritual function, cathedrals served also an important economic function: they attracted pilgrims, who, from a business perspective, played a similar role to tourists today. These cathedrals were built to last forever and create a long-term cash flow for the community. This was a way of creating abundance for you and your descendants for 13 generations! The proof is that it still works today; in Chartres, for instance, the bulk of the city's businesses still live from the tourists who visit the cathedral 800 years after it was built! A number of economists have concluded that community currency is one of the few true long-term structural measures that can spontaneously help to achieve ecologically sustainable growth within a market economy.

It can also be used on a decentralized basis to stimulate local initiatives and resolve local social and economic difficulties. This could be done independently by local decision or as a pilot project to test out aspects of the plan before it is adopted at a national level. Community currency could be introduced in parallel with existing national currency. It could be introduced in some cities or regions and not in others.

Community currency would become immediately convertible without the need for any new international monetary agreements.

I propose that we choose to develop money systems that will enable us to attain sustainability and community healing on a local and global scale. These objectives are in our grasp within less than one generation's time. Whether we materialize them will depend on our capacity to cooperate with each other to consciously reinvent our money.

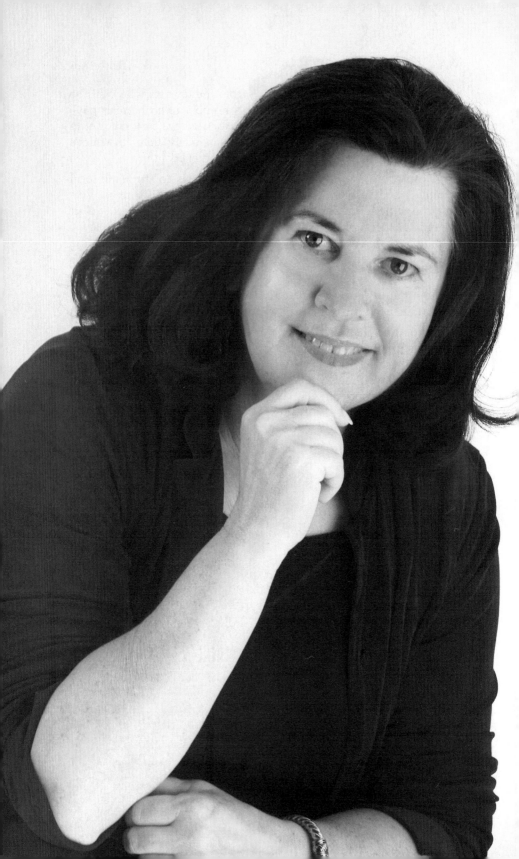

# Janet Dang:

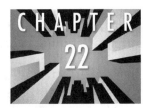

# Stepping into the Flow

As a child, I found that the only way to truly connect with my father was to participate in an activity he really enjoyed. That's how I found myself the only scrawny eight-year-old in a softball game with adults and teenagers. My dad was the pitcher for the opposing team. I was thrilled to be outside playing, and I knew that the game would be great fun. What I didn't know was that it would become a defining experience.

I walked up to bat for the first time amidst the friendly heckling of the fielders. They all moved in, assuming that the little kid wouldn't be able to hit—and I wanted to prove them wrong. My dad tossed a slow lob and I anxiously swung into empty space, the ball landing with a dull thwack right in the catcher's mitt. As the second pitch approached, however, I somehow forgot everything around me, as if I was alone on the field with the bat and the ball. Time stood still, my senses sharpened, and I was simply *playing.*

The ball floated toward me, seams spinning slowly, and I knew that I would hit it easily and effortlessly. In that moment I merged with the ball into the dance of the game. I swung smoothly, hitting the sweet spot, and it went way over everyone's head, well down the third base line. By the time the ball was thrown to the infield I had rounded the bases, joyously touching home. Only then did things slowly return to normal, so that I once again found myself surrounded by other players.

Janet Dang, Founder of Flow Practices, is a business mentor, practicing shaman, and successful executive and entrepreneur. Her breakthrough work helps people identify and step beyond their unconscious limiting patterns and beliefs to more frequently function "in the flow" while simultaneously improving their productivity and impact. Flow Practices offers a proven process to incrementally reduce stress and nonproductive action and increase energy while revealing openings to success that are hidden by our unconscious, limiting beliefs. Her promise is that clients who work with her seriously for six months will double their productivity, while improving their impact. Visit www.FlowPractices.com.

I always hoped to regain that sense of complete presence and peace during subsequent games. Sometimes it was there and sometimes not; yet the memory of that first accidental experience of peak performance — or flow — became a possibility that inspired future experiences in sports and in life.

Many years after that day on the softball field, I once again found myself in an unfamiliar and challenging situation. I had been working for seven years as an engineer for Amdahl, a mainframe computer manufacturer. We were in a contentious meeting with Perot Systems, a critical reference account who had recently taken shipment of our newest model. This new product was essential to our future revenue stream, as margins on the older product were diminishing rapidly. Everyone at our company was counting on the system working well for this key account. It was well known that Perot Systems was a demanding customer. If they were satisfied, other companies would also buy the product. The only problem was that the system wasn't working well for them at all.

The stuffy conference room was tightly packed with execs from both companies. Though everyone was talking, no one was hearing anyone else. Things were quickly going from bad to worse — it was a real lose/lose disaster. My co-worker Joe and I sat in the back of the room, petrified. We were the lucky ones who had to figure out how to satisfy this customer, so our careers and good names were literally on the line.

Somewhere in the melee, someone complained that the Perot Systems workloads were not completing every week as they were supposed to. All of our execs heard this as an accusation that our system was not as fast as we had promised. From this perspective it seemed impossible to make the customer happy.

But Joe and I were suddenly smiling. We heard the statement from a different perspective, and as a result, finally understood what they wanted. What's more, we knew how to solve the problem and were confident that we would be able to deliver, even though it required making substantial changes to our customer support software and processes. Because we had never before considered making such changes, we had never realized that there could be a better way.

By moving out of panic mode and into curiosity, Joe and I somehow stepped into the flow that was always there, hidden behind the confusion and tension. Three months later, Perot Systems gave rave reviews for that previously "unacceptable" system. The key to our success was that we remained curious and open to win/win solutions, despite the contentious environment. From that vantage point we saw the opening when it was presented.

I later left business, when the cycle of frustration and fatigue replaced any experience of flow. I felt more dead than alive and knew that I needed to recover that sense of wonder. Not only did I eventually find it, but I learned that it is always available. And I used this understanding to uncover my true vocation: coaching companies and individuals in the FlowHabit process that I developed along the way.

## Removing the Barriers to Flow

After moving on from the world of business, I was drawn to learn everything I could about consciousness and energy. With my background in science and math, I found that I had an innate understanding of some of the more complex concepts. One day, as I listened to Dr. Edgar Mitchell talking about the quantum hologram, I saw that each individual is a field of fluctuating energy and information, within a universal field of fluctuating energy and information. I was startled to realize that everything that happens in my life is the result of this universal field interacting with my own. I could clearly see how much of my time was wasted in a futile struggle, fighting this field.

Since we are one with the universal field, we can tune in at any moment. I had imagined the answer to be out there somewhere, when in reality it was inside me, ready to be accessed whenever I chose to listen to my intuitive knowing. Once I learned to stop my defensive, stressful responses to the field and just let things be, I could naturally step into curiosity. But if we never really tune in, it is no wonder that workable solutions seem out of reach.

We find exactly what we are looking for, and nothing else. When we see only problems and roadblocks, we are trapped in a limiting perspective that hides all the openings to success. As Wayne Dyer says, we can always choose to feel good — and yet we so often choose differently. Our unconscious patterns block our perception and experience of flow. In the past, I had chosen to be the smartest one, to see what needed fixing so I could struggle and make it work. In the course of my exploration, however, I have learned that it is not only possible to change perspective, but also to step consciously into that experience of flow.

As I learned to better understand the workings of the mind, I discovered that we can begin to consciously move beyond our unconscious limitations in just four simple steps:

1. **Stop the mania** to step beyond stress and non-constructive action into complete calm and mental clarity.

   • *New Perspective:* "I am the only one who is really getting in my way. Fighting the universe is a losing proposition and keeps me from the present moment. I relax in the face of stress and tension to step into my best thinking."

2. **Look inside** to see the situation as it really is. Since all the answers are in the universal field, which every cell of your body reads easily and effortlessly, look to your intuition to get a complete and accurate view. Remember, the mind creates distortions—so listen to the clear antenna, rather than to the distorted mind.

   • *New Perspective:* "The answer is in me, so stop looking out there for answers that can only be found in here."

3. **Find the opening** to inspired action by shifting to an empathetic perspective and setting a clear win/win intention. When you hold the space for possibility there is room for it to show up.

   • *New Perspective:* "I create my experience with what I look for, so why not look for what I want to find?"

4. **Choose a new compass** and you will easily see what you want to find. By getting out of the way, you orient yourself to receiving from the universe, which is already bringing you what you want.

   • *New Perspective:* "I let the universe bring it to me without resistance; there is no need to struggle to make it happen."

## The Model in Practice

As I clarified the model for conscious flow, which I called the FlowHabit process, I realized that it could benefit not just me, but anyone who felt limited by old patterns and struggled to perform more consistently at peak capability. I began to wonder whether there was a market for this kind of consulting. Would clients who were caught up in the old conflict-struggle-stress cycle be open to a new approach?

As it turns out, the unequivocal answer from the universe was… yes!

I began to work with several people who were struggling to free themselves of the limitations and ramifications of stress. Through these partnerships I learned organically about what helps and what doesn't. We discovered that the process worked incrementally, with each change bringing more peace and making it easier to identify and make the next change.

One of my early consulting jobs brought me to All-Tech, a manufacturer of custom machine parts. They had all the basics in place to make sure the business ran efficiently: standardized applications and processes, mission and values statements, effective management structure and practices, coaches, and process improvement. In short, they were well run and successful. But despite all this, in a few key areas, they were not performing at the level they wanted — and needed — to be. One of those areas was customer service and satisfaction.

Tammy, who manages customer service, had been using all the standard approaches to improve their practices. They had a defined customer quality process. Their order entry process was structured and enabled by a standardized application. They held frequent meetings to identify and try to resolve issues. Yet Tammy still received three "hot customer issue" e-mails per day. Tracking down and resolving these issues kept Tammy and her team at a high stress level, which negatively impacted her job satisfaction and enjoyment.

Tammy and I began our work together by looking at the overall context for her typical experience of life — therefore also her habitual context at work. She described her typical experience as one of "stuck gears," in which everyone must struggle and work hard to overcome the obstacles that block progress. With this compass, struggle is what she found — because that is exactly what she was looking for. Her underlying belief was that without a lot of commitment and effort, things do not work out well.

I explained to Tammy that since our personal experience of the world unfolds according to our perspective or expectations, which are a perfect reflection of our unconscious and conscious beliefs, it is on this level that we can have the greatest impact on the world.

We see only what we believe is there, and even that is distorted by our expectations, biases, subconscious desires, and fears. If I believe that only the strong survive, then I will see only your "weakness" so that I can exploit it. Since our world occurs according to our own perspective, it is actually a delusion of our consciousness. This means that the only one who is ever "at fault" is us — so there is never any point in getting mad at "them." To do so is actually a giant waste of precious time and energy that never moves us toward our objectives.

Most of the time we are caught up in our automatic, unconscious response to circumstances. These responses happen so quickly that we barely have time to stop ourselves from repeating the limiting patterns that keep us from performing at our best. There is a high cost to these patterns: They either keep us out of action altogether, or the actions we do take can tend to be destructive and require lots of recovery work. This is not a new idea; in fact, Hindu, Buddhist, and Jain teachers have long called these unconscious patterns by the Sanskrit name *samskaras*.

The FlowHabit process that I was inviting Tammy to enter into would involve making only the changes that she was ready to make in the moment; yet, those changes would have the immediate benefit of reducing stress and increasing her sense of peak performance. Changes would be made incrementally so that the value of each change could be experienced fully. Additionally, each change would make room for the next.

Tammy began to understand that she chooses how she sees what is going on and how she will respond to it. She could be calm or stressed, see a little or see more, see separate interests or shared interests, stuckness or flow. She wanted to learn how to consciously move into flow and shift her experience on the job—but first we first had to investigate her habits of perception.

## Tammy Steps into Peace in a Volatile World

The first shift focused on Tammy's perception of volcanoes—those instances when co-workers and customers seemed to erupt, and which felt to Tammy like personal attacks. In her old pattern, when Tammy experienced conflict, tension, and toxic energy she withdrew into a very defensive posture that we called "turtling." This practice drained her of vitality, sharply limiting her ability to remain present and effective. She felt as if the volcano would completely overwhelm her unless she became invisible. So, she held her breath, pulled her body back and in, clenched her jaw, and stopped listening, all in a desperate attempt to protect herself from the *perceived* attack. After one of these episodes, her "fight or flight" response often lasted for several hours, further limiting her ability to take constructive action.

Once Tammy identified her old beliefs, we were able to bring in new, more effective behavior patterns using a process I call ThetaShift. Her new pattern is to remain confident when she feels tense or attacked. She relaxes, smiles, and takes three deep, slow, calming breaths. She then checks in to see what is going on without blame or judgment. She is willing to see her part in the conflict, especially her perception of being attacked. She responds constructively as soon as it is practical to do so. This corresponds with her new belief that she is safe when she relaxes, remains fully present, and takes appropriate action to deal with the situation.

Soon after we made this shift, Tammy found herself in a volcano moment with her husband. Before she knew what was happening she found herself breathing deeply and relaxing. She was delighted that all this happened quickly and automatically, and that it completely diffused a potentially tricky situation. She is now aware of volcanoes and, more often than not, remains unaffected by them.

Over time we discovered that Tammy had a similar response whenever someone looked at her funny, criticized her, asked her a question she felt she should be able to answer but couldn't, or when she felt singled out. She now sees her "under attack" pattern more clearly and is able to respond constructively far more often.

## Tammy Tunes in to See Situations Differently

Once Tammy had shifted her pattern of response to feeling pressured, we began to work some of the more subtle issues that created conflict in her workplace. Since her department is the point of connection between All-Tech and its customers, there are many important, intersecting processes and touch points that Tammy and her team must manage. We referred to these as boundaries. But it became clear to me as we discussed the issue that Tammy couldn't really see what was going on.

Because she was relatively comfortable with grey areas, she had never really looked closely at the boundaries to see what worked and what didn't. To further complicate the issue, although she often found herself in difficult situations related to boundaries, Tammy could rarely see how she got there. This pattern of not seeing things completely or accurately is extremely common and causes much of the conflict that is experienced in business. Because it was so uncomfortable for Tammy, she spent a great deal of energy trying to avoid having to look at the situation.

As we worked together, Tammy began to see how awkward it was for her to honestly say yes or no under certain circumstances. Often she just said nothing until the situation blew up in her face. Other times, when she felt uncomfortable, she kept her ideas or opinions to herself because she felt she might not be constructive. I asked her to take a couple of weeks to see what was going on.

She realized that she had no clear standards or agreements for dealing with boundaries and boundary issues. To make matters worse, she often misjudged certain situations — so often, in fact, that she could no longer trust her responses to be appropriate. And all this was further complicated by the fact that as soon as she became uncomfortable, she stopped looking at what was going on.

Once we had identified Tammy's limiting unconscious beliefs, we used the ThetaShift technique to begin working to change them, and in so doing, change her responses. For example, we found that she believed that if she did not "see" something, she did not have to deal with it. We shifted to the new beliefs that she chooses to see everything, even if it makes her uncomfortable, that she is open and curious about all that is going on, and that she looks at everything—including her own part in a conflict or misunderstanding—without resentment or judgment. Now, whenever she is unsure or confused about anything, Tammy tunes in to her own inner knowing to get past the distortions that get in the way of her seeing things as they are.

Now Tammy has developed a powerful intuition for managing boundaries and proactively dealing with impending customer issues by listening to her body's wisdom and seeing beyond what is comfortable for her to see.

## The Bigger Picture

The work that Tammy and I did together made a big difference in her personal experience on the job; but there is always more to any dynamic system, like a workplace, than the perceptions and actions of a single person. We decided to look more closely at the larger field—including the interpersonal relationships and processes that made up the bigger picture.

Tammy manages a small team that is responsible for customer service. As with all teams, some things go smoothly for them and some are more difficult. At one point, when the volume of shipments they were processing increased substantially, Tammy and her team found working together more difficult than normal. Communication breakdowns occurred too often, and everyone became frustrated with the process and with each other. Tensions increased.

Tammy wanted to explore ways to get things back on track. I explained to her that, like everything else, teamwork is a function of the beliefs and thoughts that each of us has about our team. If we were going to be able to change the dynamic, we would need to include everyone in the process.

Once I got the whole team together, we discovered that while each of their perspectives and approaches to getting things done were quite different, their fundamental needs and commitments were the same. Each wanted to make things work well, to communicate well with the others, the rest of the company, and the customer, and to provide excellent customer service. But the differences in their individual patterns of perception stood in the way of their achieving these goals.

Tammy was comfortable with chaos, could clearly see shortcuts, and was good in difficult situations. Her thinking and explanations were complex, complete—and often difficult to follow. Too much structure felt restrictive to her. She hated to be interrupted and needed time to think situations through.

Eva liked to streamline everything and move very quickly. This meant that she became impatient when her questions were not answered quickly and simply. She did not like to wait. She wanted things presented in clear bullet points, which she checked off as she went.

Melissa, in the middle, liked order, structure, rules, and completeness. She wanted all the information in the correct order and did not like to work with ambiguity.

Compassion and shared needs are the keys to better teamwork. Tammy's team already shared needs and goals, so I wanted to help them to create compassion. This is most quickly achieved when we realize that others are just as stuck in and frustrated with their patterns as we are stuck in and frustrated with ours. So, because our individual stories are nothing more than frozen versions of our thoughts and beliefs, I suggested that we work with each team member's story to uncover her underlying patterns.

I was confident we could uncover a solution that would benefit each member of the team. Though they may not have been able to see it at the time, I knew that it would become clear once they understood one another's perspectives, quirks, and needs. I also assured them that we would only go as far as each of them was ready to go. Fortunately, Tammy was willing to be very open, which made it safe for others to do the same.

With such an extreme range of communication styles and approaches to work, it could have seemed impossible to bring these three women together. But because they were willing to work as a team without becoming competitive, we quickly found ourselves on the same page. And now that all this is on the table, they are able to work through potential conflicts in a way that accommodates everyone. Given their new perspective, they now approach one another with compassion, tolerance, and respect for differences. They also trust that each wants to do well, so they give each other more space. They share little jokes about each other's quirks and laugh at themselves easily. I helped them to see the benefits of change and what steps to take, but it was their own decision to shift their perceptions that opened the door to harmonious flow.

Much if not all of Tammy's limiting behavior was a highly conditioned, unconscious response to her perceived circumstances. Her perceptions were distorted and limited by what she expected to see, which was itself a function of her unconscious and conscious mind. As Tammy became aware of these patterns, she had more freedom to move in new directions. As she related compassionately with her community, she found actions and approaches that better aligned with what everyone wanted to achieve. The work we did together was the beginning of an ongoing, incremental process that allows Tammy to find more freedom as she relaxes and sees more clearly. Tammy is now changing her circumstances by changing her mind and allowing her response to come from her new position of intuitive understanding.

Each of us is a lot like Tammy. We promise ourselves that the next time we find ourselves in difficult circumstances, we will respond differently...but before we know it we are withdrawing, yelling, or even so angry that we might blow up. We step into a survival mode and scramble for ways to minimize our potential losses. From this perspective, it is difficult to realize that it is our own patterns that keep us from really playing fully in the flow of our own lives.

And yet, those unconscious, limiting patterns are not who we are. Because they are nothing more than old habits, we can make new choices at any moment and in response to any situation. We can consciously breathe and smile until our mind is calm and clear. We can look past our distortions, biases, and limiting beliefs to see each situation more completely. We can hold the clear intention that everyone will be heard and honored in the decisions we make and the approaches we take to working together toward a win/win reality. And we can relax in the knowing that when we have done all of these things well, the universe is already working to bring us what we really want and what is best for everyone involved.

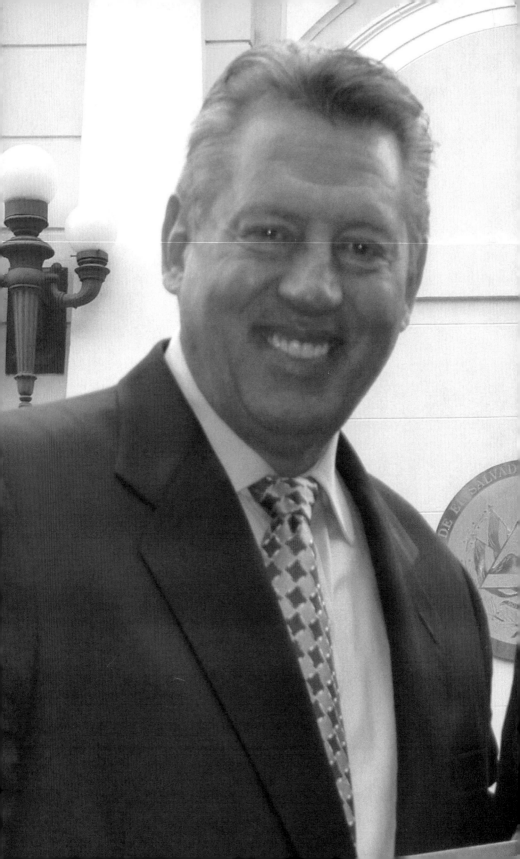

# JOHN MAXWELL:

# Servant Leadership

U .S. Army General H. Norman Schwarzkopf displayed highly
successful leadership abilities in commanding the allied
troops in the Persian Gulf War, just as he had done throughout
his career, beginning in his days at West Point.

In Vietnam he turned around a battalion that was in shambles.
The First Battalion of the Sixth Infantry — known as the "worst of the
sixth" — went from laughingstock to effective fighting force and were
selected to perform a more difficult mission. That turned out to be an
assignment to what Schwarzkopf described as "a horrible, malignant
place" called the Batangan Peninsula. The area had been fought over
for thirty years, was covered with mines and booby traps, and was
the site of numerous weekly casualties from those devices.

Schwarzkopf made the best of a bad situation. He introduced
procedures to greatly reduce casualties, and whenever a soldier
*was* injured by a mine, he flew out to check on the man, had him
evacuated using his chopper, and talked to the other soldiers to boost
their morale.

On May 28, 1970, a man was injured by a mine, and Schwarzkopf,
then a colonel, flew to the man's location. While the helicopter was
evacuating the injured soldier, another soldier stepped on a mine,
severely injuring his leg. The man thrashed around on the ground,
screaming and wailing. That's when everyone realized the first mine

John C. Maxwell is an internationally regarded leadership expert. He has
communicated his principles to Fortune 500 companies, heads of state,
the United States Military Academy at West Point, and university and
professional sports organizations. Dr. Maxwell is the founder of Injoy
Stewardship Services, and EQUIP, a nonprofit organization that teaches
leadership worldwide. He is a *New York Times* and *Business Week* best-
selling author of more than thirty books, with over 12 million copies
sold. *Developing the Leader Within You* (Nelson Business, 2005) and *The 21
Irrefutable Laws of Leadership* (Nelson Business, 1998) are million sellers.
Visit www.injoy.com.

hadn't been a lone booby trap. They were all standing in the middle of a minefield.

Schwarzkopf believed the injured man could survive and even keep his leg—but only if he stopped flailing around. There was only one thing he could do. He had to go after the man and immobilize him. Schwarzkopf wrote,

> I started through the minefield, one slow step at a time, staring at the ground, looking for telltale bumps or little prongs sticking up from the dirt. My knees were shaking so hard that each time I took a step, I had to grab my leg and steady it with both hands before I could take another... It seemed like a thousand years before I reached the kid.

-§-
How can I serve and lead people at the same time? You've got to love your people more than your position.
-§-

The 240-pound Schwarzkopf, who had been a wrestler at West Point, then pinned the wounded man and calmed him down. It saved his life. And with the help of an engineer team, Schwarzkopf got him and the others out of the minefield.

The quality that Schwarzkopf displayed that day could be described as heroism, courage, or even foolhardiness. But I think the word that best describes it is *servanthood*. On that day in May, the only way he could be effective as a leader was to serve the soldier who was in trouble.

# Having a Servant's Heart

When you think of servanthood, do you envision it as an activity performed by relatively low-skilled people at the bottom of the positional totem pole? If you do, you have a wrong impression. Servanthood is not about position or skill. It's about attitude. You have undoubtedly met people in service positions who have poor attitudes toward servantood: the rude worker at the government agency, the waiter who can't be bothered with taking your order, the store clerk who talks on the phone with a friend instead of helping you.

Just as you can sense when a worker doesn't want to help people, you can just as easily detect whether someone has a servant's heart. And the truth is that the best leaders desire to serve others, not themselves.

What does it mean to embody the quality of servanthood? A true servant leader:

1. **Puts Others Ahead of His Own Agenda**

The first mark of servanthood is the ability to put others ahead of yourself and your personal desires. It is more than being willing to put your agenda on hold. It means intentionally being aware of other people's needs, available to help them, and able to accept their desires as important.

## 2. Possesses the Confidence to Serve

The real heart of servanthood is security. Show me someone who thinks he is too important to serve, and I'll show you someone who is basically insecure. How we treat others is really a reflection of how we think about ourselves. Philosopher-poet Eric Hoffer captured that thought:

> The remarkable thing is that we really love our neighbor as ourselves; we do unto others as we do unto ourselves. We hate others when we hate ourselves. We are tolerant toward others when we tolerate ourselves. We forgive others when we forgive ourselves. It is not love of self but hatred of self which is at the root of the troubles that afflict our world.

Only secure leaders give power to others. It's also true that only secure people exhibit servanthood.

## 3. Initiates Service to Others

Just about anyone will serve if compelled to do so. And some will serve in a crisis. But you can really see the heart of someone who initiates service to others. Great leaders see the need, seize the opportunity, and serve without expecting anything in return.

## 4. Is Not Position-Conscious

Servant leaders don't focus on rank or position. When Colonel Norman Schwarzkopf stepped into that minefield, rank was the last thing on his mind. He was one person trying to help another. If anything, being the leader gave him a greater sense of obligation to serve.

## 5. Serves Out of Love

Servanthood is not motivated by manipulation or self-promotion. It is fueled by love. In the end, the extent of your influence and the quality of your relationships depend on the depth of your concern for others. That's why it's so important for leaders to be willing to serve.

# How to Become a Servant

To improve your servanthood, do the following:

§   **Perform small acts.** When was the last time you performed small acts of kindness for others? Start with those closest to you: your spouse, children, parents. Find ways today to do small things that show others you care.

§ **Learn to walk slowly through the crowd.** I learned this great lesson from my father. I call it walking slowly through the crowd. The next time you attend a function with a number of clients, colleagues, or employees, make it your goal to connect with others by circulating among them and talking to people. Focus on each person you meet. Learn his name if you don't know it already. Make your agenda getting to know each person's needs, wants, and desires. Then later when you go home, make a note to yourself to do something beneficial for half a dozen of those people.

It is true that those who would be great must be like the least and the servant of all.

§ **Move into action.** If an attitude of servanthood is conspicuously absent from your life, the best way to change it is to start serving. Begin serving with your body, and your heart will eventually catch up. Sign up to serve others for six months at your church, a community agency, or a volunteer organization. If your attitude still isn't good at the end of your term, do it again. Keep at it until your heart changes.

Where is your heart when it comes to serving others? Do you desire to become a leader for the perks and benefits? Or are you motivated by a desire to help others?

If you really want to become the kind of leader that people want to follow, you will have to settle the issue of servant-hood. If your attitude is to be served rather than to serve, you may be headed for trouble. It is true that those who would be great must be like the least and the servant of all.

Albert Schweitzer wisely stated, "I don't know what your destiny will be, but one thing I know: The ones among you who will be really happy are those who have sought and found how to serve." If you want to be successful on the highest level, be willing to serve on the lowest. That's the best way to build relationships.

# PART SIX

❧

# Inner-Directed Change

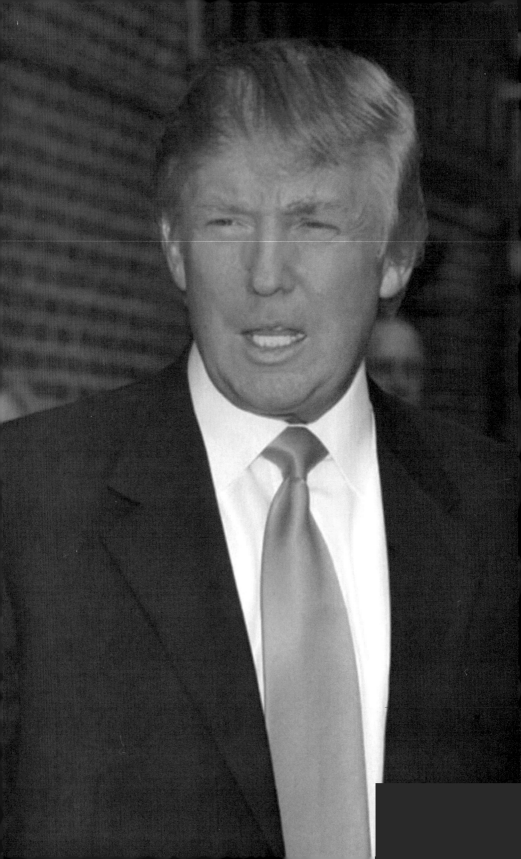

# DONALD TRUMP:

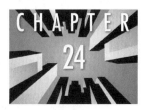

# CHAPTER 24

# Change Your Altitude

Wlhen I say *altitude,* I'm not referring to my jet. It's my own interpretation of the word *attitude.* I like flying because it gets me where I'm going, fast. Likewise, if you have the right attitude, you can get where you're going, fast.

What's the altitude of your attitude? Is it high frequency or low frequency? Having a high frequency will attune you to a wavelength that exudes confidence and clear-sighted enthusiasm. I'm a firm believer that this is half the battle of any enterprise.

I'm a tough-minded optimist. I learned a long time ago that my productivity was increased by a large percentage simply by learning to let go of negativity in all forms as quickly as I could. My commitment to excellence is thorough—so thorough that it negates the wavelength of negativity immediately. I used to have to zap negativity mentally. By now, it just bounces off me within a moment of getting near me. As you may have heard, I don't like germs. I'm still waging a personal crusade to replace the mandatory and unsanitary handshake with the Japanese custom of bowing. To me, germs are just another kind of negativity.

Negativity is also a form of fear, and fear can be paralyzing. On the golf course, I've heard great athletes tell me that they can't putt. They can hit a ball three hundred yards right down the middle of the fairway, but they can't finish the hole by putting the ball three feet into the cup.

---

**Donald J. Trump is an archetypal businessman. His interests include real estate, entertainment, gaming, and sports. Mr. Trump is person-ally involved in everything that his name represents. This commitment has made him the pre-eminent developer of quality real estate known around the world. He is also a successful author, having published sev-eral bestselling business books, including *The Art of the Deal* (Ballantine Books, 2004), *How to Get Rich* (Ballantine Books, 2004), and *The Art of Survival* (Warner Books, 1991), a generous philanthropist, and a member of several civic and charitable organizations. Visit www.trump.com.**

Recently, I played with a man who is terrified of putting. He hit a magnificent 235-yard shot and was seven feet from the cup. Then he looked over at me and said, "Now the hard part begins."

Another friend, also a great golfer, is paralyzed by his fear of losing his ball. Each time we played a hole near a lake, he would look down and say to his ball, "I have a feeling I'll never see you again."

I have told these two guys that they must start thinking positively or they will sabotage themselves.

Very often, negative thinking stems from low self-esteem. You have to work on this yourself. Maybe you've received a lot of hard knocks. I've learned to deal with them because I get knocked a lot. Quickly see them for what they are—knocks. But you don't have to open the door unless you choose to. I've gotten to the point where I see knocks as opportunities and as an insight into whoever is doing the knocking.

One way to chase low altitude away is to think about how fortunate you already are and how much you still have to look forward to. You can better your best day at any time. Very surprising things can happen, but you must—and I repeat *must*—be open to them. How can you fly if you've already clipped your own wings?

I don't have time to encourage as many people as I would like to, but whenever it seems appropriate, I recommend *The Power of Positive Thinking* by Norman Vincent Peale, one of my father's favorite books, and mine, too. Some people may think it's old-fashioned, but what Peale has written will always be true. He advocates faith over fear. Faith can overcome the paralysis that fear brings with it.

I can remember a time when I had a choice to make, when I was billions of dollars in debt. I had to take one of two courses of action: a fearful, defensive one or a faithful, riskier one. I carefully analyzed the situation, realized what was causing the uneasy feeling of fear, and immediately replaced it with blind faith simply because I had nothing else to go on at the time. Then I resolved that as long as I remained positive and disciplined, things would workout.

There was not much more I could do. I didn't know how it was going to go, but I was determined to move forward, even though it wasn't easy. Within a relatively short amount of time, the situation was settled positively. I learned a lot from that and have since had a better understanding of what courage really is. Without facing my own fear, I would not have known.

When I think of someone who is tough, I also think of someone who has courage. People who persist have courage, because often it's a lot easier to give up. Some of the bravest people I've met are children with handicaps. I'm active with United Cerebral Palsy. What those kids deal with is humbling, but they are enthusiastic and thrilled with every day they've been given.

You've been given a day, too. When you're down, look at it that way. Another day can equal another chance. Sometimes, as obvious as it sounds, we really do have to take things one day at a time. Immediately after the events of September 11, we didn't know what was going to happen, but we all kept going, one day at a time, and we're still moving forward.

Maybe you've gotten to the point where you think you can't get through another day. That's shortsighted of you. You're missing the big picture. You're on the runway, but your fuel supply is the problem. You won't get off the ground without it. Feed yourself some positive thoughts and you can take off at any time.

Ever wonder what makes certain people keep going? I do. Abraham Lincoln encountered a steady procession of setbacks but he just kept at it. Nothing deterred him. He must have had a lot of faith, because he didn't receive much encouragement along the way. He's an excellent example of someone who never gave up.

The other extreme is the person who seems to run into obstacles with the unerring aim of a marksman. I knew a guy who was remarkably accident-prone. If there was something to run into, he'd find it. If there was a hole in the ground, he'd break his foot by stumbling into it.

Once, he was in such a slam-bang accident that he was hospitalized for six months before being completely patched up. Finally, the day of his release from the hospital arrived and it was decided that he should get an ambulance ride home, just to be on the safe side. As the ambulance was taking him home, it crashed into a car—another spectacular slam-bang accident. My friend was immediately brought back to the hospital, in a new ambulance dispatched to the scene of the disaster. What can I say? Maybe he's just a really unlucky guy. Or maybe he's a loser. I know that sounds harsh, but let's face it—some people *are* losers.

The altitude level of losers is so low that they should walk around in scuba gear all day. They are below sea level on the altitude map. We all know people like that, and they might make great comedians because they have so much material—but first they'd have to learn to be funny. Honestly, I've known people who are such accomplished losers that I think that's what they devote their time to:

How can I be the biggest screwup possible?

How can I prove the born loser theory to be correct?

How can I defy the law of probability to make it an absolute disaster every time?

How can I achieve a perfect record of total wipeouts?

How far can I get at zero miles per hour?

How can I reach the lowest frequency possible?

How can I operate so that radar could never possibly find me even if I get lost, which I probably will?

These people need a new speedometer.

Get going. Move forward. Aim high. Plan for a takeoff. Don't just sit on the runway and hope someone will come along and push the airplane. It simply won't happen.

Change your attitude and gain some altitude. Believe me, you'll love it up here.

## Start Visualizing Positively

Positive thoughts will create positive visuals. Have you ever heard someone say "I can just *see* it!" when they are enthusiastic about something? I know from experience that if I can see something as a possibility, it has a much better chance of happening than if I can't see it happening.

Give your higher self a chance once in a while by giving your possibility quota a boost.

Keep a book of inspiring quotes nearby, so you can change a negative wavelength the moment it descends on you. Here are some of my personal favorites:

Know everything you can about what you're doing.

–My father, Fred Trump

I know the price of success: dedication, hard work, and an unremitting devotion to the things you want to see happen.

–Frank Lloyd Wright

A leader has the right to be beaten, but never the right to be surprised.

–Napoleon

Let's avoid subtlety on this one.
  –Charlie Reiss, *Executive Vice President of Development, The Trump Organization*

He who looks outside his own heart dreams, he who looks inside his own heart awakens.

–Carl Jung

Exciting is a dull word for the business we're in.

–Fred Trump

Imagination is more important than knowledge.

–Albert Einstein

Continuous effort—not strength or intelligence—is the key to unlocking our potential.

–Winston Churchill

I remember when *I* was the Donald.

–Donald Duck

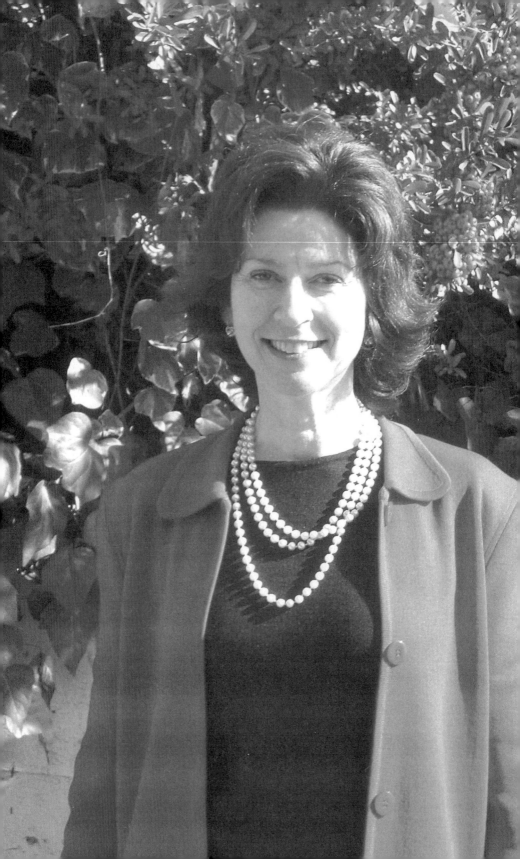

# FREDERIKA HASKELL: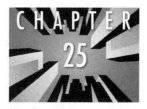

# The Highest Form of Art

When I visited Italy a few years ago, the art and the architecture, the sense of history, and the salt air of the Ligurian Sea enthralled me. Yet, thinking back on my time in Tuscany and Liguria, it is something far simpler that piques my longing and colors my vision of what life can be. It is the memory of a bakery, and of a heartfelt moment of human connection.

Not long before my trip, I had learned that, in Italy, it is considered impolite to enter a shop without greeting the shopkeeper. Having lived in urban areas on the West Coast of the United States for most of my adult life, this was not something I was accustomed to. I embraced the tradition conscientiously, however, and in return, I was rewarded with genuine warmth and numerous friendly conversations with local Italians. A bakery in Rapallo was no exception.

It was near the end of my stay, and I was hoping for one last chance to buy my favorite breakfast pastry, *pescatero*. The counter attendant didn't speak much English, and I didn't speak much Italian. Still, I managed to order my pescatero, letting her know that I would be taking it with me on the train back to Florence. I watched the customers come and go, the workers in the bakery interacting with each other and with the customers, and I was struck by the grace of friendly encounters. When the woman returned with my pescatero, I saw that she had carefully wrapped it in beautiful paper, taking the time to tie it well so it would survive my luggage banging around on

Frederika Haskell envisions a world where people work and play well together in all aspects of their lives. Her work is infused with a passion for integrity, quality, mutual respect, and enhancing the connections between people. She helps organizations reach their goals by aligning employee strengths with group and organizational objectives. With a graduate degree in Organizational Development/Human Resources from the University of San Francisco, Frederika has spent 25 years working in business settings that range from entrepreneurial start-ups to Fortune 500 companies. Find her on the web at www.TheHappyHuman.com.

the train. Thanks to the care she took, I was able to enjoy the pastry for several days, even saving some for my flight back to the Bay Area so that the memory of the encounter would linger more freshly in my mind. And as I savored those last bites somewhere high over the Atlantic, I remembered the warmth of her smile and the kindness in her voice as she wished me a good trip in a language I only barely understood.

Shortly after this trip, I migrated to a Northern California town that is just the right distance from the urban hustle and bustle. I realize now that though the seed for this move had been planted years before, it was watered by my travels in Tuscany and Liguria, where I enjoyed a slower rhythm of life and strangers said hello to each other when they passed on the street. How different it was from the self-contained, time-is-money experience of typical urban-American existence.

Nowhere was this more true than in the corporate world. In this world, I witnessed perfectly good people doing perfectly awful things with and to each other. I saw adults who had raised their own children reverting to childhood behaviors when the going got a little bit difficult. And I learned, to my horror and through hard experience, that people actually can have two sets of values, living by one code of ethics in the workplace and another in their non-work lives.

What is going on here? Why do individuals who can raise large amounts of money for their local PTA and lead entire committees to pull off a community event suddenly seem to lose their capabilities when they go to work? There are many reasons, of course. One stems from the very way we structure our businesses, produce our products, and get them out the door. The paradigm in which we conduct business — in both the for-profit and the not-for-profit sectors — has led to practices and habits that undermine the greater personal and cultural good. What can we do? We can begin to question our assumptions about how people work.

The existing paradigm has led to the creation of a society in which our education and efforts are largely dedicated to production of consumer goods, and our primary goal is to be "successful" in business. Work is broken down into discrete units and delegated to individuals and small groups, so that very few people are allowed a holistic involvement in production from conception to end. This has led to an entrenchment of organizational systems and structures that inadvertently result in perceptions and behaviors that undermine cooperation, efficiency, effective problem-solving, and even profitability. When the analysts report to shareholders and boards of directors that the numbers are not looking good, reparative measures often involve layoffs for hardworking people who have been caught up in the cycle.

This paradigm in which we work is so limited that it neglects the profound nature of our human interrelatedness. It requires that incredibly creative, funny, caring, complex, emotional, lovely, broken, amazing human beings leave their brains and hearts at the door and assume a work persona that may or may not fit. Now, this isn't all bad—we're also called on to express our better natures at work. In the interest of working well together, we have to set aside our prejudices, criticisms, and disabling behaviors that harm others and ourselves. We are frequently called on to practice skills we have not been brought up with, such as effectively navigating the ordinary conflicts that arise when people and groups depend on one another.

In the early 1990s there seemed to be a bandwagon that all the Fortune 500 companies were jumping on. They were exclaiming that shareholder value is the most important business result to focus on. Even paeans to "employees, customers, and shareholders," highlighted in corporate mission and values statements and annual reports transmogrified into a complete focus on shareholders as the primary stakeholder of concern to business leaders.

Jeffrey Skilling was recently sentenced to 24 years in prison for the various and many white-collar crimes he committed at Enron. I think of his wife and children. Perhaps he has sisters, brothers, parents who are still alive, and cousins, aunts, and uncles. I think of those relationships, how his family is affected, and by extension, how the communities surrounding these family members are affected. I have heard the litany of his illegal acts, but they are so numerous and complex that I can't repeat them all. What it boils down to, however, is that he conspired to make it look like company performance was far better than it actually was—all in the name of shareholder value.

It starts out small, usually. We know the drill, we're adults. We tell a fib, then another to cover that fib, and then pretty soon we're busy covering our tracks. But would such fibs be so tempting in the first place if the company owners (shareholders) and leaders (the C-suite, the Board of Directors) shifted their focus to the people, operational efficiencies, and profitability which ultimately lead to value for shareholders, managers, and employees?

It is time to apply our imagination to organizational structures and settings, and to imagine entirely different approaches to human systems within a capitalist-style economy. The business organizations of today have significant influence on life in our communities, in our larger society and culture, and in the world. And yet they are ultimately human systems. It's time to imagine ourselves as something more than interchangeable parts of a machine, and to envision a mode of work that nurtures fully creative, fully responsible beings with heads *and* hearts. It's time to imagine different possibilities.

We have few models of how to conduct business in such a way that everyone within an organization benefits. Perhaps this is because we've only been at this for perhaps a few hundred years out of our entire human existence. But the urgent need for change is here, now. Given the enormous impact of business on our homes, neighborhoods, and communities, the rate of technological and economic innovation and the extent of the unfortunate effects our practices have already had, we must find a way to shift the general cultural features of our workplaces.

There has been some movement toward this type of effort in organizations that are developing and internalizing the concept of sustainability, the three-point bottom line of People, Profits, and Planet. There is promise here, though my observation about the sustainable enterprise movement is that the "people" portion of the equation is getting short shrift. Attention is given to people outside the organization — to customers. Many companies highlight charitable giving and support of volunteer efforts as examples of being "good citizens" in the communities in which we work. These are admirable and much-needed efforts, and more can be done. But I think that attention to people *inside* the organization is urgently needed. This is where the greatest, and potentially most positive, community impact can be nurtured. It is these people who make the goods and services — and the organizations themselves — possible.

How do we do imagine different and better ways of organizing ourselves? We learn in freshman-level sociology and psychology courses that people naturally organize themselves into leaders and followers. Sit in a group and talk about a thorny issue, and notice the dynamics. But these roles are interdependent, and in order for either to function there must be a mutual understanding and respect. In addition to the deeply embedded organizational challenges we face, our incredibly complex legal and regulatory landscape impinges on constructing relationships that move beyond manager-employee, boss-subordinate — the old model of superior-inferior. There is, in much of the work world, an inherent mistrust of management, some of it cultural, some of it bred by years of hard experience, and some of it engendered by careless, ignorant leadership.

Beginning in the early 1990s, when waves of layoffs were sweeping corporate America, Lew Epstein was facilitating men and women to practice deep listening and to cultivate compassion, forgiveness, and a state of grace with one other. He proposed ways to be with and acknowledge fundamental fear as an incredibly strong driving force behind our action—and our inaction. In examining my own responses to various situations I could see that, when I dug deeply, I almost always found some fear. I was always afraid of losing something, be it money, approval, security, friendship, reputation, or face.

I think people are afraid. I think we worry about how we're going to pay the mortgage or get our children through school so they can make something of themselves. I think we worry about that upcoming doctor's appointment and about all the symptoms and disease we experience as a result of our dysfunctional, stress-filled work lives. I think we worry about whether we can pay for it all, because we know of so many stories, including our own, where, whoops, one morning we go to work and we get the pink slip.

What do people do when they live in fear, when their very livelihoods are threatened? It's not as if the majority of our population has been educated in how to recognize and express emotions constructively. There are plenty of stories of people who rebound, of course; but what is their experience along the way? And what about those who take much longer to rebound? Or those who never recover at all, for whatever reason—lack of self-esteem, lack of safety nets, lack of resources, lack of support systems. Even the best of us find ourselves afraid and acting out in the face of fear. Addiction is one response, as are domestic violence, depression, bullying, and withdrawal. We humans are persistently in a state of fear and compensation, whether we are conscious of it or not. And so the greatest gift we can give each other is to listen deeply, intently, with compassion, and to allow ourselves to be heard, fully and completely.

Punishment mentality is another core component of the hierarchies and structures we work in: Play the game or you'll lose your job, get a poor performance evaluation, fall out of the boss's good graces, be an outcast. All this gets taken home. Events seeded at the top of the business hierarchy affect our relationships outside of the workplace, with our friends, parents, children, teachers, neighbors, and in churches, synagogues, and temples. What does the "people" part of the three-point bottom line really mean?

The pressure that the focus on profit has brought to bear on us as individuals filters out into our communities. We don't have time to volunteer. We don't have time to connect in person. We don't have time to support our schools. We don't have time to truly understand the complex issues that require our attention, such as transit, protection of our open spaces, housing, healthcare, what it means to be a country and to protect our society, what it means to have national boundaries in a time of globalization, what it means to pay taxes and how those dollars are used. We don't have time to evaluate for ourselves the truth or falseness of the words uttered by our "leaders." We are so tired that we just want to be entertained, and so we are.

We must find a way to shift the paradigm from one that causes fear and mistrust to one that encourages trust and nurtures flourishing, healthy individuals who want to and can participate in community. We're human, and we need to work together. We need to rely on each other. Right now, at this point in our human story, business is the dominant social institution that is driving the whole show at the global level, so it is the perfect place to start in figuring this out.

I propose that a key component of the new agenda must address the welfare of people working inside the organizations, of the citizens of the communities these organizations inhabit, and of the consumers of the goods and services produced. In a world where a three-point bottom line is a reality, I imagine people at all organizational levels interacting all the time, bringing their most creative selves to work, and learning how to work together to solve problems. I imagine all people having complete, ideally hands-on understanding of the entire product or service from inception to "out the door." And I imagine the abolition of "performance evaluations," because feedback is constant and helpful, with all workers sharing in profits at livable and sustainable levels.

I envision us stretching our notions of what it means to work, of working relationships, and of what it means to create and produce goods and services while we tend our families and communities. I envision us acting from the realization that we are interdependent. Yes, we need to be individually responsible; but individual responsibility does not mean that you tend only to your own garden at the cost of your neighbor's. Individual responsibility means that as we act collectively, we are honest about our individual actions and hold one another accountable to community standards. It means that as we produce goods and services in a market economy that is about the people, we account for both hidden and visible costs of production, mindful of and accounting for the effects our actions have on the communities in which we do business, whether in our own home towns or half way around the world.

Do cooperatives have a place in our new world, or worker-owned entities? Is it possible for publicly traded corporations to move away from traditional hierarchies and the industrial-model division of work to create structures in which workers can see and touch and celebrate the outcome of their efforts up close? Is it possible to adapt the legal environment to the needs of a booming population on a small planet? We can only find out by imagining, and by trying.

What we do know is that people like certainty. They ultimately want to know what their job is, to have it clearly defined, and to know what is expected of them by their supervisors. They also want to be able to trust those supervisors, and trust can only come from human connection. We live in a world of the most unimaginable change, in which human connection is often mediated by electronic communication devices. This new reality presents both challenges and exciting options as our organizational systems evolve. It's possible to spend hours alone yet connected to others over the internet; but in the meantime, as the planet's population continues to expand and there are more and more people to work with, we spend less and less time making actual contact.

Of what can we be certain in this world of change? That we all experience the desire to be loved and appreciated. That we experience fear as we navigate the paths of change. That we experience joy in watching our children grow and flourish. That we get angry when we're disappointed and grow frustrated when, day after day, our dreams are dashed and unsupported. We can be certain that we are all anxious and afraid when asked to give up everything we know and try something new — especially when we don't know what that "something new" is. And we are angry when we have to put aside the things that really matter because some faceless, institutional shareholder wants their darn profit! Yet, we are also encouraged when the people with whom we work understand that sometimes a child is very sick and needs to be cared for, or a teenager is in trouble and needs their parent right now so that they can become a functioning adult. We share the experience of wondering what is happening to the fertile land, our blue skies, the vistas across the valleys, and mourn silently or loudly, as the case may be. We are not all alike, yet I am convinced that each of us has these things in common.

We need organizational norms that include compassion and deep listening. We need structures that support us in learning to express ourselves constructively rather than destructively. We need safe places to work so that we can provide safety for our families and our communities, and by extension, for all people on our small planet.

I recall one of my many pleasurable walks with a particularly close family member. I was talking about my political and environmental concerns, and she responded by saying that she just can't think about it because it's too depressing. More recently, after watching the film "An Inconvenient Truth," another family member said, "What can I do?" It was a statement, not a question. These comments reflect an underlying cultural belief that individual actions don't count, that they don't influence those around us, and that they don't have a larger, more mysterious effect. And yet I think back to that simple, heartfelt connection in the bakery in Rappalo, and know those beliefs are not based in truth. What might be possible if we shed this illusion?

Perhaps we can rediscover the profound nature of our world, of our relationships at work and in our communities, and of working together. Perhaps we can begin a new trend toward care and compassion as predominant cultural qualities. From this, perhaps we could build communities in which our children are safe and a planet where our humanity is more highly valued than our profits.

It all begins with conversation, with asking questions that lead to more questions and, ultimately, to action. Rainer Maria Rilke captured this intention beautifully when he wrote:

> I beg you...to have patience with everything unresolved in your heart and try to love the questions themselves as if they were locked rooms or books written in a very foreign language. Don't search for the answers, which could not be given you now, because you would not be able to live them. And the point is, to live everything. Live the questions now. Perhaps then, someday far in the future, you will gradually, without ever noticing it, live your way into the answer...

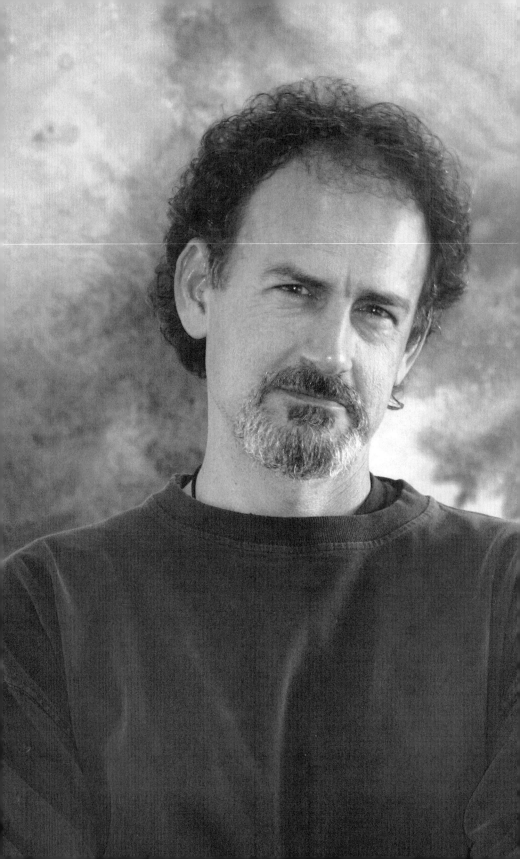

# MATTHEW GILBERT: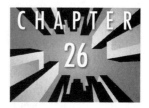

# Now Thyself

Centuries ago, the Buddha extolled the importance of the present moment. In the psychological laboratory of the 1960s, psychedelics pioneer Richard Alpert, aka Ram Dass, wrote *Be Here Now*, a free-wheeling spiritual travelogue that still sells remarkably well. But it was comedian/philosopher Mel Brooks who actually counseled his audience to "now thyself." What better authority could you ask for?

The axiom "now thyself" is an endlessly intriguing one, made all the more popular these days by Ekhart Tolle's *The Power of Now* franchise of books and tapes. It essentially suggests that the past and the future are distractions — the past is done, the future doesn't exist — and the only reality that counts is what's happening in the moment. Accepting that reality and being totally present to it empowers one to make more thoughtful and ultimately more effective decisions about life, work, and relationships. And so we need to give all of our attention to these moments, to cultivate self-awareness and awareness of what's going on around us.

But there isn't much time for *now* in the workplace, unless it's an extension of the past or a bridge to the future. In the business world, to now oneself — to embrace and live fully in the present moment — goes against the grain of nearly everything one is taught about how to get ahead, work a customer, meet a deadline, and so on: analyze, strategize, dance on the head of a pin. In that world the mind

**Matthew Gilbert is Director of Communications at the Institute of Noetic Sciences, editor of the quarterly magazine *Shift: At the Frontiers of Consciousness*, and editorial director of Noetic Press. He has written extensively about business, psychology, and spirituality, and is the author of two books: *The Workplace Revolution: How to Restore Trust in Business and Meaning to Our Jobs* (Conari, 2005) and *Communication Miracles at Work* (Conari, 2002). In previous incarnations he has worked as a book editor and publishing consultant, market research analyst, mediator and facilitator, and statewide organizer of the Green Party USA for Colorado. Photo by Kelly Durkin.**

is like a monkey desperately trying to stay ahead of some unseen menace. Slow down and you'll get eaten! Even as I type these words I find myself going faster and faster, fight or flight, missing keys, heart pumping, wondering what I'll tap in next. When life is a 24/7 marathon, moving so fast that to simply survive is triumph enough, embracing the present moment is a nearly hilarious notion.

## Inside-out, Outside-in

I recently heard a talk given by Hans-Peter Duerr, a nuclear physicist and former director of the Max Plank Institute for Physics and Astrophysics—a high church of science. He was describing the process in physics of breaking things apart into smaller and smaller pieces in order to find that one ultimate physical unit that will illuminate the source of all matter. It turns out, he noted wryly, that after decades of such finely tuned parsing, the best scientists in the world seem to have discovered...nothing. "Matter disappears," he said, "and only the relationship remains. This is the 'new physics.'"

How very interesting. It's the relationship between things that counts, not the things themselves, and that got me to thinking: If we were to organize our lives into both *being* states and *doing* states, into who-we-are moments and what-we-do moments, then it seems we spend most of our time doing and not being. Sure, our actions reflect at least some aspects of who we are, such as our creative interests or skill with numbers or wordsmithing acumen. But all of this doing—meeting deadlines, establishing goals, churning out products, and so on—represent the things of our lives, and we are more than those things. We are equally defined by our relationship to those things and our motivations for doing them, by our relationships with those we work with, and, perhaps most importantly, by our awareness of the thoughts and feelings we have as we move through the moments of each day. Such awareness can mean the difference between the constant drain of reacting to the things that arise from the conditioned mind and the empowering energy of acting from an inner *noetic* knowing.

The power of self-awareness is in revealing ourselves to ourselves, as honestly as we can, perhaps for the first time. It begins to reveal how our minds work, where our fears and desires live, who and what the buttons are. Self-aware people will often think twice before responding to a situation, taking a moment—nowing themselves—to better choose the right words or a wiser course of action. Over time, the self-aware person begins to develop a maturity and a personal ethic that is immune from outside influences, guiding their behavior and keeping them grounded no matter the circumstance. "When you are unconscious," writes Let Davidson in *Wisdom at Work*, "you remain a mechanical victim of your own subliminal mental tendencies, painful habits, and counterproductive patterns. Heightened self-awareness reveals these habits and patterns, so that you can deal with them. You can accept them, let them go, or change them. Awareness gives you the choice to respond appropriately, to channel your power in the directions you choose." Or in the powerfully simple prose of Zen, "Serenity is not freedom from the storm but peace within the storm."

I remember standing in a crowd of people after having just been given the responsibility of coordinating a major national gathering of political activists. Requests, demands, advice, and congratulations were coming at me in waves, and I felt myself going under, trying to keep all of it in some semblance of control. A small but distinct voice whispered over my shoulder, "One thing at a time, one thing at a time," then everything suddenly slowed down and I was able to connect with an inner calm that helped steer me through the noise.

Similar to self-awareness, but more outwardly focused, is mindfulness, another tool for helping us to "be here now" and approach our work in a renewed spirit of engagement. In such an attentive state we make meaningful contact with our workplace surroundings: the stress—or joy—in a co-worker's voice, the "feeling tone" of a meeting, the integrity of a potential business client. It's a matter of training oneself to be alert and responsive. The complexity of the world around us deepens as new information starts flowing in; we feel more connected and involved. Tuning in to the deeper flows beneath someone's behavior helps us to make more insightful decisions about how and when to respond, or even if a response is called for. Over time, the practice of mindfulness can turn what might otherwise be just another ho-hum irritation into an opportunity for knowledge and compassionate response. Being this aware, this present, takes us out of our isolation and into direct relationship.

I know, it all sounds good in theory because in the corporate world there is little time for the luxury of present-moment immersion. Efforts to slow down and smell the reality, to really get to know oneself, to *be* oneself, are easily undermined by the relentless pace of doing and deadlines. Meanwhile, a swarm of highly paid psychologists and consultants try to box us into movable pieces of personality shorthand. Forget the present moment, they say, we'll tell you who you are. In a spirited and sometimes subversive effort to harness the unruliness of personality in the workplace, these specialists come armed with tests and typologies designed to lubricate corporate performance by simplifying those pesky complexities of humanness. Some of the more popular include:

# Chapter Twenty-Six

# Myers-Briggs

This is the most enduring system of psychological profiling, based on the pioneering work of famed psychologist Carl Jung and developed in the 1940s by the mother-daughter team of Katherine Briggs and Isabel Briggs-Myers. The system measures personality according to four specific areas:

§ How a person relates to others (Extraversion vs. Introversion)

§ How a person takes in information (Sensory vs. Intuitive)

§ How a person makes decisions (Thinking vs. Feeling)

§ How a person organizes their life (Judging vs. Perceiving)

The MBTI—the Myers-Briggs Type Indicator—identifies 16 specific types (ENFJ, ISTP, ESFP, and so on), each one with a dominant temperament. The Briggs never personalized the different types other than to discuss their general characteristics, but others have come up with such names as Mystic, Innovator, Helper, Realist, and so on.

# Big Five

The Big Five evolved from the work of Sir Francis Galton, a pioneer in the field of behavior studies who practiced more than 100 years ago. Galton was considered the first man to investigate individual personality differences scientifically. The Big Five basically draws from the research behind the MBTI model but moves away from "types" and toward actual personality traits. It identifies five key characteristics—Conscientiousness, Extraversion, Neuroticism, Agreeableness, and Openness to Experience—each of which has six "sub facets."

# Stress Personalities

Back in the 1970s, two social work professionals, Mary H. Dempcy and Rene Tihista, came up with a typology based on how we deal with stress. Each of seven basic "stress personalities" — the Pleaser, the Striver, the Critical Judge, the Internal Time Keeper, the Saber-Tooth, the Worrier, the Inner Con Artist—represents a particular behavior pattern. Each one reacts to and in many cases creates stress in its own unique way. One type will usually be dominant, but different personalities can surface depending on the circumstance.

# Enneagram

The Enneagram, characterized by one practitioner as "an ancient teaching of mysterious origin," draws from the spiritual traditions of Sufism and Christianity. It was popularized in the West by the Eastern mystic G.I. Gurdjieff and modified over time by several others. Unlike such models as the MBTI and the Big Five, which are more focused on observable behavior, the Enneagram seeks to go deeper by classifying people according to their core motivation. There are nine basic personality types: the Reformer/Perfectionist, the Giver, the Achiever/Performer, the Individualist/Romantic, the Thinker/Observer, the Loyal Skeptic, the Enthusiast, the Leader/Chief, and the Peacemaker/Mediator. These types are further clarified by additional psychological patterning such as "compensating beliefs," "coping strategies," "driving energies," and "traps."

Is there a category for those of you who aren't confused by all this! And while we're on the subject…what's your sign?

So you're an EIFJ, a Striver, the Rebel, the Pleaser, most of one thing and part of another. How is this supposed to help you? The study of personality can seem endless, the vagaries of "typing" as numerous as people themselves. Perhaps in this process we do gain some self-knowledge, some inkling of our conditioned psychological and emotional patterning. But however helpful these models may be, I believe that they fail to reveal the essence of who we are underneath the coping and the conditioning and the behaviors. They are mostly metaphors trying to capture a very subjective condition: our essential selves—the foundational ground of being that lies beneath all the surface layering. When you stand solidly in the moment and feel into what it is like to be you, only then do you begin to get a *real* sense of your deepest, most authentic identity.

## Hardwired for Choice

In their quest for the ultimate something, physicists discovered yet another remarkable anomaly: The very focusing of attention seems to affect the object of that attention (see Schrödinger's Cat). This "mystery of entanglement" is confounding some of the best minds in science, while suggesting to the rest of us that what we think about *matters* (so to speak)—our thoughts have a literal physical impact on our environment and ourselves.

The notion of *neuroplasticity* affirms this. It suggests that our brains are capable of changing *at any age* in response to new learning, new experiences, and new behaviors. Further, the field of epigenetics, made popular by Bruce Lipton, suggests that gene expression is not fixed; it, too, is affected by changes in our environment and our thinking. In short, we are not held hostage by our conditioning or our history; we are in fact designed for choice and change, and when we "now ourselves" we can begin to control our responses and behaviors and rewire ourselves in a direction of our conscious choosing. If we can accept that the present moment is the culmination of everything that preceded it, then would it not make sense to accept that the future will be shaped by that same moment? If this is true, then we best pay close attention to it.

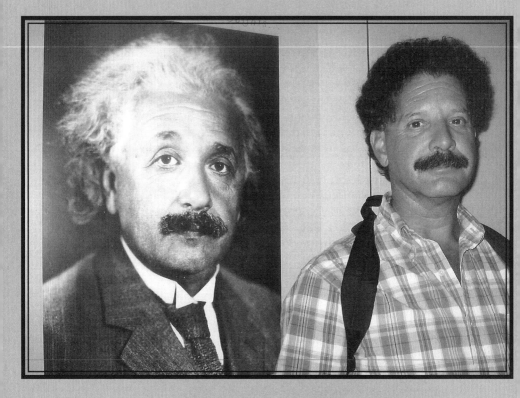

# PAUL KRUPIN:

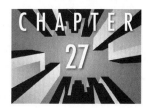

# The Magic of Business

re you ready to do business? Are you sure? Really sure? Really, really sure?

How do you know when you are really done designing and developing your products and services? When do you say "I'm done creating," and say "I'm ready for business"?

How do you know when you have what it takes to be successful? Have you reached a point where you truly know you are ready to fulfill your destiny?

It doesn't matter who you are, you'll need to pull a rabbit out of your hat. If you are an author or a publisher, you'll need to be successful with your book. If you are an inventor then your invention will need to be remarkable and sell. If you're a scholar, you have to sell the importance of your work to your peers. If you're a nonprofit, you have to sell the value of your program to funding agencies. Even if you're a parent, you have to sell your vision of the family to the rest of the family members. If you are married, you need to be effective at communicating so your marriage succeeds.

It doesn't matter what your business is, there is a way to make sure your business works and works well, indeed, whether it's on the very first try or it's your tenth or one hundredth time at bat. This involves learning how to become remarkable. All it takes is a little homespun business magic. Let's first take a look at a simple definition of business success:

Paul J. Krupin is President of Direct Contact PR, a custom publicity service. He is the author over 25 books, including *Trash Proof News Releases*. He has been described as a longtime PR Guru who has developed sure-fire proven strategies for getting publicity. He works with individuals, companies, and organizations, helping them to write effective news releases and copy, select and deploy the right tactics to reach the right media. He sends out over a million news releases each year on behalf of hundreds of inventors, authors, and publishing companies. For a free download from *Trash Proof New Releases*, visit www.DirectContactPR.com.

*Business success is reaching the people you can help the most and not losing your shirt doing it.*

This means providing people with a product or service and making a profit, after salaries and expenses, or at least not losing money as you do it. If your business maintains, then you get to live another day. This is business success.

Now, to achieve business success requires the delivery of a product or a service that people will buy. Let's say you are a publisher of books—even one single self-published book. You are in business. To be successful as a publisher, you have to sell books. That is, you have to write to sell and your job of writing isn't done until the book sells. This is where many self-publishers go astray. They publish their book without verifying that it is really ready for market. They sell very little of their product. They get no return on their investment. They may even operate their business at a financial loss because they failed to sell their product.

Yes, choke you may, to be a business success you have to *sell*. In order to be successful, you have to test your ideas and test your product on real live people. You have to identify your end users and the people who will buy the book for your users. And finally, you must learn what it takes to sell your product.

So you must write to sell and test, test, test your sales process. You do this in small doses till you get the right buy signals. Reliably. Not just once or twice, but repeatedly and reliably. Nowadays, you can do this in small quantities using print on demand (POD) technology. You can do 25 to 50 POD versions and test it with these important people.

The same is true with any business. To achieve success, you have to design your product and services so that you really and truly deliver what people want, and so that you can sell your wares. In marriage, this is called keeping love alive. In business, it's called survival.

If you can be even a little remarkable, you can sell quite easily. To be even just a little remarkable you have to use a little magic. How do you find this magic? You create it. And there is a way to make sure you create magic.

## Creating Magic in Business

But first, what is this magic?

It is the spark of energy that you create when you communicate effectively with your prospect or your customer. It is the energy-packed communication that creates the intense desire to have what you offer. It is the force that instantly converts a prospect and turns them into a willing customer.

Where do you find this magic? It is the things you say or do when you talk to a customer. It may also be in the things you hear about a product when someone else is talking about it. It is the feelings that are created and the energy that is imparted to a person when they pick up your product. It is the mental affirmation that comes with a realization that your product can make their dreams come true.

The bottom line is that it is information that galvanizes your prospective customers' attention, commands their interest, and persuades people to take an action — to buy what you are selling. Do you want to see this magic?

Look around you and you will notice when it occurs again and again. Here are three key typical examples that illustrate this magic and when it occurs:

1. You read an article in the newspaper or a magazine and it motivates you to find the source so you can buy a product, using the toll free number at the bottom or through the web site listed at the end of the article, or even through a search when the contact information isn't listed.

2. You are driving down the highway in traffic at 65 miles an hour. The announcer on the radio says something and, despite the hazards all around and coming at you, you are so galvanized by what the announcer says that you take your eyes off the highway and stare at the radio — even though it doesn't show you a thing.

3. You are shopping in a bookstore and you pick up a book. You look at the front cover, you look at the back cover, and you then open it up to look at a few pages. Done deal! Without any further hesitation, you head straight to the cashier.

4. You hear about a product or a service from a friend, an expert, or a trusted colleague or consultant, know in advance that this is what you need to have, and, sight unseen, you buy it.

Do you see the lightening spark in action? Do you see the point at which the instant realization occurs? If you are in love it is in the looks your beloved gives you when you say something or do something that makes them feel wonderful.

If you are in business, you can build this magic into your products and services. You can also design this same magic right into your promotional and marketing communications and your public relations. Here's how:

The first thing you need to do is pay close attention to your prospects and customers when they look at what you offer. Watch customers when they shop in your store. Look at their eyes. Study their body language when they interact with your sales personnel.

You must watch and wait till you see something magical occur. You will know it when you see it by what the person does. Their body language and the action they take will tell you. What signals do you see? What signals do they send that confirm to you that you are giving them what they want? How do you know when you have built a remarkable experience into the product? How can you tell when you are done? Here are some questions to ask:

§ Does your product or service give them a spark when they touch it?

§ Do they experience magic when they pick it up and hold it in their hands?

You will see something very special when you give people the magic they want! You'll know by their behavior and response whether you really have what it takes. You will also know if you don't have what it takes:

If you can't get people to even look at it, then you're not done.

If they look at it and put it down, then you still have work to do.

If people look at it and grab it, you might be done. It depends what happens when they then pick it up and peruse it. If they put it down, then you're not done.

If people walk away without taking the desired action, then very simply, you did not produce magic.

You may have to redesign and re-write until you know you are done. You have to work with your prospective audience to get real feedback, and you must listen to what people say and address the issues you receive. This may take a lot of reiterations. But one thing is for certain: There is a point that you will reach when you know that you are done. It's a wonderful thing when you get to this point and know it. This is because you will see the magic. You know when you are done...

§ When people look at it, grab it, and head to the cashier.

§ They pick up one, look at it, grab four or five of them, and head to the cashier.

§ You show your product to someone and they turn to their colleague immediately and say "get a load of this!"

§ If people look at your product, pick it up, hold it close, and won't give it back freely — you've got them.

§ You show them the product and, while they are clutching it in their hands, they reach for their wallet.

§ One person picks up the product, grabs it, and goes to show his or her friend the book — and they both buy one for themselves.

You know that you have something when kids pull it off the shelf and haul it over to their mothers and fathers with a look of desire and wanting and excitement in their eyes that says, "Please!" I call this the *clutching response* or the *hoarding syndrome*. There is no doubt that you have seen and experienced this in a variety of ways.

This occurs when people clearly indicate to you that your product has such inherent value and importance that they are willing to pay for it. They know it and you know it instantly. This is what you have to create. You have to create something that people covet when they see it, feel it, or touch it.

## Identifying Your Magic

It is very cool to observe such magic directly, and it is very clearly an accomplishment when you design your product and service so that it produces this response reliably and repeatedly. The next challenge is figuring out what it is that produces the magic. This is what you want to identify and document. And you want to do this systematically, so that you can tweak it and reproduce it — and make it better and better.

The bottom line is that you build to sell. You create to sell. You design to sell. And you must redesign to sell, and redesign, redesign, and redesign until your product sells. You don't stop revising and improving until you know it sells, and sells easily and continuously. You can prove it with small test numbers. Use the technology that is available to create and test your products, services, and processes wisely. Then move it up through the production and promotion chain level by level.

What should you do if you think your product should excite and grab people, but it simply isn't happening?

You still have work to do. You can't speculate about what's wrong, you need real data. So ask your candidate customers for feedback and advice. How would you improve this? What would you like to see? What would make this product magic to you? Ask until you are blue in the face and get the hard data and feedback you need to redesign and redo this project.

Think about other super-successful products. Learn why they are magic to people. Learn why people love products. The think about how to add magic to what you do. You are not done until people fall in love with your creation. And guess what? What those people really want turns out to be what most people in the world want! They want a remarkable experience. They want to experience a vivid emotion. They want energy, hope, vision. Yes, they want physical satisfaction—but what they really crave is emotional satisfaction. They want to feel loved, to feel your heart speaking to their heart.

This should come as no surprise. People want an emotional experience that takes them out of their boring, humdrum lives and temporarily transports them far, far away. They want information, education, or entertainment that allows them to experience the dramatic personal gain, pain, suffering, pleasure, or achievement that someone else is going through. You'll see this in the media almost everywhere. Look around you and you'll see that all news coverage is basically designed to cater to this very special goal; this is what the people want. People want to be stimulated emotionally and spiritually. Not just intellectually, but deep, deep, deep inside. They want to feel what it's like to be in someone else's shoes. Once you realize this, then you'll realize and learn how to push people's hot buttons.

## A Real Magic Spell

If you are going to be successful, then you must give people more than just what they need. You must give them what they crave, fantasize, and dream about. This is not rocket science. It is psychology.

If you hope to jumpstart your business by getting publicity, you will aim at getting coverage for your business in newspapers and magazines, or on radio and TV. Editors and producers are publishers. They produce magazines and newspapers. They are in business and survive and thrive because they provide their audiences with written, audio, or visual materials that people are willing to pay for. They are always looking for useful, educational, entertaining, and inspirational content. This is how they make a living. This is what drives them.

You can't get them excited by sending a news release that begs for a commercial endorsement. Don't write a commercial ad. Don't ask for free advertising. This is not what they want. This will not help them survive. They want education and entertainment. This is what you must provide them. You must analyze what you have that an editor that will truly appreciate. So what do editors want?

Study any publication. Listen to the radio or watch any TV show. You will find that they want distinctive, informative, remarkable, and emotion-provoking material. They want to positively affect the lives of millions of people. They want to generate or contribute to social controversy that produces beneficial social change.

In order to do this they need written materials that can produce enthusiastic thank you letters in return for their information and insights. They want to be appreciated by their audience in the form of repeat subscriptions that result from their publication providing the best information available in their field.

This is where you come in. This is what you need to provide. As a publicist or promoter of your own product, services, or creative work, you can make it to onto the page only if you provide the materials a publisher needs to fulfill his or her business needs and those of their audience.

If you study what the media actually publishes you can boil it all down to one simple, magical little formula that describes how they do what they do. Here it is: DPAA+H.

These letters stand for Dramatic Personal Achievement in the face of Adversity, plus a little Humor. If you look at almost all the media around you — from the front page of *USA Today*, to coverage of the Olympics, to the evening news, to the sitcoms on TV — you'll see that this is the magic that describes what the American public wants, desires, and craves the most.

As a culture, we crave to see the human spirit triumph in matters of the heart, and in trials of hardship and tragedy. We ask to be uplifted right out of the humdrum of our everyday reality into the exhilaration and extreme emotions of those who are living life on the edge. This is the magic that galvanizes our attention. It rivets us to our seats. It captures our attention and our hearts. And this is what the media seeks to provide. This is what works.

Now look around you and see that this magic exists everywhere. Look at the front page of the newspaper and at each and every article. Look at the TV news, shows, soap operas, and even the commercials. Look at the shows produced by the shock jocks and reality TV.

One thing is for certain: You will see these elements everywhere you look, in varying degrees. It is a rare media feature that doesn't contain most of these elements. In fact, if you think about it you will realize that the media constantly uses better and better technology to increase the assault on our senses, enhance the effect, and make our experience ever more compelling and memorable. This is how they command people's attention. And to get a piece of the action for your business, you must be memorable as well.

Describe the 5 Ws — the What, Who, Where, When, and Why — in dramatic personal adversity and achievement terms. Use a little humor if you can. This helps you cast your spell to the widest possible audience. There's a real business reason why this works: Attention results in sales and profits. So use DPAA+H.

When it comes to whether you'll be successful getting publicity, if there are more dramatic personal stories of achievement in the face of adversity, plus a little humor, available that day, you lose. If not, you win. If there is a more dramatic, more personal product or service that delivers more achievement in the face of similar adversity, and even offers more fun, then they will get the business, and you won't. One thing is for certain. If you learn how to use DPAA+H your message is more likely to reach your audience.

## Casting Your Magic Spell

It takes a little thinking and self-analysis, but you can identify the right things to say and products and services to provide. You do this by analyzing your own experiences to identify the successful sales pathway.

First, think very carefully about who your customers are. Visualize them. Identify the representative customer and create a word picture of who they are. Think about a real situation. Think about the very last time you were in front of a person like this. In fact, think about all the times you've been in front of people like this. Now ask yourself: "What did I say or do, very specifically, that resulted in them buying my product or service?"

Get this information! This is the crucial data. Document what you said. Make a list of the things you said, the order in which you said them, and think about the other person's response. Think very specifically about what you say that speaks from your heart to their heart and results in their decision to buy your products or services.

If you don't know, then you need to first pay close attention when you are speaking to your clients or customers. You may need to have someone watch you and take notes, or record what you say so that you figure out just what gets heads shaking up and down. You may even need to ask them "Why did you buy my product or service? What did you like the most about what I said or did?"

You need to identify the hot buttons that you can push to galvanize attention and get people to buy your product or service. It may be things you say or do individually, or when you speak in front of a group. Whatever it is, the crucial thing is that you must know what you do and be able to repeat it again and again. This is the essence of your potion. Get it right and you'll have very powerful magic.

You must be sure that you've identified the right sequence of statements. You must repeat the experiment till it works just about wherever you go. Once you carve a positive known reaction using your formula, you can tweak it carefully and experiment with modifications using the following criteria to guide your actions: If it works, do more of it. If it doesn't work, stop doing it. This is the essence of continuous improvement, and, even though it is simple, it is the most powerful thing you can do to create magic in your business.

So the first step is...identify what works!

The second step is to verify and prove that it works through repetition.

The third step is to apply these hot buttons to your products, services, and communications.

The fourth and last step is to improve it. When you discover something new, you add it to your potions. At any time you can always return to your basic formula.

## Sprinkling Magic Dust Wherever You Go

The amazing thing here is that, once you define the hot buttons with one person, and then with two people, and then with three people, you really have developed a truly amazing and magical tool that can renovate your business and the lives of those that you hope to serve.

What this means to you is that when you design and build and then publicize, promote, or sell your products and services, you must carefully identify those magical things you say and do that motivate people to buy. When you have discovered what you can do to trigger and produce emotional feelings on command, speaking from your heart to someone else's heart on a reliable basis, than you have figured out the key to your success.

This is why people buy what you are selling. They want to have what you have. They want to be able to experience more of what you've just allowed them to taste or experience. Sound like fun? It is! This is the magic of business.

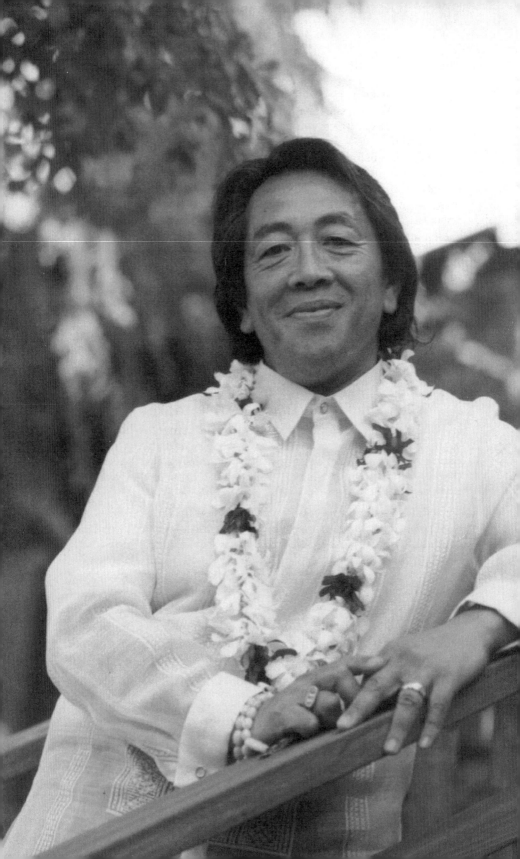

# DIXON DE LEÑA:

# Authentic Power

E ven across the phone lines, I could hear the anxiety in my client's voice. "Dixon, did you see the news yesterday?" Dennis asked. "Tell me," I responded. "At a concert last night," he said, "one of our top bands held a mock 'white mass' in which they invited members of the audience to come to the stage and declare their allegiance to the devil. Quite a few young teens accepted their invitation."

As he gave me more details of the event, the problems became clear. Dennis was CEO of American Arts and Graphics, a family-owned company based in Seattle, Washington, whose modest beginning was built on a line of industrial labeling products. The arrival of the 1960 era changed everything for them as AA&G quickly moved into licensing, producing, and distributing posters. AA&G helped create one of the ubiquitous icons of the era: flocked, neon-colors, psychedelic-style — the artful representations of rock stars and their bands, concerts, festivals, and everything else about the new counter culture.

I began consulting with the company in the early 1980s. At that point they were struggling to survive and looking for options beyond merely getting by. We worked together to help them create a new future, one that represented their heart's desires. Once they'd identified a powerful new direction, they quickly and enthusiastically brought the whole company in line with their vision. They implemented their commitment to their people, their integrity,

Dixon de Leña is CEO and Founding Partner of Integral Partnerships LLC, a consulting company whose mission is to assist business, political organizations, and civil society in the urgent need of our time: to build a wiser, sustainable, and resilient future for our planet, through vision-ary and unequivocal action. For over 25 years he's consulted leaders and their people to transform their relationship to power to ensure process improvements, reorganizations, strategies, and other positive change efforts succeed. His client list spans several industries in the Fortune 50 and 500 as well organizations in the private and public sectors.

and to making a difference through everything they did. Success came slowly at first; but they gained velocity as they succeeded in moving through the discomfort of change, challenging their past images of themselves, making hard choices, and keeping their promises to implement new strategies, improve their systems, and change their company culture.

As they transformed to reflect their vision in everything they did, they rose quickly to the top of their industry once again. And as they found success everywhere, they no longer needed the services of our company with the same frequency. We went from regular meetings to occasional engagements, and finally to working on a request-only basis. They were a precious pearl among my clients, and we enjoyed a mutual respect and admiration, grateful for what we had accomplished together.

Dennis Russell, one of three children of the founder, had moved into the role of president of AA&G shortly after the company engaged me. His appointment was one of the early mini-transformations that mirrored their unequivocal commitment to doing what was needed.

Now, as I listened to Dennis's story, he laid out his ethical dilemma. If he did nothing, he would appear to be condoning the band's behavior. If he acted, he could run afoul of other company members. While AA&G was a religiously tolerant organization that had made explicit attempts to accommodate all points of view, other team members knew that Dennis was a devout churchgoer, an engaged parent, and a responsible community member. He was disturbed by the band's actions—yet knew that he might be the only person in the company who had a problem with what the band had done.

If it was just a publicity stunt the band's popularity could shoot sky-high, leading to enormous sales of posters and other memorabilia in the AA&G product line. Dennis faced a strong financial incentive to overlook the incident. Also, if he took negative action, his staff might perceive him as preachy and moralistic.

We needed to tap the source of the wisdom that had brought the company to its current high point. The method we used was open-ended inquiry, based solely on a search for the truth in a given situation. To hope for *the one correct answer* shuts down the space of discovery. Attachment in the form of expectation or prejudice, however slight, limits what is possible. But openness to every possibility allows the truth to emerge, sometimes excruciatingly slowly, but surely. Our inquiry eventually led Dennis and me to several truths.

First, this situation presented another opportunity to actually *be* the visionary company that AA&G had declared itself to be and stand behind its values. Second, prior experience had taught Dennis and his team that for any action to be successful, they would need the complete alignment of everyone in the company. On the basis of these truths, Dennis was able to take action.

Working with the whole leadership team, Dennis eventually crafted a letter outlining the situation, and explaining to customers that they decided to recall the posters of this particular band. The company sent the letter to the CEOs of their biggest customers, like Kmart and Walmart. Then they sent their reps out to collect what used to be hundreds of thousands of dollars of saleable posters, but now was only ink and paper. Everyone at AA&G held their breath as they awaited the effects of their decision.

The response was immediate, powerful, and positive. AA&G received letters of acknowledgement and support from many of their customers. The revenue lost from retracting the posters was offset by the surprising and unexpected success of an in-house artist's teddy bear poster that suddenly became popular. A new AA&G star was born.

Gradually, the company went further. As posters came up for reprint, they replaced inventory previously chosen based on popularity with items that were in alignment with their values. The universe responded with an ever-increasing revenue stream. AA&G became #1 in their industry shortly after the "band debacle" — seven years ahead of their goal. Most importantly, they trusted the power of publicly being whom and what they had declared themselves to be.

The great need of our time is that we all must ask ourselves the big questions about the role of our business organizations and our role within them. As far as I know, we haven't asked enough of businesses or the institutions that support and enable them. For example: What quality of life are we building on this planet? What changes must be made in order to ensure resiliency in all of our planetary systems for generations to come? And, as individuals, could we ask ourselves questions such as: What kind of future does my heart long for, and how do I see my role in business changing to support that future? I'm fairly confident that many of executives and managers are not having inquiries of this depth with themselves, their employees, their stakeholders, or their customers.

We have come to realize that it is our human activity, particularly our way of doing business, that is contributing to global warming, to the growing gap between the rich and poor, to conflict between nations over depleted resources, and to mass extinctions of fauna and flora. While the data supporting the need to change our business practices becomes even clearer, the response we are getting from companies gets muddier. It appears that underneath all the financial, strategic, and marketing expertise, the majority of organizations lack the wisdom to guide them into action on the most obvious of baby steps to remedy our collective situation—let alone contemplate their ultimate transformations.

The vast majority of businesses have placed their trust and allegiance in principles such as shareholder value, market share, return on investment, time value of money, GAAP rules, the SEC, and Wall Street's fickle demands for "more, more, more!" They have become what I call *survival-driven* organizations. Survival-driven organizations have the benefit of seeing the world through the profit/ loss window of perception, but their management struggles mightily whenever they have to consider the "soft metrics" of a complex, ever-shrinking world.

Survival-driven organizations are at a significant disadvantage unless they can find their way out of the box called "if it makes good business sense, then and only then." The way to get out of this box is to become a *soul-centered organization*. But the journey is difficult, and old habits are hard to break. Is this level of transformation possible?

There are many pioneers on which to model the journey. Soul-centered organizations are showing up all over the planet. They are wiser, more creative, generous, transparent, and more responsive to the various forms of feedback coming from all quarters of the living systems in which they find themselves. They are responding enthusiastically to the urgent call to do business in the new ways. They're building their business models with strategies that respect the interconnectedness of our environment, the intrinsic value of indigenous cultures, the true cost of toxic wastes, and the inefficient use of precious resources. They ingeniously engineer, and in some cases completely re-engineer, their products, services, and processes in the attempt to lessen their impact. In fact, many aspire to have their entire operations eventually help regenerate the services that our planet provides for our comfort and sustenance. These organizations are committed to boosting the quality of life of all the members of the Commons, not just increasing the net worth of a select few.

Businesses that do good do well financially. These companies are now catching the attention of venture capitalists and Wall Street. That's because mere survival is not an effective business strategy. Even when they appear successful, survival-driven organizations exhibit symptoms of the "fight or flight" response: short-term thinking, antagonistic assumptions, bullying behavior, paranoid marketing practices, heavy-handed competition, empire-building, infighting (aka "healthy competition"), and ethically compromised choices.

Soul-centered organizations are significantly different in many ways. They naturally adopt the long view of the market. They respect and promote collaboration, see abundance in the systems, and trust in the wisdom of mutually beneficial, interdependent partnerships.

Soul-centered organizations look for truth. Truth is a core value for these types of businesses, powerfully shaping their people regardless of rank or accountability. Trust—truth's companion—is the other prized value, which soul-centered organizations recognize as Truth's companion. Soul-centered organizations know you can't ask for one without adopting the other. Even when the company's survival is threatened, they align themselves with truth, which invites the presence of soul wisdom.

"Force hath no place where there is need of skill," declared the ancient Greek philosopher Herodotus.

Open-ended inquiry is one of the key tools for inviting the soul and its wisdom to help us discover the truth of a situation. There are many different kinds of inquiry. Most begin with an explicit desire for something to happen. Open-ended inquiry does not. It guides the questioner through the treacherous currents of survival and the hidden rocks of opinions, prejudices, worldviews, and ego structures that restrict possibility.

The same holds true for organizations. Declarations of new directions and missions rarely take hold, for the survival tendency is dedicated to the status quo even though people say they desire the new mission. New strategies have to share space with the hidden reality of the old structures.

Free and open inquiry allows us to consider all the elements— those that empower us and those than lock us into the old prisons. New, soul-centered companies don't carry this baggage. But old, survival-driven companies making a transition to a soul-centered function must grapple with the reality of what they already are and then till the ground that allows a new reality to take root.

Rarely do organizations even attempt to re-invent their culture of force into one of authentic power that invites soul. The risks are very great when they do, but then so is the prize. One such organization was GTE Telephone Operations Finance. Roger Utzinger, a longtime executive of GTE and someone I'd had the privilege of coaching, called me one day to tell me that he'd taken a new job at the company's headquarters. Roger recognized that GTE had become a survival-driven organization. Deregulation, recent acquisitions, downsizing, and aggressive earning goals made for the benefit of Wall Street were only intensifying its survival-driven behavior.

Roger's boss had initiated a process of creating a new vision. It required an ambitious series of transformations by the people in his business unit, as the principal transformational resource of a financial organization is its people. For two years he had been trying to lead this change, while the people in his department seemed stuck in deep freeze.

The executives in the group engaged in a process of open-ended enquiry into their leadership, their culture, their management philosophy, their notions of power, and their values. By co-inquiring into questions normally not reserved for examination, GTE Finance created a space for a new possibility.

When the truth about coercion, manipulation, domination, repression, and other forms of force is discussed frankly, the discussion alone can transform an organization. Doing so nurtured the many new changes in the unit's organization. Opportunity began to sprout. Within a couple of years, GTE Finance went from near the bottom of the rankings of desirable places to work within the company, to near the top. Roger's boss was ranked the number one executive in the company.

Authentic power invites soul presence, while survival sucks the life out of people in such organizations. Columbia University now offers a course based on the ancient Hindu scripture the Bhagavad Gita called "Creativity and Personal Mastery." Columbia instructor Srikumar Rao says that many of the attendees are "fast-track managers who, though highly successful at work, are still miserable."

In this kind of cultural landscape, rarely are there authentic invitations for the soul to preside. Studs Terkel remarked, "Jobs are too small for people's spirits." Soul presence is immune to force, particularly the new, well-intended, benevolent forms of mentoring, coaching, and management designed to "help" us find our way. We cannot coerce the soul, as most of us who have an established meditative or spiritual practice have discovered. Our ego cannot command soul to show up in one sitting! Many people get frustrated with such practices because they discover they can't manipulate the results. In addition, we cannot coach someone to contact their soul presence, at least not in the conventional sense. We cannot "manage" for soul either, and we certainly aren't able to stand on a soapbox spouting dictums about the importance of soul, as it becomes the new, fashionable leadership style.

Our task, then, is to commit to creating the time and space necessary to engage in the conversations that invite the soul into the workplace. In order to do this, we must invite the wisdom of the heart. A good starting point is the question: Tell me a future your heart longs for. If we relax into the inquiry and stay vigilantly curious, soul will provide access to our own inner wisdom as the inquiry unfolds over time. We'll end up being reminders for each other that far more is possible—a miracle in our world, where too many of us have fallen into a stupor, completely convinced that what we hold in our hands or see with our eyes is what's real. Soul is much more subtle than what we perceive with our ordinary senses. Practices that invoke the presence of soul support our other senses to develop more fully, and we come to taste, feel, and even see soul presence as obviously as we do outer reality. When we live in that state, reminding others by our living presence that soul is all around us, just beyond the next turn of the conversation, we will spontaneously invent models of business that effortlessly embody the highest truths of Being.

# PART SEVEN

# Engendering Evolution

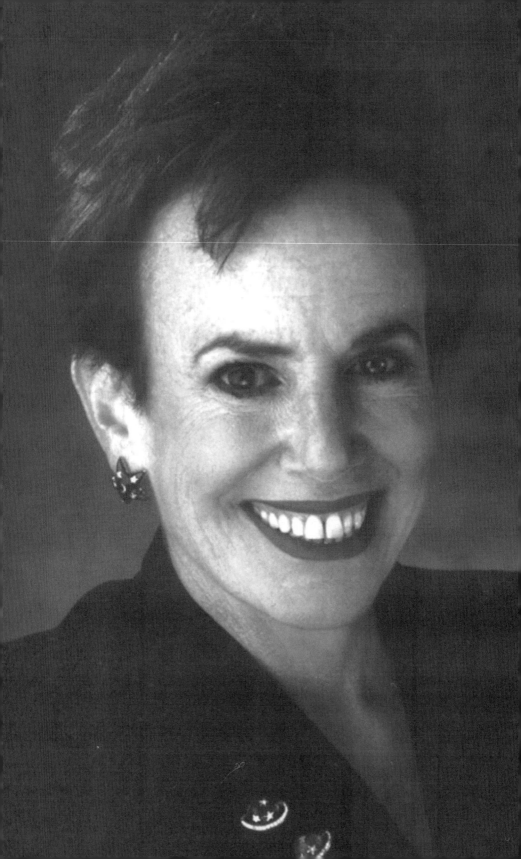

# FAITH POPCORN:

# EVEolution

**N**ever try to deceive a woman. She has X-ray vision. Eventually, she'll see right through you.

You *might* get away with it once. But it'll never work twice. Remember Shakespeare's warning, "Hell hath no fury like a woman scorned." Once she's on to you, you've lost a customer forever.

Which is a long time.

If you think a famous logo, clever ads, a Fortune 500 ranking, even that the expertise of your sales reps will protect you — think again. When it comes to marketing to women, there's nowhere to run, nowhere to hide.

Women do business with people they trust. Trust happens when you're open about your actions and act with a conscience. Therefore, responsibility is no longer just a good public relations idea. It's a necessity for doing business.

If your company is accustomed to business-by-spin, you'll have to either reform now or find another line of work. It's that simple.

Your new EVEolutionary goal: A reputation — built and maintained over the long term — for honesty, integrity, ethical behavior, community give-back, and a maniacal attention to detail.

While men and women alike are both tuning in more closely to

Faith Popcorn, author of *EVEolution: Eight Truths of Marketing to Women* (Hyperion, 2000), is a top forecaster of consumer trends and key advisor to many Fortune 500 companies. She is the founder of Faith Popcorn's BrainReserve, a New York-based marketing consultancy whose clients include Bell Atlantic, BMW, Cigna, GE Capital, Hasbro, IBM, Lipton, McDonald's, Nabisco, and Procter & Gamble. She is author of the national-al bestseller *The Popcorn Report* (Collins, 1992) and co-author of the national best-selling *Clicking* (Collins, 1998). An internationally known speaker on consumer trends, Popcorn lives in New York City and Wain-scott, NY. Visit www.faithpopcorn.com.

a company's ethics and practices, women especially care about the details.

A few months ago, the son of a friend of mine came home from college and announced he'd met the girl of his dreams.

His father asked, "What's her name? What's her major? What does her father do?" And, because he couldn't help himself, "Is she a looker?"

His mother (my friend), on the other hand, annoyed her son by asking seemingly irrelevant questions. "How many siblings does she have? Is she the youngest, middle, or oldest child? Does she have any pets? Where was she born? Where were her parents and her grandparents (on both sides) from? Does she believe in God?" And, because she couldn't help herself, "What size does she wear?"

Why does this sound familiar? Because it's happened to you. I'll bet if you thought about it, you could come up with dozens of examples of how women evaluate people, events, even institutions, in a way that's completely different from men. Because women tend to view everything as related in some way, they need all the details to connect the pieces.

You could write off this female behavior as "nosy," "prying," or "who really cares?"

Or you could seriously consider the way in which this gender difference, this affinity for detail affects the way women view your brand. (Here's a tip: Only one of these ways of thinking will be a positive influence on your business.)

If you decide to dismiss women's holistic thinking, consider this: Suppose you've convinced your female consumers to bond with your product without giving them the full story. Suppose their relationship with your company or institution stops at product performance, and doesn't go all the way to Corporate Soul.

Now suppose something goes wrong with the product. Suppose an unavoidable defect is discovered, a recall is mandated, tampering occurs, or a consumer is just plain disappointed. Where does she turn for information, help, comfort, or some kind of restitution?

Certainly not to you. Who are you? No one she's ever had a relationship with before.

I'll tell you where she turns. To your competition.

## The Five Ps Of Marketing

Women are driving a new millennial marketing model. Getting

women to join your brand is not only about the traditional four "Ps" of marketing (sorry, MBAs). Product, Pricing, Promotion, and Place are not enough. *Today you need to add a fifth "P" to the marketing mix: Policy.*

Because things you would never have thought to focus on ten years ago *matter*. Issues that are normally banished to obscure corners of corporate communication *matter*. The things that management do *matter*. The things that the companies you do business with do *matter*.

In other words: *Everything Matters.*

*Because marketing to women today isn't just about value. It's about values.*

What I'm suggesting is an EVEolved marketing model that women will respond to. Products that follow this model will rely less on standard marketing tools like commercials (the hype means nothing) and point-of-purchase materials (it's what's inside the package that matters). And the "badge value" of these products will come not from whether they were expensive, or exotic, or cool. The new "badge value" will be based on values like conscience, responsibility, openness.

Think of this new model as the *transparent brand.*

Transparency means inviting your female consumer to see all the way through your brand to the company behind it—back to its origins, its roots, its founder. Transparency means there is no room for inconsistency of mission, strategy, execution, and communication. Transparency means no secrets.

I was talking about this with Gail Evans, CNN Executive Vice President, who added her own take on the subject: "Women care about integrity, but not in the sense of not telling a lie; more in the sense of understanding everything about a person or a product, including fallibilities. They want everything out there."

What are the "everythings" that women want to know? What is transparency made of? Beyond the quality of the products and services that you deliver, the components include:

§ The personal ethics of your owners and managers.

§ How you treat all your employees.

§ How you treat women and minority employees.

§ The number of women and minorities who hold corporate offices.

§ How much money top executives make.

# CHAPTER TWENTY-NINE

§ What kind of perks top executives receive.

§ The salary gap between the highest paid man and woman.

§ How much money your CEO gives to political campaigns. And to which candidates.

§ Who you give charitable donations to and how much.

§ Your environmental record.

§ The origin of the materials you source and how you source them.

§ Your distribution policies (for instance, not opening locations in tough inner-city neighborhoods).

§ The policies of your outside resources, like your bank and law firm.

§ Whether you give reporters and consumers on-demand access to inspect your factories and offices.

The good news is, you don't have to rely on your product alone to create a joinable brand. Every other business component offers your company an opportunity to show your female consumers that this is, in fact, the kind of company she can live with.

This might sound like a dangerous amount of exposure. Who doesn't cringe at the thought of the klieg lights of public scrutiny shining on his or her every move? But in the end, the fact that Everything Matters actually turns out to be a very healthy (read: good for your business) thing.

Because if every company, every brand, every board member, and every brand manager believed that they had to be prepared to explain everything about their brand, believe me, their businesses would be better off for it.

If you think your female consumer doesn't look past the surface to read the fine (or even the not-so-fine) print, you might be surprised to learn that she's got a few questions for you. And be prepared. Women are likely to have noticed things about your brand that may raise some awkward questions.

"Why are your 800-number phone reps so rude?"

"How come Jay Leno was making fun of you last week?"

"How can you permit discriminatory practices by your franchisees?"

"What's up with that sex scandal concerning one of your division presidents?"

None of this is her business, you say? Well, she's made it her business. And if she doesn't like what she sees, it'll be bad for your business.

The Internet has taken access to a whole new level. Female consumers will be using it more and more to find out minutiae about a company. And to trade information with other consumers in a way that no corporate public relations program can control. So you'd better have a clean act. And shout about it. By creating a complete ethical biography in virtual space, a company is giving the female consumer what she feels she's entitled to know. Added benefit: If you get your ethical ingredients list cleaned up, she'll not only buy your brand, she'll buy your stock.

Howard Schultz, CEO of Starbucks, put it succinctly: "If people believe they share values with a company, they will stay loyal."

Who else lives and breathes the concept that absolutely Everything Matters?

Clue: It's a division of General Motors.

I know what you're thinking. "Oh, God, not another Saturn case history!"

Entire forests have been cut down to make paper for the articles and chapters in marketing books praising this four-wheeled phenomenon.

There couldn't possibly be anything left to say about Saturn's successful launch or its unique marketing strategy.

Well, maybe just one more thing.

In all the dissection of the Saturn marketing model, nobody has pointed out what, to me, is the most important factor in its success. *Women love Saturn.*

Maybe it's because I've been obsessing on this subject for the last few years, but it seems pretty obvious that the way Saturn behaves — both as a brand and as a company — is perfectly designed to attract women.

And this in an industry that does a really good job of ignoring and offending women. I can't resist relaying horrifying stories from two turn-of-this-century meetings I had with the Marketing Directors of two huge car companies (one American, one Japanese). Both acknowledged strong sales to women, yet after hearing me explain the Truths of EVEolution, the director of the American outfit said in front of a conference room filled with women reporters: "Advocacy groups. I'm sick of advocacy groups: Hispanics, blacks, women, gays. They all buy my cars anyway."

The second guy, an American director of the Japanese company, wasn't so John Rocker-ish, merely dismissing the particular needs of women buyers: "Look, we don't thread our marketing through a needle that way." Some big needle — 50 percent of the market.

Conversely, Saturn is such a highly EVEolved company. Let me start with its chief, Cynthia Trudell, President. In a *U.S. News & World Report* article, Trudell was quoted as saying, "If I have to get involved in the heavy-duty, top-down decision making, something is wrong." It went on, "For her, managing means working on relationships and understanding 'interdependency.'" That's pure EVEolution.

Take the Saturn theme line: "A different kind of company. A different kind of car." When is the last time you heard a car — or any brand — lead with a focus on the company *behind* the star product? That's a transparent brand.

From the very beginning, Saturn urged the car buyer to look beyond the hardware to the behavior of the company and the buying experience — something women are naturally inclined to do anyway.

Then there's the experience of buying a Saturn. From the beginning, the brand revealed its EVEolutionary leanings with a no-haggle policy, the famous "no-dicker sticker." (Meanwhile, the rest of Detroit is still arguing over fake imagery, nuts and bolts and price and miles-per-gallon. Yawn.)

Here's an example of a piece of corporate behavior that's so powerful, it almost defines the brand. With this one small step, Saturn broke ranks with an industry that had institutionalized the awful buying experience — especially awful for women. In fact, research shows that a woman typically pays 28 percent more than a man pays for the same car.

The more you look at the Saturn strategy, the more you see the Everything Matters scaffolding supporting all that the company says and does.

Ironically, even Saturn wasn't prepared for the female consumer's response. Apparently neither was its ad agency.

Steve Morrissey, account director at Publicis & Hal Riney, admits: "We were really surprised. I mean, I knew we were resonating well with women, but when I first saw the breakdown of the gender statistics, I thought, 'Holy cow! Nobody has done that.'"

Women are demanding customers, and are becoming more so as the EVEolution marches on. From measures as lofty as values and morals, to those as prosaic as cleanliness and courtesy, Everything Matters to women.

To start you on your way to practicing the Everything Matters

Truth, ask yourself:

§ If my consumer knew every single detail about my brand, from the process to the product, would I still be selling as much of it?

§ Am I doing as much as I personally can to better every aspect of my brand? Can I sleep at night?

§ Does my brand have a soul? And can my consumer see right into it?

§ Does she like what she sees?

When you come to realize the power of the transparent brand, you suddenly see that the opportunities for gaining her trust and keeping it are infinite.

Just remember: Everything Matters.

And Matters.

And Matters.

And Matters.

And Matters.

And Matters.

And Matters.

And Matters.

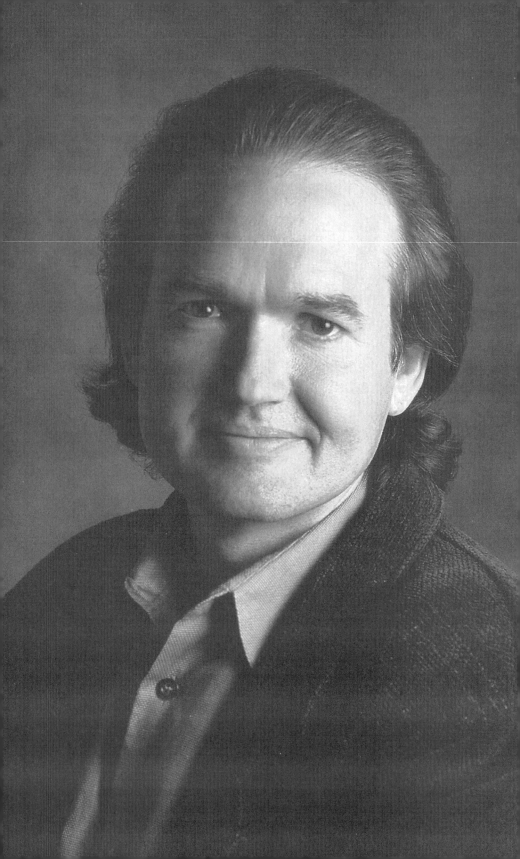

# JOHN GRAY:

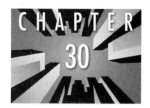

CHAPTER
30

# Feelings in the Workplace

B oth men and women have feelings, but how they express their
feelings in the workplace is very different. When two people
speak the same language, sharing feelings is a way to strengthen
the bond of trust and connection. Communicating feelings, when done
appropriately, can increase cooperation and confidence at all levels
in the workplace. By building trust, productivity, and job satisfaction
increase as stress and tension decrease.

Feelings are conveyed not just by words but by gestures,
facial expressions, and tones. It is estimated that only 20 percent
of communication involves the choice of words. While words are
important, it is the communication of unspoken feelings that is more
important. A happy smile, a delighted giggle, an understanding
"mhum" sound, a confident tone of voice, or the nod of the head
can be much more potent than a well-organized presentation. The
feelings you convey will evoke similar feelings in others. Most
decision makers will consider all the facts, figures, and logic, but
when it comes to signing on the dotted line, a feeling or hunch makes
or breaks the deal.

## Sharing Feelings on Mars and Venus

On Mars, the sharing of positive feelings builds trust and
respect, while on Venus, the sharing of *both* positive and negative

John Gray, Ph.D., is the bestselling relationship author of all time, and an
internationally recognized expert in communication and relationships.
He has conducted personal growth seminars for 30 years and is the
author of 12 bestsellers, including *Men Are from Mars, Women Are from
Venus* (Harper Paperbacks, 2004). He is a Certified Family Therapist, a
consulting editor of the *Family Journal*, a member of the Distinguished
Advisory Board of the International Association of Marriage and Family
Counselors, and a member of the American Counseling Association. John
lives with his wife and three children in Northern California. Visit www.
marsvenus.com.

feelings builds relationships. Men readily respect positive feelings like confidence, joy, satisfaction, pride, humor, happy relief, and relaxation, but they often don't respect negative feelings.

A man will tend to focus on expressing positive feelings rather than negative feelings. When he does express negative feelings, if he is to earn the respect of other men, he is careful to make sure they are expressed in a manner that is not personal. He may be frustrated, but he will not express "personal frustration." For example, he might indicate that he is frustrated that a delivery is late, but he will not show that he is frustrated because he is having a bad day.

On Venus they don't favor positive or negative. Nothing is black or white.

For women, any feeling, positive or negative, expressed in a respectful manner can be an opportunity to share and connect with another. They do not discern between personal or impersonal emotions. There is no big taboo about revealing vulnerable feelings or negative emotions. Unlike men, they do not view expressing personal feelings as a form of weakness.

## Personal versus Impersonal Feelings

It is easy to distinguish positive from negative feelings, but to separate personal and impersonal feelings takes some training. Most men automatically filter out their personal feelings but can freely express the nonpersonal ones. On the other hand, women tend to filter out impersonal feelings and freely express personal feelings. The problem that emerges from this difference is that men and women misinterpret each other and feel blamed.

Here are some examples of personal and impersonal feelings. In each example, the phrase "The letter was lost, I don't know what we are going to do" is expressed with a different emotion. While the emotion is the same, the meaning is different on Mars and Venus. This chart helps make clear the distinction between personal and impersonal reactions.

In each of the above examples men and women tend to misunderstand each other. A man hears personal feelings as blaming statements, while a woman hears impersonal feelings as blaming statements.

Without an understanding of how men and women express emotions differently, women often feel attacked by men or take their emotional expressions personally when that is not how they are intended. Another man in the same situation would not take it personally.

## Impersonal Feelings

When he says, "The letter was lost. I don't know what we are going to do," he means:

He is frustrated that the letter was lost and as a result an opportunity was missed.

He is disappointed that sales were down in the third quarter.

He is worried that the project will not be finished in time or he will not have time to do it.

He is embarrassed that the work was not very good because the letter was lost.

He is angry because without the letter the job will not get finished.

He is sad because so much time was wasted and the project will not be recognized.

He is afraid because he does not know how they will make up the time lost.

He is sorry the letter was lost because the project will not get done in time.

He is furious that the letter was lost because the other company will get the deal.

He is hurt because he worked hard on the project, and now it has failed.

He is scared that the company will look bad and not have another chance.

He is ashamed that the project failed and the company really looks bad.

## Personal Feelings

When she says, "The letter was lost. I don't know what we are going to do," she means:

She is frustrated that the letter was lost, she had asked for it, and now she feels that she is not being heard.

She is disappointed that her efforts to improve sales were not implemented.

She is worried that she will be blamed if the project is not finished in time and lose her job.

She is embarrassed that others may see her as inefficient and uncaring.

She is angry because without the letter she may lose credibility.

She is sad because she disappointed others and she wasted her time.

She is afraid because she may lose respect from her peers.

She is sorry that the letter was lost and she feels powerless to do anything about it.

She is furious that the letter was lost because she worked so hard and to no avail. She may not get her promotion.

She is hurt because she has worked hard on the project and her participation was not recognized.

She is scared because the company looks bad and she now feels that she can't trust others in her department.

She is ashamed that the project failed and now she looks very unprofessional.

It is quite common for two men to argue with a lot of feeling in the tone of their voices, and neither feels personally attacked or gets personally defensive. A woman listening to the conflict may become alarmed, but men listening recognize that no one is being personally attacked and so all is OK. If it gets personal, then other men listening would feel the need to intervene to avoid escalating tension and conflict.

In a similar manner, when men hear women express their feelings in a more personal manner, although a woman would not feel attacked or blamed, a man will. The most well-known example of this concerns anger. On a music album, Barbra Streisand popularized the message that men are respected when they express anger, but when women express anger they are seen in a negative light. She was correct. This is unfair for women, but fortunately there is a way to understand each other better.

Not all women who express anger are seen in this light. Some women who express their anger are seen as strong. When a man or woman is able to express anger in an impersonal manner, then men listen and respect what is being said. When a woman's anger is personal, resulting from her feeling personally attacked, hurt, or wounded, it is then that she is viewed in a negative light. On Venus, there is nothing wrong with expressing personal feelings of anger, but on Mars it is heard as a personal attack.

When a woman's anger is personal, men mistakenly conclude that she is blaming others and taking no responsibility for what happened. When a woman's or man's anger is respected by men as an expression of strength and conviction, it is because the anger is about a situation or circumstance. Personal feelings in the workplace are often viewed by men with less respect.

What determines whether something is appropriate is the context in which it is expressed. If you are attempting to win the respect of someone from Mars, expressing personal emotions in the workplace is inappropriate because they can be so easily misunderstood and misinterpreted unless the man is adept in understanding Venusians (and most men are not). When a man hears women express personal feelings, the man often interprets their behaviors as selfish, self-pitying, or as finger-pointing. When women hear men express impersonal feelings, they often feel men are cold, inconsiderate, and indirectly blaming others.

In his Academy Award-winning role in the movie As *Good As It Gets,* Jack Nicholson explains how he is able to portray women so intimately: "I think about my male friends, take away all reason and sense of accountability, and I am left with how women think." Though this is not accurate, it is how many men, at times, misinterpret how women think and feel in the workplace. With a better understanding of our differences, this can be corrected. Understanding impersonal and personal feelings helps both men and women to see through the illusion of blame and more effectively realize our true intention to be more professional in the workplace.

# Who's Blaming Who

One of the biggest problems with personal emotions in the workplace is that men tend to react defensively. When a man reacts defensively, his emotions become more personal, and he starts to blame others. In a similar manner, when a man expresses impersonal feelings, a woman will withdraw and react in a more impersonal manner. At this point, she will begin to blame him for his lack of sensitivity and consideration.

Men have personal feelings just like women, but as a general rule, unless he feels *extremely* mistreated, he will keep his personal feelings to himself. This is the Martian code of professionalism. It is similar to the idea that the customer is always right. To be professional, one doesn't think so much about oneself but focuses primarily on what it takes to get the job done and provide the best service.

On Venus, there is a similar but different code. As a general rule, unless a woman is feeling *extremely* mistreated, she will try to stay personal and not become impersonal. Blaming others is also considered inappropriate.

Many times men feel unfairly blamed and women claim they are not blaming. Women often say, "I am not blaming you, I am just telling you how I feel." Likewise, women claim a man is blaming when he is simply upset and explaining why he thinks he is right. As a result women feel "men just want to be right" and are therefore "unapproachable." A woman will conclude that a man cannot "hear her" when really he can hear much more than she thinks and will consider her comments.

# Giving and Receiving Support

When a woman expresses personal emotions she is looking for support and giving it. Her openness to share personal emotions is a sign of her willingness to trust another. At such times, a man can make a few small adjustments and strengthen the bond of trust in their working relationship.

A man does not instinctively give reassurance, because when he expresses his negative emotions he is not looking for emotional reassurance. For example, when he is disappointed, he doesn't want to hear a woman empathetically saying, "I know you must feel really disappointed." On his planet this kind of support is considered demeaning and condescending. At best it would make him feel uncomfortable, but most of the time it would be offensive.

Yet these same words could make most women feel supported. Let's look at a variety of ways a man or woman could respond to personal emotions in a supportive manner. When a man correctly identifies the tone of a woman's emotions without distancing himself, she already feels supported. By adding a supportive, reassuring comment, she feels even more support. Let's look at a few examples.

## Giving Reassurance on Venus

When a woman says, "The letter was lost. I don't know what to do": different personal emotions and corresponding meanings are listed in column one; a corresponding reassuring response is listed in column two.

At times of distress, a Venusian appreciates that someone else knows what she is going through and cares. On Venus, when you really care for someone, their joy makes you happy, and their sadness makes you sad. This matching of emotional tone makes your message assuring. In addition, by making a few validating comments and acknowledging statements, a woman will feel even more support.

These same comments could easily backfire when talking to a Martian. On Mars, they assess themselves based on their competence. To offer help when he has not asked for it is to convey the message that he is somehow weak. Most of the time a man doesn't want a reassuring comment. His feelings are not personal, but impersonal, and require a different kind of support.

| She feels: | How he can give reassurance: |
| --- | --- |
| Her tone is frustration. She is frustrated that the letter was lost; she had asked for it, and now she feels that she is not being heard. | He says, "This must be so frustrating, you had specifically asked for that letter...maybe next time they will listen to you." |
| Her tone is disappointment. She is disappointed since her efforts to improve sales were not implemented. | He says, "It must be very disappointing, you had so many good ideas, and they just didn't listen...maybe now things will change." |

Her tone is worry. She is worried that she will be blamed if the project is not finished in time and lose her job.

He says, "Are you worried about keeping your job? Everyone is so upset about this. Even if it doesn't finish on time, everyone knows it wasn't your fault...you are doing a good job."

Her tone is embarrassment. She is embarrassed that others may see her as inefficient and uncaring.

He says, "You seem embarrassed. It wasn't your fault. We know how much you care and put into this project."

Her tone is anger. She is angry, because without the letter she may lose credibility.

He says, "You have every right to be angry about this. I know it certainly is not your fault. It is so unfair...you have done a great job."

Her tone is sadness. She is sad, because she thought it would have turned out better, but instead she wasted her time.

He says, "It makes me sad, too. I know you thought it was going to turn out better. You did your best, and that's all you can ever do."

Her tone is fear. She is afraid, because she may not have enough time to correct the situation, and others will be disappointed in her.

He says, "I can understand if you are afraid. Everything is happening at once... I think it's going to be OK."

Her tone is regret. She is sorry that the letter was lost and feels powerless to do anything about it.

He says, "I know you feel sorry. No one expects you to make it reappear magically...it's OK."

Her tone is outrage. She is furious that the letter was lost, because she worked so hard and to no avail; she may not get her promotion.

He says, "I would be furious, too. You have worked so hard and then this. I can appreciate how much you have done and how difficult this must be for you...you still deserve a promotion."

Her tone is hurt. She is hurt because she has worked hard on the project, and someone else may get the deal.

He says, "It must really hurt a lot. You worked so hard and now you may lose the deal. You didn't deserve this... I know it will eventually work out."

Her tone is anxious. She is scared that the company looks bad and she now feels she can't trust others in her department.

He says, "This is scary. Everyone is so busy. How can you trust anyone to remember anything?... Things will get better."

Her tone is shame. She feels bad that the project failed, and now she looks very unprofessional.

He says, "I know you feel really bad. You did all anyone could do. No one expects perfection... you handled this whole project in a very professional and competent manner."

At such times, a man supports another man by not directly offering any reassuring comments or direct empathy. Instead he gives a special kind of encouragement. This is done in a manner that allows him to save face. This encouragement recognizes that he is somewhat distressed, and trusts in his ability to handle the situation in the best possible manner. Venusian reassuring comments can easily be interpreted as a lack of trust or criticism implying he can't handle the situation without her emotional support.

On Mars, it is a mistake to directly acknowledge impersonal negative feelings. To a certain extent, these feelings are to be overlooked or ignored. Putting attention on his feelings gives the problem more importance, thus increasing the sense of failure. For most men, it would be completely inappropriate to say, "I know you must be hurting, let me help you."

Responding in the emotional tone of another in distress works on Venus, but not on Mars. If a man is disappointed, it doesn't work to feel disappointed "for him." If he is worried, don't express the tone of worry for him. When he is happy, you can feel happy for him, but when he is sad, it's not appropriate to feel sad for him. That can make him feel worse.

Often men don't even understand this. They just know that after a woman expresses empathy they just want to shake it off. This explains why men don't share feelings with women and also why men have no idea how to give an empathetic comment.

This does not mean that all men will be turned off by emotional reassurance, but when they seem to pull away, a woman can correctly assess the situation. It is not that he doesn't want her support, it is that he doesn't want emotional empathy. With this insight she will not take his withdrawal personally. She can then easily undo her mistake with a simply apology. She could simply say, "Excuse me for getting so emotional." The less said the better.

One little apology can quickly mend the mistake. Without this understanding, a woman would never even consider giving an apology for either getting emotional or being empathetic. In this manner she can make light of it and give a brief apology. He will be able to easily let it go or release any resistance he has to her.

## Giving Encouragement on Mars

Just as women appreciate reassurance at stressful times, a man will appreciate encouragement. Men love being appreciated and cheered on. To acknowledge what a man does encourages him on. If he is under stress and expressing negative emotions, there are ways a woman can be most supportive by making comments that sound encouraging on Mars.

An encouraging response, unlike a reassuring response, gives the message "I trust you can handle this, you clearly don't need my help." An encouraging message on Mars contains trust, acceptance, and appreciation.

Keep in mind that the words alone are not enough. The tone is very important. To give encouragement, make sure the tone is not an empathetic, "I feel your pain" tone. It needs to be more upbeat, sometimes jovial. Empathy tends to have a heavy tone, while encouragement has a light tone. Imagine you were responding to the world's greatest expert. The last thing you would do is "feel sorry" for him. Let's look at some examples.

| He feels: | She can say to support: |
|---|---|
| He is frustrated that the letter was lost and as result an opportunity was missed. | She says in a tone of relief, "I'm sure glad I don't have to do your job." |
| He is disappointed that sales were down in the third quarter. | She says in a neutral tone, "Sometimes you win, sometimes…you lose." |
| He is worried that the project will not be finished in time, or he will not have time to do it. | She says with a confident tone, "I'm not worried, you'll figure out something." |
| He is embarrassed that the work was not very good, because the letter was lost. | She says with a casual tone, "Well, you can't win them all." |
| He is angry, because without the letter he can't prove his competence. | She says in a playful tone, "Well, I guess that's why they pay you the big bucks." |
| He is sad, because so much time was wasted and he will have to start over. | She says in a matter-of-fact tone, "You can only do what you can do." |
| He is afraid, because he does not know how they will make up the time lost. | She says in a hopeful tone, "It's not over till it's over." |
| He is sorry the letter was lost, because the project will not get done in time. | She says in a carefree tone, "Well, it won't be the end of the world." |

By role-playing and giving this kind of playful, matter-of-fact encouragement, a woman can learn to give the kind of support a man appreciates. By experiencing her resistance to this kind of support, she can begin to glimpse the kind of resistance men have to making reassuring gestures that are appreciated on Venus.

## Expressing Feelings in the Workplace

The best way to stand out in the workplace is by expressing positive feeling. When you are confident, people have greater confidence in you. When you feel good about yourself and your job then others feel good being around you. When you feel calm then you are an oasis of peace and others will be drawn to you. When you are able to appreciate the opportunities before you then you naturally attract more.

Feelings can be shared directly with words, but most often and most powerfully they are shared through the tone of your voice and your physical mannerisms. For example, after completing a task, there is big difference between a "big sigh of relief" and a "big sigh of exasperation." The actual behavior of taking a deep breath is the same, but the feeling conveyed through the tone and facial expression is entirely different. A sigh could convey positive feelings, neutral feelings, or negative feelings.

### Containing Negative Feelings

On Mars negative feelings are a sign of weakness and are processed privately. Healthy men have a healthy sense of privacy regarding their inner demons. When personal feelings of frustration, anger, disappointment, etc., arise, he skillfully holds back or contains these feelings until a later time when he can process and release them. This is often accomplished by doing something that is fun, relaxing, or challenging that is not directly work-related. Once he feels more relaxed and peaceful he is able to casually reflect once again on what happened at work from a more positive perspective.

Unmannered, weak, insecure, or dysfunctional men will readily display negative emotions and as a result will be subjected to the same disrespect that a woman would. On Mars a professional is someone who can do the job regardless of what he is feeling inside. In show business this is reflected in the popular expression "The show must go on."

When it comes to expressing negative feelings in the workplace, both men and women are judged by men with the same set of rules. The inability to contain negative emotions is unprofessional. When men, not just women, are unable to contain negative feelings they lose the respect of other men. Unless a man has some special talent that makes him indispensable, an inability to contain negative emotions will block his success.

One important distinction in this example is that on Venus, healthy and well-mannered women do not have this sense of privacy regarding their inner negative emotions. On their planet it is not offensive to display negative emotions. To the contrary, it is a symptom of healthy self-esteem. As we have already explored, sharing negative feelings on Venus is an efficient way to minimize stress while strengthening connections and building trust.

On Venus, however, a woman will discern when and with whom she will share her feelings. Strong women, like men, also have the capacity to contain negative emotions. A well-mannered Venusian doesn't readily share her negative feelings with someone who is not her friend or supporter. She will often contain them until the right time and place. When she feels more trusting she will begin to open up and share. This explains why sometimes you can ask a woman what's wrong when clearly something is bothering her, but she will insist it is nothing.

A woman, however, will mean, "Something is wrong but I don't know if this is the right time to talk about it. If you care and you have the time, then ask more questions and I will tell more."

In this example the difference between men and women is that when a man says "nothing is wrong," he is not only containing his feelings but he doesn't want to talk about them.

Making this shift toward containing negative emotions is actually not such a stretch for women. A woman is not required to deny her fundamental feminine nature. Women are already experts in "containing" feelings in situations where they don't feel supported. To succeed in the workplace she can now apply this same skill and "contain" her feelings to more successfully give support. With this insight, instead of wondering why she is losing the respect and support of men, she can do something about it.

By applying the discipline and restraint necessary to give support, both men and women can learn to contain their negative emotions and reactions in the workplace. This on Mars is called professional behavior. Some women mistakenly conclude this is unhealthy when it is actually a healthy discipline for both men and women. It would only be unhealthy if a woman didn't take time outside the workplace to discharge her stress. Suppressing feelings is unhealthy but "containing" feelings and then dealing with them at a later time outside the workplace is very healthy.

Besides creating more success, containing negative emotions exercises the muscles of emotional control. When you practice holding back and then freely expressing emotion, at an appropriate time, then you gain a greater control of them. This increases your ability to manage stress. Instead of letting your emotions control you, you gradually learn to control them.

Because it is helpful to take time to explore upsetting feelings in therapy, people mistakenly conclude they should do this in the workplace. The workplace is not, nor should it be, therapeutic. Likewise, it is inappropriate to use business time to support your own personal needs to process your emotional distress. By making sure that you have a personal life outside of your work life, you will have the time and support needed to handle "contained" emotions.

If one is not getting the emotional support they need from their personal life outside the office then they should look to a therapist and not their job for that kind of support. Learning to contain upset feelings and then taking time to process them at a later time is one of the healthiest things a person can learn to do.

This adjustment of containing feelings is like a new kind of makeup to bring out a woman's best characteristics in the workplace. Holding it in this light is helpful because some women resist having to hide a part of themselves, when the truth is they are already doing it in many ways. Many women willingly put on makeup to hide a blemish, put caps on their teeth or use whiteners, or wear clothes that will particularly flatter their figure. Containing negative emotions is just another way a woman can accentuate her best characteristics.

This doesn't mean she can't be herself. It just means she cannot be all of herself all of the time. Successful people have learned how to authentically express different parts of themselves at different times. They understand that you can't express all of who you are at all times. There is, however, a time and place for each part of who you are.

It is not just women but men as well who are required to hold back from freely expressing whatever they feel. Men are generally more receptive to this idea because they have to work on it all the time. Although women are often seen as more emotional, it is not an accurate generalization. Differences in one's tendency to react emotionally are based on different temperaments and are not gender-specific. What is different between men and women is how we process emotions differently.

Men have a much greater tendency to act without thinking when they experience negative emotions. A man in combat may feel enormous fear but he learns to contain his fear and not act on it by running away. He contains his anger and ensures that he doesn't act impulsively. He learns to contain his sadness and get the job done regardless of how he feels. Men are already more familiar with the need to contain feelings, and so with the added awareness of what women need they can more easily put it into practice.

When men and women take time to process their contained feelings at home or in more personal relationships it is easier to make this adjustment in the workplace. When, however, there is no outlet for feelings in our personal life this small adjustment can seem impossible.

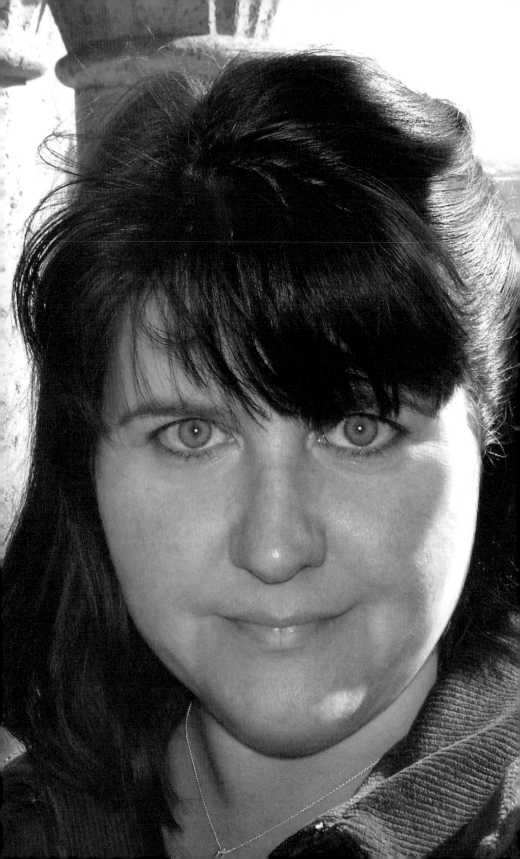

# BONNIE SARKISIAN:

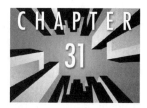

# Tend Your Garden

I learned the single most important concept of my corporate career not in a boardroom or a busy office, but on a warm summer day when I was six years old. My parents had gone on a day trip, leaving me in my grandmother's care. Though I loved her very much, my grandmother and I were not close. She had little interest in my toys and games, and my constant energy exhausted her. And because she had grown up in a very different time, we had almost nothing in common and little to talk about or share.

On this particular day, there was a street fair in town. Some of our neighbors had offered to take me along with them, but when I asked my grandmother, she said no. I spent the rest of the day feeling miserable. While we never said much during dinner, this night the silence was heavy and awkward. Then, as we were clearing the table at the end of the meal, she looked at me with warm eyes and softly said, "B, tend your garden." In that moment, I took her comment to mean, "Just drop it."

I heard those words from her many times as the years went by. Eventually, I came to understand that "tend your garden" was her way of encouraging me to focus on those endeavors that would bear fruit. Little did I know on that miserable day that my grandmother had given me a compass to guide my life and an instrument for leadership that has benefited me for decades.

As I developed and grew, this metaphor became my philosophical

Bonnie Sarkisian is an exciting, emerging voice with a fresh point of view and irrepressible wit. Bonnie has an eclectic background that includes the arts, life coaching, and corporate experience in the fields of manufacturing, health care, and entertainment. She is a lifelong student of strategic applications and patterns, seeking to understand life cycles, design and form. As a result, natural balance and respect is central to both her writings and visual art. Currently she is the Human Resources Director, Operations, Disney ABC Media Networks. She currently lives in Los Angeles, California. For more information about Bonnie, visit her website at www.BASarkisian.com.

touchstone. Not only is this garden a place to remind me to focus on that which will bear fruit, but it also represents the benefits of respecting the nature of things. It is a place of simple natural lessons. A gardener cannot expect a plant to produce if the soil is depleted, if weeds are allowed to takeover, or if there is no light. In the many times when I have been unclear about which path to follow, I have looked to the concept of my garden to help me determine which option would bear the best fruit and which elements were needed for that fruit to develop.

This concept of the garden continues to give me a perspective on my challenges as a leader, as well. As I work to meet corporate needs, I also seek ways to respect the nature of people and situations. Being a great leader is an aspiration, not a destination. Leadership at its best is organic, starkly human, and personal. Lance Secretan says it so well: "Great leadership is about human experiences, not processes. Leadership is not a formula or a program, it is a human activity that comes from the heart and considers the hearts of others. It is an attitude, not a routine." This is the perspective I seek to bring into my life and my career, and it is my grandmother's voice that continues to inspire me.

In a rich, healthy garden all things grow together—inseparable, interrelated—and yet each plant is independently perfect and complete. Some plants thrive in full sun, and others in shade. When you get the placement right, they provide rich fruit in return. When you have a healthy garden, the variety keeps the soil fertile. A blue ribbon gardener knows from experience the elements, patterns, and secrets that make him better than the others. He is better because he optimizes the natural strength of the garden through intuition, observation, and respect.

For a leader to bear the best fruit in business, there must be this same balance. Just as the gardener has a vision for his garden and the plants grow to fulfill his vision, the leader and the team also have distinct roles. As the gardener must respect the landscape and protect his garden from frost and weeds, the leader must meet management needs and protect the team from internal and external pressures. The gardener seeks to optimize the potential of his garden, manage situations, and act on ways to improve the garden; the leader does the same.

In today's teams, the leader might not be the person with the most experience, corporate knowledge, or technical skill. This is in contrast to earlier generations, when management was developed from within the company. In those days, a person with management potential was mentored, came up through the ranks, and was well versed in the processes and history of the company. That is no longer the common practice. Now leaders, more often than not, have developed their skills outside of the company in which they hold leadership responsibility. This creates a problem with the traditional top-down leadership model. To be successful, leaders must create an environment that leverages group intelligence for the good of the group and the company. This requires a new kind of interdependence between the leader and the team, much like tending a garden. Take care of the garden and the plants will provide you with rich fruit. Neglect the garden, and you will starve.

Even with the role of leadership changing, one thing will always remain true: Leadership requires *vision*. Vision is the strategic destination of a group. Developing and keeping the vision is the single most important role of a leader. Without a destination, all of the group's energy will be wasted on reactionary transactions without hope of a better outcome. To optimize the group strength, this vision must be so clear and complete that the end picture can be conveyed in a way that enables everyone to see the destination. To leverage the strength of all the team members, every person must know, understand, and own the journey.

Having a clear vision first requires that you believe in an idea. To lead you must be genuine, and to be genuine you must make the idea your own. Making the idea your own and creating a vision requires discovery, reflection, and seeking to find something to be passionate about. It requires discovering what is compelling about the new idea, and forming a belief in the need to take action. It takes time to develop vision, and the courage to take that time. This vision must then be communicated, supported, and at the center of the team's actions. Only when the vision is clear will the team create ways to bring the vision to fruition. If this isn't done initially, there will be confusion and frustration for everyone involved. The hardest thing to do is stop momentum—even misguided momentum—in order to get it right.

A few years ago I was working for a California health care company when it decided to move from multiple vendors to a single vendor for temporary labor. This was a large project with several problems. First, the project manager left just prior to the contract being signed. Another issue was that, even though the implementation had not yet been planned, the Human Resources department had been asked to encourage all departments to use the new vendor. The vendor was not ready for the increased orders, which created missteps and misunderstandings. This in turn created additional resistance from departments that were already upset that they had to give up their favorite vendors.

The battle lines had already been drawn when my team inherited this project. As we plowed through the original project plan, everyone on the team became more and more unhappy. The whole company relied on temporary labor, and this mess was affecting the business. My team became the target of this frustration, and the problems increased by the day. Before long, everyone on my team had been pulled from other priorities to react to the flood of complications.

Finally, it occurred to me that we were floundering without a communicated vision. The purpose of the change to a single vendor was clear: cost savings, better reporting on temporary usage, and better quality control. I had mistaken *knowing the purpose* for *communicating a vision*. It wasn't until I declared that we own this project and the team heard me state the vision that we were able to gain some control. In that same meeting, one of my team members pointed out that we might be able to get somewhere if we could just get everyone to talk to each other instead of yelling, and at that moment it all came together.

That revelation lead to our team doing something unheard of in this company: talking to each other in person. We created a new way to implement the change by addressing the major concerns of both the vendor and the internal clients *in person*. My team would go on the road with the vendor to present and to learn—and until every department was ready for the switch, they would continue to use their current favorite vendors. This gave my team something to strive for, took the pressure off our clients and the vendor, and demonstrated that we were dedicated to making this happen the right way. We were on the road for two weeks creating a foundation for collaborative change.

It takes great courage to stop, refocus, and start again. We all want to believe that we got it right the first time, or that we can change the wrong answer into the right answer. When everything is going wrong, frustration is high and everyone spends time reacting; this is a clue that there is something fundamental that is not being tended to. But when the leader focuses on vision and tends to the garden, adversity becomes an opportunity to succeed.

Every professional career presents difficult situations. Even with all the vision in the world, if a team is to be set up for success, the leader must understand the difference between *situation* and *opportunity*. In nature, the situation may be that there hasn't been rain in weeks and there isn't a cloud in the sky. For the gardener, opportunity may be a water hose, or maybe a watering can. While this is obvious for anyone tending a garden, this is not as well understood in business. The situation is the current reality, while an opportunity is a path to a better future reality. Time is wasted and frustration created when energy is expended on trying to change a situation. The current reality is what it is. It is simply the place you start from. In contrast, an opportunity is a chance to make a strategic change.

For example, in my first corporate job, my department lacked consistent leadership at a time when recruiting was being moved from a decentralized to a centralized Human Resources function. In a five-year period, I served under two directors for one year each, with a contractor in the role for the other three years—creating a pattern of director, contractor, director, then contractor again. There was a similar pattern with the leadership above the director. During this same time period, the company hired three different vice presidents to manage this department.

There was a lot to be done. Yet no one wanted to begin new initiatives or make improvements for fear that they would have to start all over when the next new leader showed up. Work became exhausting, as we all toiled away at the administrative tasks. One day while playing around on my computer, after months of frustration, I happened on a new way to manage vacant jobs. Suddenly my exhaustion faded and I was energized, thrilled by this small improvement. I sought out ways to continue this path of improvement.

Under the existing system, it took two weeks from the time a job candidate was selected for an offer and benefits letter was generated and furnished to the candidate. I spent time with the six people involved, and we brainstormed for ways to improve this process. As they saw new possibilities, their excitement began to grow. The prospect of change began to feel like fun. A team spirit developed, and within a month we were generating new hire documents in 30 minutes. Because we acted on opportunities, the situation improved.

Both leaders and teams are most effective when their roles are clearly defined. The leader is the keeper of the vision. The team owns the journey. By keeping these roles separate, the team is less likely to be distracted from the destination or derailed due to micromanagement. If everyone is mired in details and unable to relate small decisions to the larger vision, you will wind up lost the whims of immediate pressures. The leader must be focused on the relationship of the progress to the destination—and be prepared to correct course if necessary.

Micromanaging is the outcome of a leader trying to do the work of the team instead of leading. This is much like a gardener standing over a tomato plant demanding that the plant grow faster. Instead, a blue ribbon gardener is deeply engaged with the garden—feeding, watering, protecting from frost, and weeding as she goes. By keeping the vision and letting go of the journey, you allow the team the opportunity to create something even greater than the original vision. A one-size-fits-all approach only gives you only one size. Mix it up, create variety, play, and most importantly, facilitate connections. The best thing to hope for is a movement. This can be a change in thought, priorities, or values, but it is always a change in perspective. Let the team move and grow, and they will make you proud.

Something magical happens in a diverse group that has trust, mutual respect, and focus on a single outcome. When the members gather in a safe environment, planning turns to silliness, which turns into craziness, which turns into outlandish ideas—one of which just might work. The outcome is a group creation, and that creates solidarity. This is much more powerful than the concept of gathering "buy-in" for a new idea. Creation is a natural human process, while "buy-in" is a management construct designed to minimize the negative impact of predetermined changes.

When you ask a team to trust and take risks, you must protect them in return. Two threats endanger a healthy garden. The first is *weeds*. In business, weeds are threats from within the team, including all the things that destroy morale, productivity, or energy. Like anything else in nature, people adapt and produce best in supportive environments. If there is a behavior that is inappropriate, weeding as you go means addressing things in the moment. Weeds can strangle and deplete the soil. They spread quickly and can overtake the garden when you're not looking. By not allowing weeds to take root, you not only protect the vision, you gain trust. Many of us have worked on teams that have deteriorated through slow suffocation. Weeds always start with a single unchecked moment; the longer that weed has to take hold, the harder it will be to recover.

As a leader, weeding as you go means being very present and not letting things slip through the cracks or waiting until a pattern has developed. For instance, when time is precious, it can be extremely frustrating to have to wait for a team member to finally show up. Weeding as you go means that, as the leader, you address this issue in the moment. When someone is late to a meeting, to respectfully ask that everyone be on time is a powerful correction. Not only will that person be unlikely to be late again, but everyone in the meeting understands the importance of being respectful to the group.

The second, equally powerful threat to a healthy garden is *frost*—those negative influences that come from outside the team. Examples of frost include undue criticism from management, or a negative company or department culture. This damage is hard to recover from.

In a garden, it can mean losing not just the fruit, but all the plants as well. There will always be outside factors beyond the team's control. Companies go through layoffs, periods of poor leadership, and poorly managed change. A good leader recognizes a frost warning and acts to protect her team. This can mean many things, but most important among them is being present and openly discussing issues as they occur. No news is no longer good news. Where information lacks, weeds grow.

Frost can also be the impact of honest mistakes or underestimations. Change is a pendulum that swings both ways. The greater the change, the bigger the mistakes the team will make—and they *will* make mistakes and underestimations. The underestimation is the unexpected byproduct you create along with change.

When I was working for the health care company, my team spent a year replacing a manual process with a technological solution. The result was great: We were able to gather data faster and reported it with a shorter turnaround time. But we didn't anticipate the byproduct of this change: As people in the company began to use the new data, they wanted more of it. They demanded more reports. We didn't foresee this increased demand. Suddenly, we needed a full-time person just to create reports. Plan as you will, these are the things that blindside you late on a Friday afternoon with no budget to make the problem go away. Great leadership isn't measured by the ability to avoid these situations, but by the rate at which you can recover from them. The key is to protect the team while they recover. This is the responsibility of the leader, who must protect the team by addressing the criticism—while continuing to deliver on the vision. If you have a healthy garden without weeds, you will recover.

Communication is key to minimizing frost. It is important to keep in mind that, as a leader, your garden is part of a larger landscape. Alignment and agreement are essential to the protection of your garden. A great leader manages up as well as down, setting expectations and resolving issues with their superiors before they affect the team.

The best way I have found to keep my garden healthy is to be very present and available and to freely share information. One way I do this is by meeting with my team on a daily basis. Whenever I have taken over the leadership of new teams, the initial reaction to daily meetings has been negative. We all have too many meetings already. Yet, as the group turns into a team and the team becomes empowered as a result of leveraging group intelligence, they eventually realize that this time is essential for success.

In teams that don't hold frequent meetings, team members

tend to hear about important updates in passing conversations and may seek out other team members to confirm the information. As a result, they often have different understandings and will seek further confirmation to find out who has the correct information...and so it goes. Someone acting on outdated information may go for days working counter to the project. Difficult issues that may be quickly straightened out with group support can overburden and frustrate a team member who is unnecessarily trying to go it alone. Remember, wasting energy is a weed.

Some leaders speak with team members individually, but this approach also has limitations. The manager must decide who needs what information—and there is no opportunity to leverage group intelligence.

My meetings are scheduled for 30 minutes, but if we are done in 15 then that is all the time we take. By meeting frequently, everyone hears the same thing at the same time, and we leverage group intelligence. Everyone watches the leader act and react to information. Everyone laughs, learns, and contributes. No one is left behind. The leader can measure morale and respond if necessary. As a group, team members recognize even the smallest of victories, rally together to recover from frosty issues, and learn about their company through shared stories. The leader can weed, nourish, and refocus the group, and the team members are guaranteed time with the leader and each other that is solely dedicated to giving them what they need to be successful. I call this *transparent management*. It's transparent because the light can pass through unfiltered and free of distortion. It's management in the sense that the team is watching and directing the journey as a group, and I am watching and directing the vision.

As a result of the team's frequent interaction, the team creates a distinct identity and personality in a short period of time. Interdependency supports different behaviors than those that are stereotypically corporate. While individual contribution is still recognized and appreciated, the method of individual success cannot undermine the vision or the journey. This means that the stronger or more skilled team members focus their talents on the delivery of the vision and often help to develop other team members, which leads to greater success. Peer mentorship is often a natural byproduct.

Other benefits of daily meetings have surprised me. One of these is a natural kind of career development. Imagine how your early career might have been boosted if you were able to hear managers and analysts share information and watch the journey unfold one day at a time. Another benefit is group marketing and support. When every member is well versed on the team projects and initiatives, they all have the confidence and pride to share the progress with co-workers outside the team. The team reaps the benefits of their own great press. They also correct misinformation and can support team efforts with ongoing education. This greatly reduces gossip and misunderstandings within the larger department.

Great leadership grows organically from within the leader. We can learn a great deal about this from nature, which is resilient, fearless, and ever evolving. Nature lives in eternal patterns, like the seasons. They pass yet always return. Nature is also protective, providing its creatures with highly evolved defenses and ways to regenerate. When we talk of work-life balance, we are usually referring to a balance between work and home; but another kind of work-life balance also needs to be established within the workplace — that between the corporate reality and the natural human.

Joy and unbridled creativity spring from having a vision and giving your team ownership of the journey, from respecting the situation and acting on the opportunities, from managing upward as well as downward, from protecting the team, and from practicing transparent management. I look forward to the day when every company creates the balance that allows individuals to contribute in their entirety. This would give the term *human resources* new meaning; I can only imagine how great this resource might turn out to be.

In the meantime, I will continue to tend my garden.

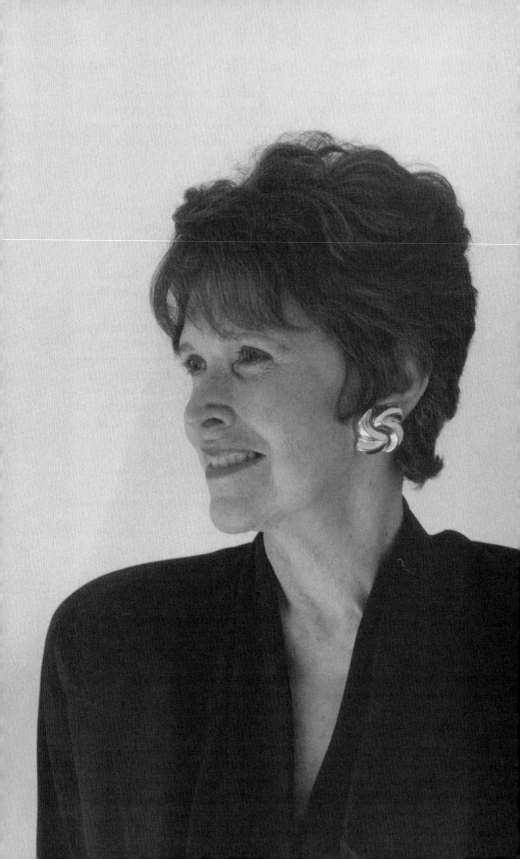

# RIANE EISLER:

# The Caring Business

The corporate scandals of recent years—Enron, WorldCom, and others—did not happen in a vacuum. The business executives who defrauded their companies, cheated their shareholders, and ruined their employees' livelihoods and retirement funds were able to accomplish these arrogant feats because of the system under which most of society functions. The reach of this system is far deeper than most social researchers have explored or, like fish that do not know what water is because they are immersed in it, than they even suspect.

Using a new method of analysis over the last thirty years, my research has identified an alternative that can help us resolve the growing host of problems that now threaten our continued existence. While our entire society calls out for this alternative, the business world could use its immense power to lead the way, both bestowing and receiving many benefits.

To identify this alternative, I had to use an approach that examines our current configuration of society from a larger perspective. This approach, which I call the study of *relational dynamics*, goes far beyond the typical studies of society that focus on conventional views of politics and economics.

Most studies of society are still bound by old conceptual frameworks, such as secular vs. religious, capitalist vs. socialist, right vs. left, and industrial vs. pre- or post-industrial. They generally

Riane Eisler, Ph.D., is best known for her international bestseller *The Chalice and The Blade* (HarperSan Francisco, 1988). Her new book, *The Real Wealth of Nations: Creating a Caring Economics* (Berrett-Koehler, 2007) is also widely recognized for its innovative and practical proposals, as are her other books, including *Sacred Pleasure* (HarperSan Francisco, 1996), *Tomorrow's Children* (Westview Press, 2001), and *The Power of Partnership* (New World Library, 2003). Dr. Eisler is president of the Center for Partnership Studies (www.partnershipway.org) and co-founder of the Spiritual Alliance to Stop Intimate Violence (www.saiv.net). She keynotes conferences worldwide and consults to business and government.

look at only one nation or period at a time. Moreover, they draw from an incomplete database that gives scant if any attention to the cultural construction of the primary human relations. That is, they do not factor in the importance of how a society constructs the foundational relations between women and men and between parents and children—the relations where people first learn what is considered normal or abnormal, moral or immoral, possible or impossible.

The study of relational dynamics draws from a larger data base than conventional studies: the whole of our history, including our prehistory; the whole of our lives, including both the so-called public sphere and the private sphere of family and other intimate relations; and the whole of humanity, both its female and male halves. This approach that makes it possible to see patterns or connections that are not visible otherwise.

Because there were no names to describe these patterns, I called one social configuration the partnership system and the other the domination system. I want to clarify from the outset that the partnership and domination systems don't describe conventional polarities such as hierarchic or hierarchy-free organization. Nor do they describe cooperative or competitive patterns of behavior. What they describe are two very different configurations of beliefs and institutions (from the family, education, and religion, to politics and economics) that support two very different kinds of relations in all spheres of life—including businesses.

## The Domination System and The Partnership System

In the *domination system*, there are only two alternatives for relations: dominating or being dominated. Those on top control those below them—be it in families, workplaces, or society at large. Economic and business structures in this system are designed to benefit those on top at the expense of those on the bottom. Trust is scarce and tension is high, as the whole system is largely held together by fear and force.

The core configuration of the domination model consists of: top-down rankings in the family and state maintained through physical, psychological, and economic control; the rigid ranking of the male half of humanity over the female half (and with this, of traits and values labeled masculine over those labeled feminine); and a high degree of culturally-accepted abuse and violence ranging from child- and wife-beating to chronic warfare.

On the other hand, the core configuration of the *partnership system* consists of a democratic, egalitarian structure in both the family and the state. Gender relations are based on equal partnership between women and men. Violence is not institutionalized or idealized, since rigid rankings of domination, which can ultimately be maintained only through violence, are not part of the culture. And since women have a higher status than in the domination system, stereotypically feminine values, such as nonviolence and caring, can be given social priority.

While the domination system supports top-down rankings, the partnership system supports mutually respectful and caring relations. There are still hierarchies, as there must be to get things done. But in these hierarchies, which I call *hierarchies of actualization* rather than *hierarchies of domination*, accountability and respect flow both ways rather than just from the bottom up. Leaders and managers facilitate, inspire, and empower rather than control and disempower. Economic and business structures in this system are designed to support our basic survival needs and our needs for community, creativity, meaning, and caring—in other words, the realization of our highest human potentials.

No society is a pure partnership or domination system. It's always a matter of degree. But the degree of orientation to either end of the partnership–domination continuum profoundly affects all aspects of society. It determines whether a society is violent and inequitable or peaceful and equitable. In the case of business, it determines, among many other things, whether the business environment will or will not be conducive to Enron-like deceit.

We are all accustomed to the domination system, since that has been the primary human model for the last several thousand years. We tend to accept it as the natural way of things, but, in truth, it is simply a system humans created and which humans can transform.

In recent centuries, there has been movement toward partnership, as seen in the creation and spread of democracy, more equality for women, the move to eliminate slavery and racial discrimination, and so on. While the Taliban, for instance, can be seen as an extreme example of domination systems, the Nordic nations are an excellent example of an entire society moving toward partnership.

Nordic nations such as Sweden, Norway, and Finland have made a great deal of progress towards much more political and economic democracy in both the family and the state. With the rise in the status of women in these countries has come a rise in the status of traits that, in the domination system, are stereotypically associated with women, such as caring, caregiving, and nonviolence—qualities that both men and women can embody and embrace. These nations pioneered policies in line with these values, such as universal healthcare, childcare allowances, and very good paid parental leave.

These more partnership-oriented countries aren't perfect. But they have also taken the lead in removing traditions of violence from their cultures, passing laws making it illegal to physically punish children and creating a strong men's movement against men's violence against women. They pioneered peace studies and are involved in nonviolent conflict resolution and international mediation.

They are more in partnership with Mother Earth, as shown in the Swedish "Natural Step," a way for businesses of all kinds to work together to create a sustainable world based on three tests: Is it good for the organization, good for society, and good for the environment?

But the movement toward partnership structures and beliefs has been slow and uneven. It has been fiercely resisted by some and punctuated by periodic regressions. A major obstacle to the shift to partnership is that we inherited the domination system from earlier generations, and are often still taught that it is inevitable, even beneficial. And business is not excluded from that heritage.

If we look back to the early industrial workplace, it was very much a top-down structure governed by "hard" or stereotypically "masculine" qualities (which, I want to emphasize, are not inherent in men but in the domination system's definitions of masculinity). There was little or no attention to workers' safety or health, to their families, or to any aspect of their lives outside of work. Workers were simply disposable cogs in the industrial machine, and caring was generally considered "soft" or "feminine" (that is, associated with the "inferior" half of humanity), and thus not considered important or appropriate for business operations.

Even now, many people still cling to the notion that this kind of disregard for workers as human beings is the most efficient way to operate a business. But of course it isn't.

## The Effectiveness of the Partnership System

We have a wealth of evidence today that the domination system decreases an organization's effectiveness, particularly in our post-industrial era, where what economists call "relational resources" are so critical to success. There is also a lot of empirical evidence disproving that so-called soft behaviors are impediments to productivity.

Studies show the obvious—that when people feel cared for, they feel fully alive and become more productive and creative. Studies also show that this is very good for business success and economic development.

For example, Intermedics, Inc. decreased their turnover rate by 37 percent with on-site childcare, saving 15,000 work hours and two million dollars. Johnson & Johnson found that absenteeism among employees who used flexible work options and family leave policies was an average of 50 percent less than for the workforce as a whole.

As these and many other statistics show, we're already seeing movement towards partnership in business. While in some companies talk of caring and partnership is still more rhetorical than real, in others it's becoming a reality.

If you look at today's organizational development and management literature, it too shows the benefits of more participatory and caring business policies and practices. Of particular interest is that this literature also increasingly describes the effective manager, not as a controller, but as someone who inspires, who nurtures others, who facilitates, who elicits from others their highest potentials.

The movement toward this more stereotypically feminine, even motherly, management and leadership style is not accidental, nor is the movement to humanize the workplace. It's part of the cultural movement toward a partnership rather than domination system.

A major element in this cultural transformation of the business environment is the critical mass of women entering the workplace. Here I want to emphasize that the fact that women have brought more relational values to the workplace is not a matter of women being better than men. It is largely due to the fact that women are socialized to value relationship, empathy, nonviolence, and caring.

Again, I want to be clear that this is not a biological issue. For example, in what might be called the Maggie Thatcher Syndrome, some women accept and promote the domination system to the hilt, climbing the domination hierarchy because they demonstrate every inch of the way that they are not "soft" or "feminine."

I also want to make it clear that caring for people doesn't mean mollycoddling them. It simply means having empathy for people and not treating them as disposable, easily replaceable cogs. This caring for people, as well as for our natural environment, is a core element of the caring partnership philosophy that is beneficial not only to the companies that adopt it but to society at large.

## The Economic Value of Caring and Caregiving

Many people fail to understand, and hence devalue, the benefits of caring and caregiving. We see this devaluation in the workplace, where professions that entail caring such as childcare and elementary school teaching are lower-paid than those of plumbing or engineering. But this devaluation of caring and caregiving has not only affected the workplace; it has affected the way our entire economic and social system has been structured.

Consider that conventional economic models and indicators give no value to the work of women (and increasingly also men) who work in the home raising children, producing the "human capital" that economists insist is so important. These models and indicators also fail to give value to the work done by those women and men who volunteer their time in charitable or social welfare organizations, which are so necessary in caring for various needs of society that government or other systems cannot or will not take on.

But not only do conventional economic indicators like GDP and GNP fail to include this essential life-supporting work without which there would be no workforce or economy; they include activities that destroy life, such as making and selling cigarettes, without accounting for the health costs and funeral costs of the harm these activities cause.

This kind of economic bookkeeping makes no sense. It is just the result of a way of thinking in which caring and caregiving is devalued.

Of course, some people will insist that we do value the work of caring and caregiving. But if this were so, U.S. official statistics would not show that older women in the United States—most of whom spent their lives caring for children and others in households—are twice as poor as older men.

Another misconception is that these unpaid contributions cannot be quantified and therefore cannot be counted as part of the economy. It's true that we can't quantify all the benefits we humans receive from caring and caregiving, but much of its economic value can be—and actually has been—quantified.

A recent national survey by the Swiss government, for example, found that the unpaid work performed in households has an annual value of 162 billion Euros, or $190 billion—70 percent of the reported Swiss GDP! So, the issue is not that the work of caring and caregiving cannot be quantified, but rather how we look at economics.

If we don't change the devaluation of caring and caregiving, we can't solve seemingly intractable problems such as chronic poverty and the devastation of our natural environment. Consider that today GDP gives value to the cost of cleaning up toxic oil spills, but not to caring for our environment so we have clean oceans, forests that are not clear-cut to turn trees into toothpicks, and air fit to breathe.

In our time of global warming and other unprecedented environmental problems, it is more urgent than ever before that we recognize the value of nature's life support systems. It is also essential, if we are to remedy the fact that 70 percent of those living in absolute poverty in our world are women, that we recognize the value of the life-sustaining activities still primarily performed by women in households.

Once we recognize these activities as economically valuable, indeed, as essential for our survival, we can move toward more sensible economic bookkeeping as well as to more sensible, humane, and sustainable rules of the economic and business game.

## Toward a Caring Economics

We can change dysfunctional and irrational economic policies and practices once we recognize that economic systems are human inventions, human creations based on certain beliefs. In my new book, *The Real Wealth of Nations: Creating a Caring Economics*, I am proposing that to move forward we need a new economic system that takes into account the life-sustaining activities of households, communities, and nature.

This Caring Economy recognizes that economic systems actually have five sectors. The core sector is the household, where care and caregiving are performed, which, as the Swiss and other surveys demonstrate, offers a vast amount of value—monetary and otherwise—to society, and without which none of the other sectors could exist or function. The second sector is the unpaid community economy, or volunteering and civil society activities. The third is the market, which is the primary, indeed almost only, sector considered in today's economic models and indicators. The fourth is the illegal economy, which would shrink as caring and caregiving are given more value. And the fifth is the natural economy, our Mother Earth, which is the foundation and source of all of life.

This Caring Economy is based on a completely different paradigm from our current system, and on an essential expansion of what we consider to be economically productive. This paradigm leads to business structures, policies, and practices that, as already shown by many studies, are good for all stakeholders: business owners, shareholders, employees, communities, and the planet.

In a Caring Economy, within the partnership system, the crimes committed at Enron or WorldCom would not be facilitated by the rules and structures of the system. In companies like that, with their hierarchies of domination where accountability flows only from the bottom up, the executives at the top could get away with fraud and other crimes without being held accountable. They were the dominators, the people at the top with no felt obligation to care about the people underneath them in the organizational chart. Regardless of whether the executives were evil, the rules of the game were bad.

I should again emphasize that changing the rules of the game does not mean moving to a completely flat system where all decisions are made by consensus. There are still leaders in partnership structures; in fact there are more leaders, as everyone's ideas and creativity are valued. There are, of course, still managers in businesses, teachers in schools, and officials in governments.

So, as I noted earlier, in the partnership system, hierarchies still exist, but they are hierarchies of actualization. This means that accountability, respect, and benefits flow not only from the bottom up, but also from the top down. Such a hierarchy would have prevented the crimes that are today revealed by so many business and government scandals. Indeed, in an economic system that values and rewards caring and caregiving, business norms would have prevented such crimes because of the harm they inflict on workers and shareholders, which in some of the above cases were one and the same.

Let me also add that we should not misunderstand the place of competition and cooperation in the partnership system, as often expressed today in the belief that competition is bad and cooperation is good. Again, the reality is much more complex, and largely depends on what you're competing or cooperating for. People cooperate all the time in the domination system—terrorists do, armies do, monopolies do. And people still compete in the partnership system. But here competition is more about being spurred on by the excellence of others—you're doing something well and I want to do the same, or even better—than about killing your opponents or putting them out of business.

Competition in business has come to be seen, wrongly, as meaning the survival of the fittest, who have been defined by the domination standard as the most ruthless. This is a misinterpretation of Darwin's *Origin of the Species* through the lens of the domination system.

If we follow this interpretation, the Janjaweed militia who are slaughtering people in Darfur are the fittest. That's absolute nonsense in terms of human evolution, which again and again has required mutuality and caring.

In this connection, many people ignore Darwin's second book, *The Descent of Man*. In his groundbreaking work and reinterpretation of Darwin, evolutionary scholar David Loye explains that Darwin demonstrated how, at the human level, we have to look at more than natural selection and random variation. Darwin wrote about the importance of moral sensitivity and mutual aid in human society, both of which are characteristics of the partnership system.

## The Implications for Business Leadership

The implications for business leadership of what we have been examining are huge. Corporate leadership really cannot be changed as long as the system dictates hierarchies of domination; the people who make it to the top will not be the best leaders from an effectiveness or human welfare standpoint. Nor will their policies be adaptive in our time, when the once-hallowed dominator "conquest of nature" combined with high technology could take us to an evolutionary dead end.

Once business leaders understand the domination system and how inefficient it is, and the partnership system and how efficient it is, they can make a gigantic difference not only in their own companies but in the world.

For instance, why do American corporate executives not demand a national healthcare system? They are going broke paying for employees' health insurance and seem to be blind to the fact that our current patchwork healthcare system is harming their global competitiveness. But so strong is the prejudice against caring, "feminine" policies that they don't do this—in fact, may not even be able to see this.

When they recognize the unconscious power of this belief system and how we have all been taught to think in terms of dominator vs. dominated, they can begin to make much more rational choices, including a more humane healthcare system and more respect for Mother Earth. When they realize that the domination system is only a belief system—and a very harmful system at that—not anything inherent or "natural" in humanity, they might also begin to understand that our current system of education, with its mindset of No Child Left Behind and high-stakes testing, is inefficient and harmful. It is a regression to the domination system, in which children (and teachers and schools) in the bottom ranks are humiliated. Even worse, it does not produce lifelong learners or creative thinkers eager to find new ways of solving problems or going out on a limb intellectually, which is what leads to innovation and success in business, and in life.

As I show in *The Real Wealth of Nations*, ours is a time that calls for innovative, unconventional thinking. It's not realistic to expect more caring practices and policies as long as caring and caregiving are still devalued as soft, feminine, unimportant, and even counterproductive.

Since business and economics are embedded within the larger culture, we cannot change them by focusing on them alone and ignoring the culture as a whole. We must investigate and examine the domination elements we've inherited — the assumptions, practices, policies, and rules.

The good news is that this reexamination is already in progress, as the evidence mounts that our present economic, social, and environmental course is not sustainable. From all sides we're told that what we must reexamine and restructure our institutions, from the family, education, and religion to politics and economics.

This, too, has been the conclusion I have drawn from three decades of multidisciplinary, cross-cultural, and historical research. One of the findings from this research is that for this restructuring to be successful, we must pay particular attention to how society structures the primary relations between women and men and parents and children.

It's not coincidental that in virulent modern regressions to the domination end of the partnership–domination continuum, policy-makers have paid particular attention to pushing women back to their "traditional" (read, subservient) place in a rigidly authoritarian, highly punitive "father-headship" family. These were top goals for the Nazis in Germany and Khomeini in Iran, and when Stalin came to power he reversed earlier gains for women's equality. The reason is that families are microcosms of the larger socio-economic system. One foundation of domination systems is that children learn early on to divide humanity into "superiors" and "inferiors" — beginning with the ranking of the male half of humanity over the female half. Another foundation is that they must painfully learn that it's dangerous to question authority, no matter how brutal or irrational it may be.

These are systems dynamics that are unfortunately still ignored in conventional social and economic categories such as capitalist vs. socialist, religious vs. secular, rightist vs. leftist, Eastern vs. Western, and industrial vs. pre- or post-industrial. They are dynamics that are relevant not only for government leaders but for business leaders, as the authoritarianism and violence resurging in our world today threatens the social stability needed for businesses to function.

The domination system and partnership system offer new social categories that can help us make the changes in our lives — and in the social and economic rules that govern our lives — that are needed for a more secure, equitable, and sustainable future.

We have a good deal of work to do. It won't be easy, and it won't be quick. But once we understand that many beliefs and traditions about how we can structure society are simply our heritage from earlier, much more rigidly domination-oriented times, we have a chance.

As Einstein said, we can't solve problems using the same thinking that created them. As we break free of the mental fetters of dominator beliefs, we can join together to create a caring economics –and with this, a way of living and making a living that meets human needs and aspirations, and preserves the beauty and bounty of our planet.

# PART EIGHT

❧

# Business as a Sacred Activity

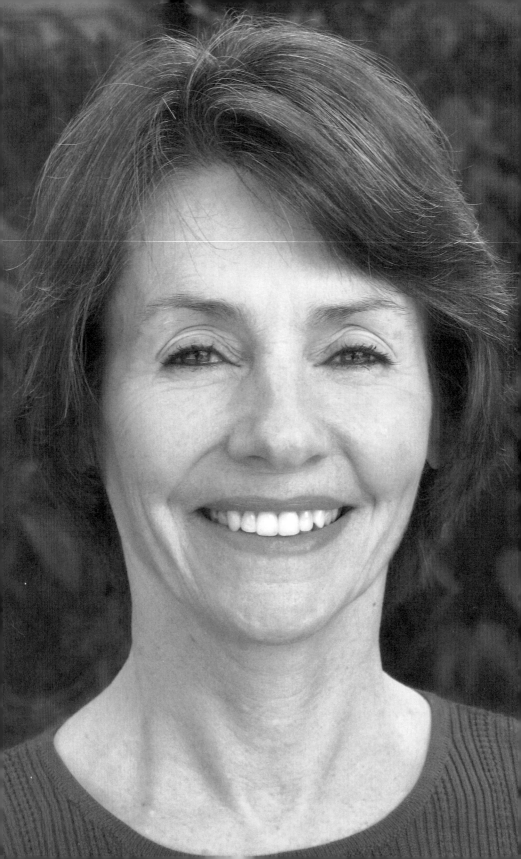

# LYNNE TWIST:

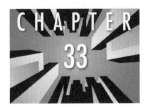

# The Soul of Money

For my first 25 years as a global activist, mentor, and fund-raiser to end hunger, I assumed that the world of business was far removed from me and my work. In those days the words "business" and "philanthropy" or "social responsibility" didn't often show up in the same conversation. I didn't routinely ask businesses for money. Then, as is largely true today, the lion's share of giving came from individuals like you and me, not from companies.

When I first began writing my book, *The Soul of Money: Transforming Your Relationship with Money and Life,* several years ago, I wanted to share what I had learned about living with integrity in our relationship with money: how we earn it, spend it, save it, and give it away. I assumed I was writing mostly to people concerned about money at a personal level. I didn't assume that my message would carry far in the corporate realm; the world of day-to-day business just seemed more over there than right here.

I was in for a surprise. It wasn't long before I realized that many of the people who encouraged me the most were (and still are) among the most successful entrepreneurs and business leaders in the world. They were pioneers on the frontier of socially responsible business, creating strategies for business success with conscious attention to integrity in product development, manufacturing and pricing, labor and management, and the consumer experience. They *knew* that the business world's relationship with money could be transformed,

Lynne Twist is an activist, fundraiser, speaker, consultant, and author who has dedicated her life to global initiatives, including ending world hunger, protecting the world's rainforests, empowering women, children, and indigenous peoples, advancing the scientific understanding of human consciousness, and creating a sustainable future. She is the author of *The Soul of Money: Reclaiming the Wealth of our Inner Resources* (Norton, 2006), among other publications. Lynne founded the Soul of Money Institute to express her commitment to supporting and empowering people in finding peace and sufficiency in their relationship with money and the money culture. Visit www.soulofmoney.org.

too, for even greater prosperity—sustainable prosperity—and they wanted the word to get out. Socially responsible businesses are everywhere now, breaking new ground and demonstrating new practices that generate profits responsibly.

My ongoing experience as a consultant and collaborator with those enlightened business leaders, and the many more that followed, has opened me to a new appreciation of the exciting, dynamic, evolving nature of business, and the power of the individual as a catalyst for positive change in the workplace and the marketplace. In that constantly changing arena of business, it is the individuals who challenge the "business as usual" traditions of the past who hold the key to the future.

Wherever I travel in the world, one of the most dramatic and promising challenges to "business as usual" that I see and actively work to support is the emergence of women into their power as community and business leaders, valued workers, and enlightened consumers. Whether these women are CEOs of giant companies or independent basket-weavers who will never step foot in an office building, they are changing the face, the mind, the heart, and the soul of business throughout the world.

What do I mean by that? In global and historic terms, looking back through the history of our human community, we see that women, both in their biological and social roles as primary nurturers, have been natural practitioners, carriers, and advocates of life-affirming values. That doesn't mean they aren't corruptible or uneven at times. But as my work has placed me in the company of women around the globe, I have been moved again and again by the extreme resourcefulness and enduring strengths that so many women carry within.

Wherever they live or labor, I have seen that as women fully inhabit their intuitive wisdom, they seem to possess an inner compass that lets them know when their behaviors and the behaviors of others are contrary to truly ethical, soul-based values. Questionable or blatantly immoral business practices, rules, or laws raise a red flag for these women, stir them up, and whether they act alone or together, they are drawn to act for the higher good. It shows up in dramatic ways when you think about Rosa Parks, whose refusal to sit in the back of a bus was a galvanizing moment in the American Civil Rights movement of the 1960s; or Elizabeth Cady Stanton and Susan B. Anthony, who broke through the "business as usual" of American political life and led the way to wining voting rights for women in 1920.

In families, women are not only the primary caregivers, but also the whistle-blowers and advocates for equity, whether it is in response to sibling squabbling or snags in healthcare, education or interpersonal relationships and communications. Countless times a day women act as mediators, collaborators, managers, and social entrepreneurs who balance expectations and ethics to clear a responsible path to prosperity.

Likewise, in the business world in the U.S. and worldwide, more and more women are awakening to a sense of moral and ethical urgency. Although they are at risk of being overly influenced by the mainstream corporate culture, where values of competition and profits-at-all-costs are still present, many women are courageously leading with integrity in their workplace.

For some of them, the call towards a new, radical integrity often comes through the doorway of their personal lives. It may arise out of a desire to do what must be done to increase the odds that their future grandchildren can enjoy their life and the natural world without the threats of extreme environmental destruction, pervasive toxicity, and total resource depletion. Or it may be that their focus is more immediate—doing the right thing for no other reason than the fact that circumstances call for it—and the support they find for ethical behavior comes reliably from the collective wisdom of women in their family or circle of friends.

A powerful example of that is Sherron Watkins, who worked for the Enron Corporation and found the courage to reveal the lies and treachery she had seen. Her information launched the investigation that uncovered the infamous scandal that eventually shut the company down and held key executives accountable for the dishonest practices. At a Fortune 500 women's conference I attended, Watkins explained to us that when she began to talk with her colleagues about the wrong-doing she had witnessed, the co-workers became mostly concerned about losing their bonuses. In collusion with the double-life of the company's executives, some of the co-workers wanted the problems to be ignored. But it was Watkins' mother who supported her daughter's integrity and her decision to do what was right and speak up. When Watkins blew the whistle on Enron, she ended the dissonance and discord within her and preserved her invaluable foundation of moral principles.

Women are showing up as leaders, entrepreneurs, and partners in increasing numbers of innovative, socially responsible businesses that transcend national boundaries and establish new frameworks for global collaboration. I love to share the example of my friend and colleague Shauna Alexander Mohr and Lucina, the company she launched after the birth of her daughter in 2004, when she was inspired to create a meaningful business collaboration with women and families in developing and war-torn countries.

In Shauna's previous work as a fair trade coffee buyer and strategy consultant, she had come across skillfully handcrafted materials from fair trade workshops in Africa, Latin America, and Asia. As a social entrepreneur she saw the opportunity to partner with American designers to transform these components into an elegant, upscale collection of jewelry.

As Shauna tells it:

"The old 'business as usual' practice of not paying people in the developing world what they need to live, saying 'that's too bad, but that's how it goes'—I just don't buy it. So I created a business that aims to contribute to a world that works for everyone with no one and nothing left out. This approach to business automatically calls into question the insatiable hunger for sky-high profits, massive salaries and bonuses, and the winner-loser mentality.

"When we're making decisions at Lucina, we ask the question, 'If we approach this in a way that works for everyone—suppliers, customers, investors, ourselves—what would that look like?' Many of our suppliers are single moms in Colombia, Rwanda, and Afghanistan, or families in Ethiopia and Ecuador. Our customers want the highest quality products. And we need to sustain our own families. So answering this question takes us immediately to our soul and our mission as a company—it informs our approach. Our commitment is to the highest good and that naturally attracts people who want to do business with us."

Shauna describes Lucina as the culmination of her experiences and passions in a business model that expresses her philosophy that smart, soulful business can transform lives and be an engine of world benefit. Shauna and other women who share her philosophy of business are encouraged by statistics that show a boom in start-up companies led by women, and women's growing voice in established companies that are re-tooling to reflect a deeper commitment to the goal of business success and social good.

Another wonderful example is Hands to Hearts International, the brainchild of social entrepreneur Laura Peterson. Hands to Hearts International (HHI) works through orphanages to provide women who have had limited access to formal education or secure employment with the training necessary to fill important developmental care-giving gaps common in orphanage care. HHI transforms the health and development of babies in orphanages by training orphanage caregivers, as well as local women in need of employment, to provide a child-centered system of care. Trainees learn the language, social, cognitive, and physical skills necessary for healthy early childhood development — how they can promote a child's growth in each area — as well as the vital importance of attachment and bonding. Additional women are then hired as caregivers with the support of HHI, and the orphanage provides individualized nanny-like care to the babies and young children awaiting their adoptive families.

Laura's inspiration to launch Hands to Hearts International came from a decade of working with profoundly troubled children identified through social service programs, and from the realization that many of them were so damaged by their earlier experiences that getting help at age five was already too late. For children like that, she tells me, their predictable future was failure, and likely a long struggle through the juvenile court system.

"We kept pulling these kids out of the river as they were drowning," she says. "I decided I wanted to go further up the river and find out why they were drowning, how they're getting thrown in the river in the first place, and do something about it." Her research showed the gap in early care that led to serious problems in normal development and predictable problems as the children grew. She set about to create a program through which she could reach the greatest number of children with the simplest and most cost-effective preventive care to support their development. Hands to Hearts International was born, and today has completed successful pilot programs and is expanding with programs at orphanages in India and Africa.

Hands to Hearts International began operations in February 2006, and in the first year trained 200 women and reached almost 1,000 children. The orphanages reported that results were noticeable and measurable. Children were healthier and happier, got sick less often, and when they were distressed, were easier to soothe. The women caregivers became more responsive, eager to pick babies up, and developed personal pride around the health, growth, and developmental milestones of the children they tended.

Laura describes herself as, "a businesswoman trapped inside a humanitarian," — a fitting description, as the same principles apply in both realms: solid research, careful program development, measurable goals, and successful outcomes. "I don't think there is anything new in the world. It's all about collaboration and taking good ideas and putting them together in new ways," she says. "The pieces aren't original, but how you put the pieces together is how you get the new creation."

This is the story I hear repeatedly in my conversations with women in diverse circumstances around the world. Whether they are working tirelessly to provide the most basic necessities to feed and clothe their families, or their work is in the corporate boardroom developing policies that care for employees' families and community life, they think, plan, and act from these common, life-affirming values and are willing to question the way things are in service of the way things should rightly be. They have something unique and valuable to contribute in every facet of the world of business, commerce, and global economics.

Einstein has reminded us that "the important thing is not to stop questioning". As my experience and the stories I have shared here illustrate, women have a wealth of soul, experience, imagination, and collective intelligence to contribute to a climate of inquiry, equity, and creativity in business. While this century is still in its infancy, I have a visceral sense that we are witnessing an evolutionary movement in business, a leap of consciousness that has been occurring in our world and is emerging today in more felt ways. Sometimes invisibly, this movement is making inroads into the corporate world, eroding away the greed-driven paradigms from which many businesses have been operating. Sometimes visibly, we see it in new business ventures and the restructuring of existing ones. The triple bottom-line concept of striving for profits while also caring for people and the environment is gaining ground.

This conscious evolution of business invites us all to both question what is and to take the leaps of faith needed to launch purposeful actions, with confidence that actions grounded in integrity have enormous transformative powers. As we continue to strive as individuals and in business, to use our minds in the service of our hearts, integrity gains traction and, I believe, can prevail in our world.

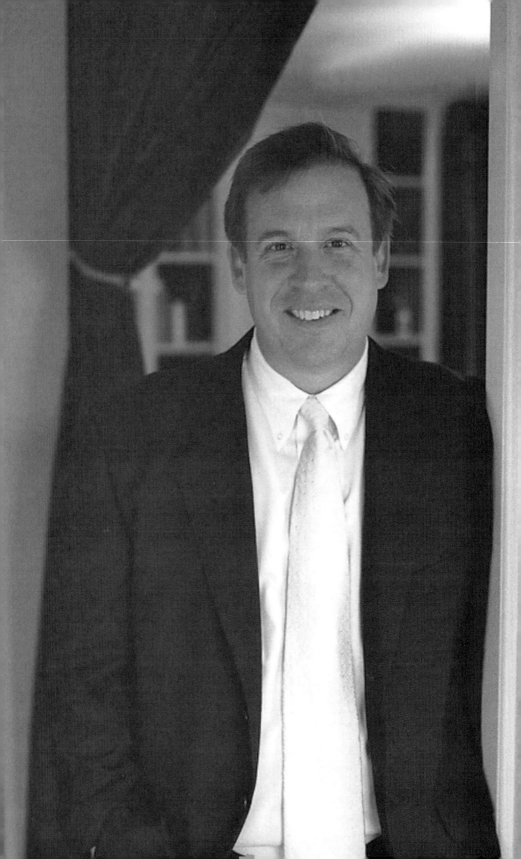

# DAVID FREES:

# CHAPTER 34

# The Language of Abundance

B usiness is a sacred undertaking. If this idea rings true, then you are well on your way as an evolved and spiritual thinker. If this concept seems shocking or counterintuitive — great. You are officially on the verge of a valuable and potentially transformative new way of thinking.

Business is a source of abundance, not scarcity. And, if business is a connection to the source of all abundance, then better communications yield better, more profitable businesses. In the right hands, better businesses can, in turn, lead to the manifestation of abundance, new ways of thinking, and new realities. Shocking? Just wait, there's more.

## Business Transforms the World and Creates Wealth

There is no true scarcity. Decades ago, in *Unlimited Wealth,* Paul Zane Pilzer, an Ivy League economist, called our attention to the unlimited power of humankind to overcome scarcity and create new wealth through our thoughts. Pilzer described how, at each historic phase when a resource was apparently disappearing, a new resource was discovered, resulting in abundance. In the 1960s, for example, when international experts declared that our worldwide oil resources would be exhausted within decades, advancements in automobile technology doubled gas mileage for cars. New technologies also

David Frees has been called a "Grandmaster" of enhanced communication skills by Steve Forbes, Editor-In-Chief of *Forbes* magazine, and a "communications skills genius" by Cheri Hill of Sage International. He is an internationally known speaker on the topics of Leadership, Persuasion, Enhanced Communications, and marketing. David has helped individuals, businesses, corporations, academic institutions, and nonprofit organizations around the world to become more powerful, creative, and profitable. He is author of *The Language of Parenting* (Red Wire, 2003), and lives in Pennsylvania with his wife and three children. To receive email tips, strategies, tactics, and alerts, visit www.davidfrees.com.

allowed us to discover and tap previously unknown oil fields. Suddenly, the oil resources were able to sustain us for many more decades even as worldwide demand soared. That was human ingenuity at work.

Think about it. Throughout history, business has functioned to transform ideas into reality and, in so doing, create wealth and a better quality of life. Businessmen and women have broken boundaries previously thought to be permanent and altered reality for the better.

§ In the 18th century, it appeared that the world's population was on the verge of mass starvation. Technology and business transformed the world, however, and our population has doubled again and again since that time. While there is still hunger in the world, human thought and technology are now working to solve the real problem, which is distribution, not the production of food itself.

§ Small pox and polio once threatened the lives of children and adults worldwide, until scientists and business, political, and religious leaders committed themselves to the eradication of those diseases. In recent years, the businessmen and women of Rotary International have funded and carried out the eradication of polio though the Polio Plus program, which they branded, promoted, and funded using their business skills and models. The eradication of polio began as an idea. It became a shared reality.

§ At one point, it looked as if North America was in danger of becoming deforested and that we would never have enough trees to meet our building and manufacturing needs. Forward-thinking businesspeople, however, developed and executed a plan to preserve our remaining forests and to develop sustainable and renewable forests for commercial use.

Business is also capable of creating human benefits from thin air. Only recently the software and computer industries arose from pure thought. There is no physical reality to the algorithms that make up computer codes. Software is just a mathematical expression of human thought. And, computer chips are essentially made from sand—an abundant resource. It was the idea of transforming sand into silicon chips that made this technology possible, and it was business that made the computer industry a reality.

Now, computers and software, which didn't even exist until very recently, allow us to make profound changes in the way we do business, design our world, and bring about change. They allow us to model storms and auto crashes, and to create other tools that can avoid or limit human and animal suffering. And the computer industry created hundreds of billions of dollars of wealth — billions of it being used to transform the world through the Gates Foundation, which has now partnered with Warren Buffet's foundation to create a historically unparalleled opportunity for private philanthropy to change the world.

## A Surprising Tool for Abundance

Charitable and business-based foundations have a greater ability to target problems and to spend for solutions than many nations. As a verse of the Upanishads sates, "They took abundance from abundance and all that was left was abundance." Ignore that tool and you may be ignoring a profound spiritual experience of co-creating your world. Ignoring your business success and your clients or customers borders on the immoral. Achieving business success is a sacred duty.

If that astonishes you, you're not alone. Many people have been conditioned to believe that business is materially focused and selfish, if not profoundly evil. That belief is a lens that profoundly alters the ways in which you may have interpreted the world, up until now. In that worldview, business creates wealth based solely on the concepts of scarcity and uses up human capital without regard to the spiritual affects it has on the world and those of us who live here. Look around you. When the world is viewed through that lens, there are plenty of examples to support this belief.

But usually, it is not that business fails to create wealth, abundance, and opportunity, but that people fail to allocate wealth or allow themselves to enjoy the new quality of life. We fail to take advantage of the opportunities that business has created for a better life. As labor saving devices are developed, we most often use them to simply make more time for work rather than using this time for our loved ones, to improve the world, or for spiritual development. Does owning a dishwasher and a car allow more time for meditation, religion, and spiritual practice? Yes, it does. In practice, do we use our time in that way? No. We make choices about the opportunities that we are given. And for some time now, many of us have been making bad choices.

But business has an undeniable sacred and spiritual quality. It is one of the most profound and prolific sources of abundance in the world. You can use this tool to transform your life and the world, to manifest original ideas as physical reality, and to eliminate scarcity.

When a new idea is developed, the world and the universe

reward the creator of this new wealth as a way of saying thank you. People buy a product or service. They use their dollars, for which they have worked hard, to say, "I value what you have done." And if financial reward from business effort is a gift, then it should not be forsaken.

For years I always picked up the tab when a meal was over. I gave gifts, made charitable pledges, and shared my wealth—but, I was unable to accept gifts from others. For whatever reason, I had to be the giver. Then someone told me that when I refused her gift, I deprived her of the happiness of giving. I was simply being selfish. This realization made me happier, pleasantly surprised those around me, and cut my dining and entertainment budget substantially.

Business success comes from the creation of an improvement in the life of others. And when you achieve that goal, you have to be able to accept the rewards. You must stop being selfish by denying the abundance that you have helped to create through your business efforts. You must stop being a barrier to the flow of greater wealth and abundance into this world, and instead become a conduit.

It is your sacred duty to improve your business, to manifest more for yourself and for others, and, in improving your business, to accept that gift of wealth and abundance. You deserve it, so welcome this duty into your life, practice it, and make a habit of using the tools to help you to do more, make more, and share more.

## The Secret of Abundance: Enhanced Communication

Communications strategies are the foundation of co-creating abundance and happiness for yourself and others. Fortunately, they are also skills that can be acquired and intentionally honed throughout life. Communications mastery is demonstrated every day in the spiritual world, in the business world, and in the worlds of politics and sales, among others. If you are interested in becoming a master of abundance, then focus your efforts on whatever spiritual practice you desire; but draw on the skills of master communicators wherever you find them.

When you begin to pay attention to these masters, you will discover that great communicators share certain values, traits, and beliefs. They all seem to use certain tactics of communication. These skills serve their masters well. How? When you are an accomplished communicator, you become more creative and you shorten the time from conception of a new idea to reality. You create and communicate ideas or help others to be more creative. You implement more quickly. You convince others who would benefit to discover, to share, and to help you to realize your new reality. When that happens, you are rewarded more abundantly than ever before. And because master communicators share and develop teams and excite those around them, their new wealth enhances the lives of others. The better, more transformational, exciting, or helpful your idea is, the more it improves people's lives — locally, or around the world.

The strategies of great communicators are few but essential. The good news is that you're likely already using these skills in some area of your life. The magic comes when you begin to apply these principles more often and in new contexts, like in your business or profession.

The following six principles and qualities define the master communicator and seem to lead inevitably to business success:

1. Master communicators are flexible, charismatic, and generous. In every undertaking, they want you to receive something that is important to you and in which you find happiness.

2. They understand the limits of language and how to overcome those limits. They know that the words they use do not have the same meaning to all listeners. They understand that as humans we each experience language in our own way. And, they use this knowledge to improve life.

3. They are forgiving of themselves and others. As a consequence, when things go wrong, as they always do, they honor the effort and move on. This, in turn, endears them to those around them — including customers, clients, and employees — so master communicators are often forgiven when they make mistakes. They keep going and make success in any undertaking more likely.

4. Leaders who derive their power and energy from great communications skills are creative and inspire creativity in others. Clarity of communication is essential to creativity. Because they truly know what it is that they are seeking, they can work with those who share that clear vision toward realizing their goal even more effortlessly. Clarity of intent yields results.

5. They are congruent in their communications and their actions, and communications are aligned with their values. This gives them an unflagging faith, confidence, and energy. It connects them with the part of themselves that transcends the purely physical.

6. They have a plan. Great communicators are outcome based. They know what they want, and what they intend — not only in the big picture, but in each and every aspect of communication. They always know the intended result before they start to speak.

# CHAPTER THIRTY-FOUR

Now let's examine each of these characteristics in a bit more detail.

## The Power of Flexibility

If you want to succeed in the spiritual aspects of business, then you must cultivate flexibility. Reality often evolves much differently than we originally anticipate. I was originally trained to have a plan for everything, and mistakenly believed that things would actually go as I expected them to. But this does have a purpose. What I learned was that having a plan gave me the human courage to begin the process of actively making my business better. Since I had faith and a plan, I wasn't afraid to act. I was able to start bringing ideas into reality.

The true purpose of a plan is to attain clarity of intention. If you then let go of the outcome, you have enhanced your connection with the universe and success becomes more likely. Flexibility allows us to adjust when a particular aspect of our plan or our communication isn't working. Instead of giving up, great communicators simply adjust and try something new, trusting that the clarity itself has set in motion the forces that will bring their idea into physical reality.

## Enhancing the Happiness of Others

Great communication also arises from a selfish unselfishness. When we look for something that brings happiness to our team, business partners, co-creators, or customers, then we also gain. Great business leaders consider what interests, fulfills, inspires, and motivates those around them. They seek to bring others into their illuminated world in a way that gives the other parties something important to them. Great communicators also help those around them to achieve clarity, because once there is clarity and shared vision, the rest is much easier. Richard Branson became a billionaire in just this way. He has made a fortune treating customers and employees very, very well. *Fast Company* magazine recently quoted Branson as saying, "The reason I went into business originally was not because I wanted to make a lot of money, but because the experiences I had with business were dire and I wanted to create an experience that I and my friends could enjoy." This man profits wildly from caring about others.

## Forgiveness as a Key to Business Success

No business undertaking is without problems, and no leader

is without fault...so, great communicators develop a practice and a habit of forgiveness.

When things go wrong, an enormous amount of human energy is often used in recrimination. Projects are left undone and relationships are disrupted. Customers, clients, and employees leave. Forgiveness allows the business of transformation to proceed. And great communicators know that by modeling forgiveness they are likely to be granted forgiveness by those around them. They even forgive others when forgiveness is not forthcoming in return. If you can't do it for the other person, simply do it for yourself. Then you can move on to the spiritual fulfillment of your business.

## Creativity and Inspiration

Truly great communication often results in a heightened level of personal creativity. Even if you're not personally the creative force of your business, it is certain that you will develop ideas capable of transforming your life and the lives of others. It happens to all of us almost every day. The problem is that we fail to act. How many times have you had an idea and failed to act, only to see another business develop and profit from it? Did that product or service improve the lives of those who bought it? Is it OK just to let others do the work of transformation?

Creativity is inspired by clarity and great communication skills coupled with flexibility and openness. People have radically different ways of being creative and implementing their ideas. Great communicators notice these traits, encourage them, and facilitate them.

## Congruency Makes it All Happen

Finally, the business leaders who achieve greatness and transform the world are those who speak and act congruently. They do this in two equally important ways. At the basic level, great communicators use language effectively, in part because they make sure that the words they chose match their tone of voice, body posture, and facial expressions. Word choice probably makes up less than 10 percent of overall communication. Tonality, posture, speed of voice, facial expressions, and many other factors are actually more important. When there is a conflict between the words and the overall expression, the tone of voice and other factors are what win out.

Next, great business leaders act in a way that is congruent with their beliefs and their basic values. If your plan is contrary to a value that you hold, you cannot achieve true transformational results. That is why it is so important to remember that business is not about scarcity. It need not be selfish—business success does not come at the costs of another's business failure. True business success expands the possibilities and can transform the world. Discover what your values are and build your business practices in a way that is true to those values, and you cannot fail. You will create a new reality that may exceed your wildest expectations.

This congruency has produced many startling examples of positive change and enrichment. John Eastly, founder of the Amazon Herb Company, was plundering the Amazon. His business methods were far from sustainable, and by his own admission, less than noble. Yet, in a moment of spiritual and business inspiration he transformed his business and created a company that was truly aligned with his inner values. Today, that company pays indigenous people of the Amazon to harvest valuable and renewable herbs and plants. They make more money than they would if the jungles were clear-cut. Their lives are better, John's life is better, and our lives are better.

But, this is not a story in isolation. In addition to the innumerable individual and small business transformations, there are thousands of such stories at the corporate level, such as those of Anita Roddick of the Body Shop, Oprah Winfrey, Richard Branson, Warren Buffett, Suze Orman, Bill and Melinda Gates, and so many more. Remember that these people didn't start wealthy. By aligning their values, they and their companies grew beyond their own expectations. The world was a better place as a result of their gifts, and it rewarded them financially.

You see this happening over and over again at the local level when small stores fundamentally change the way they do business in order to compete with Wal-Mart. They are rewarded by loyal customers who love the extra attention and personalized services. You see this when a medical, dental, or legal practice finds a new way of serving its clients, patients, and customers. Suddenly, they become radically more successful and more in demand. Do they raise their prices? Sure. But can they do even more good for the world? Yes. Chances are, the changes they made were fundamental, profound, well intentioned, and in alignment with their values. These businesspeople are rewarded with abundance, so they can meet their own needs as well as investing some of their wealth in socially responsible funds, in their own businesses, or in the form of donations of time or money to worthy causes. That investment may create new jobs in new places.

But, to make this work you must be willing to accept payment—

from customers or clients *and* from the universe—for your innovation, care, and concern. The world is full of well-intentioned business people, doctors, veterinarians, massage therapists, allied healthcare practitioners, and others who want to make life better, but whose businesses fail because they equate accepting significant payment as a betrayal of their principals.

I learned as a young lawyer how misguided this can be. When families fought about wills and trusts I would feel sorry for them and discount my fees. What was I doing? Instead of helping them—or myself—I was allowing and facilitating bad behavior. When I began to charge properly and fairly, family members were forced to truly examine their positions and find solutions to expensive problems that had previously seemed insurmountable.

Many doctors have observed that patients who don't pay at least something for their services treat the doctor's staff badly and fail to take the actions necessary to get well. They simply don't value the free advice. And, as I am fond of saying, you cannot take care of the world when you haven't taken care of your spouse, your kids, and the college tuition payments. So, build a better business. Build a business in alignment with your values that enriches your life and the lives of those around you in some way. Take the proceeds to the bank, and if you must worry about something, start worrying about how to spend, share, enjoy, and use that wealth. If you are serious about taking any business to the next level of success then this should interest you.

## Putting it All Together

Many of us who are socially conscious, spiritually motivated, and self aware have mistakenly come to believe that businesses are bad, selfish, and uncaring. But, despite the misalignment of many individual business, business itself can be a sacred undertaking, a means of co-creating our world in accordance with our own deeply held values and beliefs. Only when you are aligned will you truly succeed. When we allow our perspective to shift, however, and master the arts of intention and communication, any reluctance to accept the wealth and bounty of our efforts gives way to a new sense of duty to create, to receive, and to share abundance.

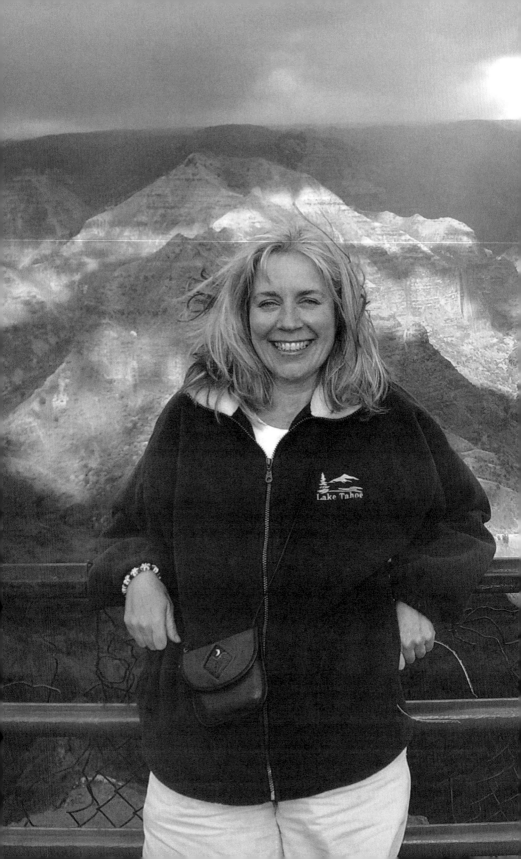

# JEANNE HOUSE:

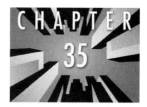

CHAPTER
35

# Defying Gravity

In the musical Wicked, adapted from Gregory MacGuire's book, *Wicked: The Life and Times of the Wicked Witch of the West*, the Wizard of Oz is starting to get out of hand. The Land of Oz has become repressed and lifeless, its citizens having forgotten who they are as they project all of their personal power onto the wizard. He, in turn, is so full of himself and devoid of respect for the people of Oz that, when they come to him with a concern he bellows, " *I am Oz, the Great and the Terrible! Whooooooo Areeeeeeee, Youuuuuuuu?"*

All of this takes place long before Dorothy and her friends come along, during the time when the Wicked Witch of the West and Good Witch of the North are growing up. Unlike in L. Frank Baum's original rendition, *The Wonderful Wizard of Oz*, however, the two witches are not inherently wicked or good from the start. Rather, when they are in school together, Elphaba, the future Wicked Witch, is very unpopular while Glinda, the budding Good Witch, is very popular, indeed.

But because Elphaba doesn't care what people think of her, she listens to her inner guidance and finally breaks free of the repressive atmosphere of the Wizard's Oz. Glinda, on the other hand, who does not want to lose the adoration she receives for being so "good," chooses to stay right where she is.

The most riveting part of the story comes when Elphaba realizes that she is beginning to know less and less—and that this is being

Jeanne House, M.A., has headed up the marketing and sales efforts of two book distributors, Summit Beacon and Associated Publishers Group, as well as holding prior positions with NBC-TV and Miami University. She has a postgraduate degree in Consciousness Studies, and is completing a second degree in Transformational Psychology. She is currently the President of Sol Communications and the Marketing and Sales Director of Elite Books. Her passion and specialty is *soul communication*—communicating directly to the soul needs of her clients and bringing their messages to their readers. For more information, visit her online at www.SoulCommuncation.com.

encouraged throughout the Land of Oz. In order to escape, she swings her legs around a broomstick and, lo and behold, it lifts her way up into the air in a spewing kaleidoscope of violet, aqua, and teal. Little did she know that by defying Oz, she would also be defying gravity! Elphaba sings:

I don't want it; I can't want it anymore...
Something has changed within me, something is *not the same*.
I'm through with playing by the *rules* of someone else's game.
Too late for second guessing...too late to go back to sleep.
It's time to trust my feelings, to close my eyes and leap!
It's time to try defying gravity,
I think I'll try defying gravity,
And you can't *pull me down*...

Elphaba is ready for a new experience and takes a big leap into the unknown. We all crave these new, fresh, vital experiences. In fact, they keep us from getting rusty or stuck in our ways. We just forget that we always have this choice to make a leap into a new idea, a new concept, or to replace an old way of being with a new outlook. Like Elphaba, we have the option to see the world that we live in with fresh new eyes on a daily basis. Then, and only then, can we experience the freedom that Elphaba does when she leaves her outworn perceptions and behaviors behind.

In *The Reflexive Universe*, physicist Arthur Young proves theoretically that we as a species have formally been evolving entirely unaware of our own evolution. But in this current time period, we now have the unprecedented opportunity to become conscious of our own evolution and take back the controls. The first syllable of the word evolution is *love* spelled backwards. We can view this as attachment to our circumstances and our inability to pull away from them in order to make wiser choices. This is what happens anytime we are attached to our present circumstances and resistant to change. But we can defy gravity by losing our attachment to matter and turning inward to define what really matters to us first, before we take any action.

Now this is a horse of a different color. These new rules suggest at best that we take time out for reflection and not get caught up in fantasies of perfection—because there is *no such thing* as perfection in the time and space universe. The rules of the past encouraged us to be in constant action in order to get traction on our projects and our personal worlds. But this left us little time to be fully present in what we were doing, and we easily become hostage to our "to do" lists and our spreadsheets. This didn't allow much room for directing our own lives moment to moment.

The Wizard of Oz is correct; he is both great and terrible—great in that he serves as necessary reminder that we are the rulers of our own universe; and terrible in that he denies that same right to the individual. The Wizard of Oz does not respect the right of individuals to have power over themselves, nor does he respect the collective intellectual capacity or interconnectedness of the whole. Consequently, the entire Land of Oz is devoid of joy and spirit.

When Elphaba makes the leap, she makes a claim to the universe that she has the right to do be doing what she is doing. No one escapes this part—not even the great avatars. While meditating under the Bo Tree, Buddha himself made the earth-touching *mudra,* or hand position, that signified his right to be seek enlightenment, even as an apparition was tempting him to believe in all of these time, space, and matter things. Jesus, too, was tempted in the wilderness, and he challenged these erroneous notions also.

No outside thing can hold power over us *unless we let it.*

Elphaba leaves her world of limitations. Her new world has infinite possibilities! She finally realizes that it has been she who creates her own reality all along. In a classical theory such as general relativity, objects have definite locations and velocities—but this excludes *our free-will choice* from the equation. In a quantum world, everything is in a state of constant flux. The problem with devising a quantum version of general relativity is that particles do not have definite locations and velocities. Therefore, they can be shape-shifters and shape our reality when we signal them to do so via our thoughts, feelings, and intentions.

Attitude is everything in our lives and our projects, because the quantum universe is susceptible to our every thought, word, and deed. Our beliefs—true or false, positive or negative, creative or destructive—do not simply exist in *our minds;* they also interact with the infinite possibilities of the quantum universe. These energies ultimately show up in our physical lives and even in our bodies. So it is critical to focus on what we *do want* versus what we *don't want.* Then all of the energy of the universe goes to work to manifest our desires.

Even our cells are intelligent, responding to everything we are thinking, feeling, and doing. When we experience a thought or feeling we send a signal to the membrane of our cells, which in turn signals the DNA to read a specific blueprint that correlates directly with our command. It is like having a *genie in our genes* who responds to our every thought and says, "Your wish is my command!"

Cell biologist Bruce Lipton, who has pioneered the application of the principles of quantum physics, says that energy in the form of beliefs can affect our biology. He also says that each cell is an intelligent being. Single cells are capable of learning through environmental experiences, and they are able to create cellular memories.

Our emotions and behaviors shape our brains as they stimulate the neural pathways to either reinforce old patterns or initiate new ones. Our gene expression has a lot to do with our subjective experiences; in fact, researchers show that 90 percent of all genes are in some way engaged and cooperating with signals from both the inside and the outside environment.

So, if we believe in ourselves with every cell of our being, then the universe responds accordingly. This opens the doors to the all the power of the universe! It sets the stage for both our inner universe and our outer universe to reflect back to us and ultimately manifest our dreams, wishes, and desires. The only requirement is that we do not get attached to how it unfolds or how long it takes — because those are simply time and space issues.

Scientist Vladimir Poponin performed an experiment in 1992 in which he took air out of a container in order to create a vacuum. What remained were photons, or particles of light. He measured the distribution of these photons within the container and found that it was a completely random. This was no surprise. But then he put some human DNA into the container and measured the distribution of the photons again. This time he discovered that the photons all lined up along the DNA. After adding the DNA, the photons became ordered. He then took the DNA back out of the container and the photons *remained* ordered.

This means that even without physical matter of DNA, the energy of the ordered photons was still present. This energy permeates all of existence. It is the stuff of magic! It is our energy source. What we do with it is our choice.

So, why is Elphaba the only one able to defy the gravity of her situation?

String theory tells us that parallel universes can exist at the same time. Like these parallel strings, each of us is operating from our own vantage point, depending on the view we have from our own personal universe or string. This viewpoint governs all of our actions, but what we often don't know is that there are infinite realities and infinite perspectives. Every person chooses to see life from one perspective; no one of us has the whole picture.

In 1957, Princeton physicist Hugh Everett, III, suggested that at every level of our lives there are many, many moments, possibilities, and outcomes playing out simultaneously. Though we are not necessarily aware of them, they are all happening at the same time. He called these parallel possibilities.

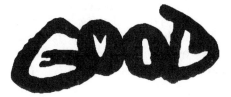

For example, what do you choose to see: good or evil? *It's all relative.* The theory of relativity is relative to whoever perceives reality at the moment. For instance, one person's good could be another persons evil, depending on their point of view. All I see is up to me. Albert Einstein said: "Reality is merely an illusion, albeit a persistent one."

If we don't realize that it is actually we who make the choice in how we perceive reality, then when our circumstances change and our inner reality is no longer congruent with the people, conditions, and situations surrounding us, we ask ourselves, *"Who Moved My Reality?"*

We are movers of our own reality. We ourselves are the mighty work of the ages. Trials, betrayals, tornadoes, and meltdowns all are designed to loose us from our rigid programming. These powerful events in our lives clear the cobwebs from our minds and hearts so that Spirit can emerge unencumbered and we feel desire once again. Desire is really *deity siring* through us. In order to pull way from the gravity of the situation, we need to get *wicked!*

## Our Inner Broomstick

Separately, all of the original characters of The Wizard of Oz were powerless until they got together and joined forces. It was as if they helped one another to overcome each of their shortcomings and fears of the unknown. They didn't know that these fears were simply illusions. As long as they gave their power away to ghosts and illusions of their minds, they were powerless.

They created their own fears by affirming, *"I do believe, I do believe, I do believe in spooks,"* and then they were off to find a wizard to save them. But they couldn't reclaim their own power until The Great and Powerful Oz assigned them the collective mission of getting the broomstick back from the evil witch. Of course, this was really taking back the power that they had originally given away. This mission forced them to come up with *brand new solutions*, which they never would've been able to achieve with their previous attitudes and beliefs!

Was the wicked witch evil, or is evil something like free-floating gravity? Unlike in Baum's original story, in which the Good Witch is a representative of the highest good of all the land, Wicked's Glinda cannot have an evil — or inspired — thought or feeling without running the risk of losing the power of her popularity. Elphaba sings:

Glinda come with me...
Think of what we can do together...
Together were unlimited!
Together we will be the greatest team there's ever been.
Because we were made to defy gravity
with you and I defying gravity they'll never bring us down!
I heard it said that people come into our lives for a reason,
bringing something we must learn,
and we are lead to those who help us most to grow
if we let them and we help them in return.
Well I don't know if I believe that is true, but I know
I am who I am today because I knew you.

Most of the people of Oz believe that Elphaba is wicked because she doesn't play by their rules. But not Glinda. She knows deep down inside that Elphaba is taking back the power that she once projected onto the Wizard of Oz. Glinda also knows that she, too, should defy him, but is paralyzed with fear and cannot move. She cries out:

*Elphaba, why couldn't you have stayed calm for once, instead of flying off the handle? I hope you are happy!*

Most of the time "flying off the handle" is not a good thing, but this time it is. This time Elphaba doesn't have a meltdown. Instead, she pauses and takes control of her emotions, listens deep within, and then follows the inner guidance that advises her to take the leap of faith.

Glinda represents the old guard, corporate model, playing by the rules that she knows are wrong in order to climb the ladder to power and "success." Elphaba represents new vision and paradigm change in business.

## Balancing the Broom: New Laws of Relativity

If we see the broomstick as a seesaw, then we can imagine two sides moving with a steady center. We must become this center between the opposing poles. But this center is different for everyone, depending on how out-of-alignment their energies might be against the backdrop of the universal ebb and flow.

Balance is always a moving target and always relative to what we have previously experienced. We can measure ourselves by sensing how much we live from *time* in our lives and how much *space* we are giving ourselves. We align ourselves with the universal currents by taking the necessary time out when our energy gets stuck in gravity. Conversely, when we have too much space and we are not galvanizing the necessary gravity to keep us tethered to our projects, we need a bit of tightening up. We may need to establish daily routines that can become a part of the larger practice in our lives.

## Gravity Busters

1. It's easy to get caught up in the experience of "too much to do, too little time." One way to steal time is to catch ourselves just as we are starting to feel overwhelmed and make a psychological reversal from a negative reaction to a neutral one. We can do this by using one of the many Energy Psychology techniques. Most of us live in a "try harder" world, but maybe we should just get smarter. What used to take up a lot of our time in the past can now be handled in just a few short sessions of Energy Psychology.

   For instance Psych-K, created by Rob Williams, is a tool that is effective at reprogramming our subconscious mind. Many of our self-defeating habits and thoughts can fail to shift because our subconscious programming runs on a different program than our conscious mind. In order to reverse this, we can harness its power with a few short exercises that reverse the patterns in both our right and our left brain simultaneously.

2. When we are stuck in a mood or a violent thought, we can visualize violet fire encapsulating that mood or thought so that it raises its vibration and frees us up from the gravitational energy. Ultra-violet light is like fire because it is emitted by stars and is full of energy.

   This light is composed of particles of magnetic energy preconditioned to remove the magnetism of old conditioned beliefs. It demagnetizes energy patterns that have accumulated in us over the years. The light coalesces around the muck that has accumulated from our paying too close attention to mundane life and living in strife. So now we can simply pass each particle of density through this flame and let go of blame.

   Fire is the core of everything, and since fire vibrates higher than our physical mind and body, it helps us to make the necessary leap out of our own limited perspective and into the cosmic solution to the negative thoughts and ideas that tend to sit our mind, our subconscious, our feelings, and our bodies.

When we visualize the violet light and affirm its power to transform us, it responds to our affirmation, dissolves the sticky substance between our cells, and frees up our energy for our work in the present. After doing this for a while, we buy some time so that, when our emotions start to act up, we can easily say, "Oh there are my emotions doing a dance. They expect me to get upset and mentally attached so I become uncontrollable in my thoughts, actions, words, and deeds."

3. Forgiveness is another key to emotional mastery. When we judge ourselves and those around us, we not only freeze a portion of our own energy with these thoughts, but also put an energetic hex on those we are judging. This is ultimate witchcraft.

When we experience mercy or compassion for ourselves and others, we tie right back into the universal flow. When we let go and let the spirit flow through us unimpeded, our desired outcomes move toward us at the speed of light.

4. We can also save time by using our intuition and not just our heart or our head. Intuition is a system-wide process in which the heart and the brain are involved together in responding to intuitive information. Rollin McCraty, chief scientist at the Institute of HeartMath, wrote in regards to a recent study he performed on intuition that the dilemma over intuition (whether it is based on past experiences or involves actual perceptions of some things apart in space or ahead of time) is comparable in many respects to the dilemma of physics in the early twentieth century. A number of now famous "anomalous" experiments in quantum physics repeatedly demonstrated that the subatomic world is a domain in which there is virtually instantaneous "communication" of information between particles separated by vast regions of space, and in which particles act as if they have "knowledge" of events before these events actually happen. In fact, the research revealed that our hearts detects future events seven seconds prior to our experiencing the event. It alerts the brain, which in turn alerts the body.

Although this defied explanation by classical physics, these phenomena of non-local communication are now accepted as established scientific fact and have led to the revolutionary understanding that such space/time-defying communication of information is the result of the inherently interconnected nature of the quantum world.

We all have billions of cells in our bodies, but until we master these, how can we become masters of our outside world? How can we make leaps of faith beyond the limitations of the fear-based, time-crunched, status quo? By defying gravity, of course! Using our free will to shift perspective, we can reclaim our power to create meaningful change in business and in our own personal lives.

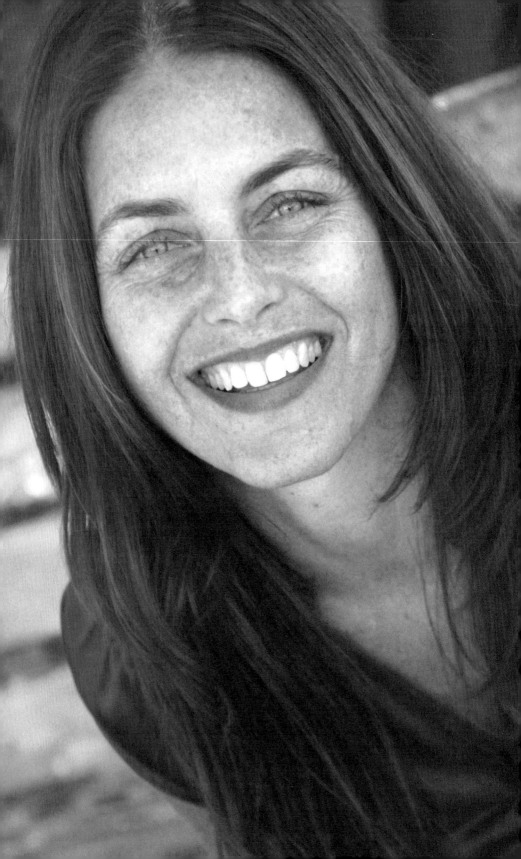

# Bari Tessler:

# Three Gateways to Money Initiation

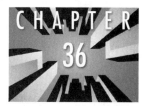

I t's a bit odd, don't you think, that our daily lives as adults are tightly interwoven with the reality of money, and yet the majority of us are never taught how to work with it — much less have a *conscious relationship* with it? No, it's more than a bit odd. It's crazy. As crazy as it would be to do away with driver's training requirements. Imagine if our parents simply bought us a car at age 16, handed us the keys, and said, "Hop in and just figure it out as you go." Though it is often unspoken, we unfortunately get this same message with respect to money. That, to me, is insane; and because collective insanity on a widespread scale undermines our true potential as humans, I felt a pull from deep within my heart to do something about our relationship with money.

Do you remember your formal initiation ceremony into adulthood? How the candles and firelight flickered on everyone's faces, lighting them with a warm reddish glow during the part where the leader of the ceremony presented you with challenges that would teach and test you about the ways of money? Well, I definitely do not have any memories of a rite of passage into relationship with money, and from what I am seeing in my work, almost no one else in our culture does, either — because such an event is simply not a part of our cultural fabric. For the most part, the whole realm of money is very much a shadow, a taboo of sorts, and seems to be one of the last unexplored frontiers in our lives. Fortunately, however, a noticeable shift is beginning to occur.

**Bari Tessler has a Masters in Somatic Psychology from Naropa University. She is a teacher, therapist, and speaker, and founder of Conscious Bookkeeping. After many years in the Psychology Field, Bari jumped careers and moved into financial and bookkeeping services. The Conscious Bookkeeping organization is an integration of these two fields, providing a financial support team for individuals, couples, families, and businesses. The team consists of financial therapists, financial coaches, and bookkeeping trainers who offer services and education to help people transform their relationship with money on a practical, psychological, and spiritual level. Visit Bari online at www.consciousbookkeeping.com.**

In the history of humanity, when something has held a place of great importance in the daily life of people in a given culture, it has often been directly taught and addressed during initiations or rites of passage that function to provide support during awkward but natural periods of transition into new life roles. They facilitate the completion of one cycle and the beginning of another. In addition, initiation rituals offer the chance to learn how to live in society and can help infuse mundane day-to-day activities with a sense of the sacred.

While pursuing my master's degree in Somatic Psychotherapy, I did my thesis work on creating space for young women to go through an initiation regarding their relationship with body image. Then, after several years of work as a counselor and psychotherapist, I began going through my own rite of passage: an unscheduled, unexpected initiation into the reality of money. There was a large, ominous, $60,000 dark cloud of a school loan that I had ignored while in school. The payments were about to begin, and the loan ultimately became the catalyst for my awakening within the realm of money. Until then, I had been the kind of person who threw away every bank statement that came in the mail. I never even opened them, and never reconciled my bank account. Feeling the weight of the school loan on my back, I realized that I would never successfully continue onward unless I learned how to work with and relate to money.

## The Meanings of Initiation

When you think about initiation, what comes to mind? For some people, it can be a grand turning point in life that involves going through some kind of challenge or test—a gateway, if you will—leading to a profound transformation into a higher level of awareness, action, and consciousness. For some, this test is uncomfortable and feels like a trial by fire. In a sense, this is true—they're burning through old layers of beliefs, behaviors, stories, and experiences. For others, an initiation is a coming of age. I've heard people as young as 18 and as old as 70 say that they would like to become adults in terms of their relationship with money. For others still, initiation is defined as a shedding of old ways and parts of ourselves that are no longer serving us. Conscious Bookkeeping, the work I created with my mentor, Tamara Slayton, incorporates qualities of each of these to guide people through an intentional initiation regarding their relationship to money, finances, and economics.

The path of Conscious Bookkeeping has been intentionally and carefully designed to lead people into challenges at the edge of their comfort zone—the kind of challenges that can lead to profound transformation. This transformation often results in five valuable gifts within people's experience of life: They walk away with more clarity, intimacy, knowledge, ease, and success.

## The Three Gateways

On this path, the process of initiation into conscious relationship with money begins by passing through three gateways: financial therapy, values-based bookkeeping, and life visioning. It doesn't matter which gateway a person enters through first, as each of them lead naturally into the others. The three gateways are interrelated in such a way that each supports the others in a dynamic, symbiotic process. For example, though it is a unique way to do one's books, just using a values-based bookkeeping system alone could never produce the greatest potential results without being part of a dance that includes a process of inquiry into our innermost beliefs, wounds, and hopes around the concept of money. And it would be a nearly lifeless and mechanical process without being wedded to the process of life visioning, in which goals, plans, and passionate life dreams are clarified and outlined. In this way, each of the gateways works with and supports the others. When clients and students of Conscious Bookkeeping are presented with our framework, it's up to them to choose the gateway they feel most drawn to walk through first.

## Financial Therapy

Many people have done some form of inner healing work, be it psychotherapy, coaching, or individual self-inquiry. Often, however, even people who have done significant self-exploration have never directly faced their relationship with money. In a sense, they have never shared their money story.

Because money plays such a key role in day-to-day living, it is often closely entangled with our core psychological issues, challenges, and wounds. To free ourselves of constraints in relation to money, then, is to seek healing for these core wounds in our psyche. And to heal these core wounds, we must inquire into their nature with gentle courage.

At the gateway of financial therapy, our challenges, frustrations, fears, and joys around money are like a red tab on the wrapper of a gift package within our mind. When we pull the tab, the packaging unravels to reveal what lies within: the real issues beneath our surface emotions around money. When we see what's really driving our frustrations, fears, and struggles with money, however, it certainly doesn't look like a gift. In fact, it looks more like an old, black, tangled ball of psychological yuck. For most of us, it isn't until we have gone through the process of psychological and emotional healing that we can see the reward. It can be challenging work, this process—but then, most initiations involve inherent challenge. In the end, we come out with skills that allow us to begin polishing up not only the yucky mess of our limitations around money, but other recurring tangles, as well. This is because the way we relate with money is often the way we relate with most everything in life. If you heal your relationship with money, you will very likely heal other parts of your life, also.

Within the Conscious Bookkeeping method, this process of bringing awareness and understanding to our inner relationship with money is the central focus of the gateway of financial therapy. It begins with inquiring into your past experiences with money, starting with what you learned from your parents and grandparents. For example, when you look back on your memories of when your mom or dad paid bills, do you remember them as being calm, joyful, and happy, or stressed out, frustrated, or even angry? Oftentimes, the most powerful lessons about money are taught through behavior and emotion, rather than words. These unspoken, often unconscious lessons then guide us in how we earn, spend, save, borrow, and invest money. And because they are unconsciously delivered, integrated, and put into action in our own lives, they are also unconsciously passed along to our intimate partners, children, friends, and co-workers. Financial therapy is one way to end this perpetual cycle of unconsciousness around money.

This unconsciousness can show up in another area of our inner realm as well, as the secrets we hide around our money issues. From borrowing money that we never pay back, to inheriting large sums of money, to never tracking our spending and never reconciling our bank statements, there are plenty of stories about money hidden in the basement of our mind. When the stories, beliefs, and feelings we have about money are brought into the light of consciousness, however, we see that we can edit them. And that is the essence of the goal in financial therapy: to transform our unconscious stories about money into conscious tales that illuminate our path to a greater sense of freedom and happiness.

## Values-Based Bookkeeping

There is a myth out there that bookkeeping and accounting are dry and boring, but this is far from true! Bookkeeping is actually a fun and very dynamic system. You just have to use it in a way that makes it more enjoyable.

The first step in passing through the gateway of creating a values-based bookkeeping system is learning the language of accounting. This important step can empower anyone and everyone who ever believed that they were incapable, that it wasn't creative, or even simply that they should already know this stuff but for one reason or another hadn't yet learned it. And all it requires is a willingness to come face to face with things you may have heard of in passing, but avoided learning anything about: a chart of accounts, which includes reports on assets, liabilities, equity, income, and expenses; financial statements, like a profit and loss or balance sheet; and that stale cracker of bookkeeping—budgets.

In order to teach people about how to use these reports and statements, we change some of the names, and, more importantly, invite students to name categories within the reports themselves, so they more clearly resonate with a deeper sense of personal meaning. The act of renaming engages us in a process of first becoming intimate with our intentions and passions in life—our deeply held values—and then expressing those intentions, passions, and values right in the very structure of our bookkeeping system.

For example, when most people hear the word "budget," the feeling that arises in their body is one of constriction. I don't know many people who love the word budget so much that they find themselves running home to do one. The resistance most of us feel is directly related to the unconscious lessons we learned about what budgeting is: scrimping, clamping down, and generally holding tightly onto our money while we let small, precise amounts of it squeeze out into predefined categories such as rent, utilities, credit card bills, entertainment, and so on. The word budget, and the concept it traditionally represents, tends to induce an often-unnoticed attitude of fear and constriction.

We can, however, take another perspective on budgeting. We can look more deeply into this aspect of bookkeeping and ask, "What's really going on here?" What we find is that—though most people don't use it consciously in this way—a budget is a tool designed to help us align our spending patterns with our intention. The second thing we notice about budgeting is that it tries to help us map out a future plan for spending patterns that are supposed to be an expression of our intentions. From this perspective, we can see that budgeting involves a map and some intentions. So why don't we call it a "Map of Intention"? Much better, yes?

Creating a Map of Intention is more than just assigning a new name to an existing model. It is a new approach to planning how we'll spend our money in the future—an approach that is based not in fear and constriction, but in excitement and joy. Through this process, we discover where our values are being met and expressed—or unmet and unexpressed—through both our spending and making of money.

We begin by looking deeply inside and coming up with a list of all of the things that feel important to us. This can include anything that we feel is of value, such as keeping our body healthy by eating organic food and practicing yoga, donating money to a nonprofit, or going on a meditation retreat once a year. The list of values is then compared with the categories in our Map of Intention. We see immediately if all of our values are being represented in the Map, and if not, we can add categories or rename ones that are already there. For example, when one of our clients was going through this process, she asked herself: "Okay, Rent, what is that really? Rent feels like a bag of bricks tied around each of my feet. What is that money really providing me? Home…safety…love shack…a sanctuary. Ahh, much better. I'll call this category Sanctuary." For her, the word "sanctuary" reminds her of the deeper meaning of what that money brings her each month: a feeling of home, of safety. She realized the value in having a home that is a safe sanctuary, and that value is now expressed in her Map of Intention. Rather than sending off a big check each month to her landlord with fear, constriction, and some sadness that all that money is going for nothing, she shifted her perspective on what this check brings into her life. She actually began to notice as sense of happiness and gratitude when she sent it off each month. The rent check became a sanctuary check.

The value-expressing categories that are created in the Map of Intention then appear across the board in all of the other reports and financial statements. In this way, the path of Conscious Bookkeeping leads us to create an entire bookkeeping system based on our values. That just makes sense, doesn't it? But the first time people see what were once boring, dry financial reports now filled with their personally meaningful categories, they feel unexpectedly excited. These reports actually become rather fun to look at. Such a system truly empowers us in the areas where we touch the world, where we meet life and have the chance to share our gifts. This is because our values are represented directly in the system. When we use a values-based bookkeeping system to look at our current financial situation, or to plan for future saving and spending, we get direct, immediate feedback on whether or not we're spending our money in ways that align with our values and goals.

This system supports us in living true to our own highest vision for our life — but it can't work unless we use it, and use it often, which is why we invite everyone to engage with this type of bookkeeping every few days, or at least once a week. Making this into a practice involves continually cycling through a number of simple stages that turn this into a working, dynamic, life-giving system that generates frequent financial feedback. This is what the practice looks like: When we go out into the world and purchase things, we put the receipts in a little accoutrement, or wallet, or bring them home and file them in a special box. Then, every few days we enter the receipts into our Quicken or QuickBooks register. Afterward, the receipts are stored in folders that have the same names as the expense categories in our Map of Intention. This process is repeated often so that it becomes a habitual practice. When we get our bank statement each month, we reconcile the statement, print out reports, and look through them to see how well our spending behavior matches up with our Map of Intention. This is essentially a check-in process to see how well we're doing in terms of spending our money in ways that express our values.

Along the way, different people will tend to "fall asleep" at different steps. Some people check out at the grocery store and don't bring home receipts. Others fall asleep when they get to the step of printing out the reports because they're terrified to see the reality of their spending patterns. Whenever we lose awareness of what we're doing in relationship to our money, we have an opportunity to begin the process of self-inquiry into the underlying thoughts and feelings. If we're having strong feelings around seeing our reports, for example, we place our attention on the sensations and feelings that arise in our body, seeking to gain insight into what may lie beneath them, or what their true nature really is.

This cycle of steps is repeated every month, and once a year we review all of our financial information for the past year. The intention in creating a dynamic bookkeeping system like this is to help us become aware of where we go unconscious in relation to money, and to help us remain awake and aware throughout the entire cycle.

Sometimes people feel resistance when they imagine bookkeeping as a regular, ongoing practice. When this comes up, I ask them to imagine what they would feel like if they didn't exercise every couple of days, but waited, instead, to do the entire month's worth of exercise all in one day. Or if they waited until the end of the month to do a whole 30 days' worth of brushing their teeth. The consensus is always that they wouldn't feel very good at all. Unfortunately, many people wait until the end of the month to take care of all their financial business, such as gathering receipts, entering them into their register, and reconciling. Others don't even do that, choosing to wait for several months, or even an entire year, letting all of this bookkeeping work build up as they go about their lives in a state of financial unconsciousness.

Many people find that creating a little ritual helps them make conscious bookkeeping a practice. One client, for example, lights a candle, eats some chocolate, puts on her favorite music, and takes a deep breath to slow down a bit. Just stay present and in your body, and you will find the right way to make the practice special and enjoyable for you. Often, people who initially have some resistance to making bookkeeping into a regular practice end up telling us that, while it took a little time for them to adjust, the process soon started to be fun. They find themselves continuing with the system out of their own natural desire.

## Life Visioning

Why are you here on this planet? What is the real purpose of your life? What burns in your heart with a passionate glow? What things must your soul absolutely do before facing the inevitable reality of death? These are big questions, which we humans have been asking ourselves for tens of thousands of years. This is why they are a foundation to the initiation process of the Conscious Bookkeeping path. In fact, the ultimate goal of this practice is to discover and live true to the answers to these questions. Each of the elements of Conscious Bookkeeping is intended to help us create a life in which the dream answers to these questions become the lived experience of our day-to-day life.

So, why the "conscious" in Conscious Bookkeeping? Simply put, each aspect of the path is intended to help us raise our level of consciousness in relationship to money, so that we can use the positive power of money to realize our highest aspirations. And when we raise our level of consciousness in relationship to money, it is almost inevitable that we will naturally become more conscious and awake in relationship to other aspects of reality. The limitations of the system are defined only by your own investment.

While visiting India, a friend of mine was introduced to three Buddhist monks. During their conversation, my friend learned that each of the monks had memorized the entire Pali Canon, which contains hundreds of discourses, or teachings, given by the Buddha. My friend asked the monks, "What is the essence of the Pali Canon?" One of the monks leaned slightly forward for emphasis and calmly replied, "Know what you're doing." To me, that's another way of saying, "Be fully conscious and awake in relationship to all aspects of reality." Conscious Bookkeeping helps us to begin that process by initiating us into conscious relationship to money. Like any good initiation, this process can be both challenging and rewarding. We are brought face to face with our shadows around money, and in the end emerge into greater clarity, intimacy, knowledge, ease, and success. Through this financial rite of passage, we can begin to relate to all of life with the same kind of awareness.

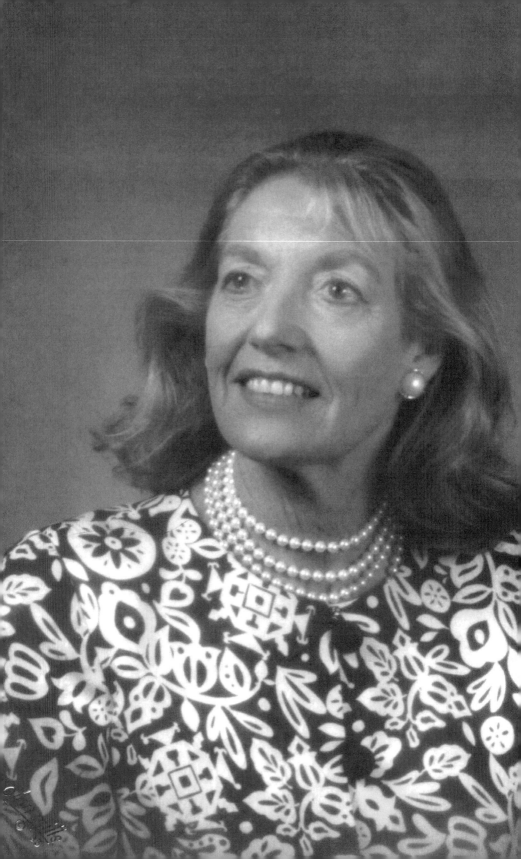

# HAZEL HENDERSON:

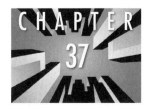

# Gross National Happiness[1]

Traditional economists are finding it increasingly difficult to defend their profession as a scientifically based system operating in a value-free fashion. As the gap yawns ever wider between the world's rich and poor, as environmental assaults continue to degrade the health of the planet, and as the grab for dwindling fossil fuels drags nations into war, the reality of economics is becoming clear. In truth, it is a political ideology designed to protect and maintain the narrow interests of a powerful few. Rather than being ruled by Adam Smith's metaphorical "invisible hand of the market," by which the supposed rational self-interest of all economic players also lifts up the poor, economics helps to replicate a social system that preserves the status quo.

The story of modern economics began with a confluence of events in Britain during the late eighteenth century. Until that time, peasants had been able to farm and graze their animals on open land that was used in common; but when landowner aristocrats enclosed their acreage with fences, the peasants were forced to find another way to support themselves. This enclosure was allowed under acts of the parliament. As factories needed workers, formerly self-reliant artisans and peasant farmers were pushed off the land into the factories and the Industrial Revolution got underway.[1] The rural population did find work in the new factories, but these were horrific places where the peasants were, in reality, little more than slaves.

Hazel Henderson, futurist and evolutionary economist, has authored eight books and over 100 articles in refereed journals. Her latest book is *Ethical Markets: Growing the Green Economy* (Chelsea Green, 2006-2007), the companion volume to her PBS series (also seen in Brazil, Australia, and China). She co-created the Calvert-Henderson Quality of Life Indicators with the Calvert Group (www.Calvert-Henderson.com). Her editorials are syndicated worldwide by InterPress Service. She has advised the National Science Foundation, the National Academy of Engineering and the U.S. Office of Technology Assessment and is listed in *Who's Who in Finance, Who's Who in America, Who's Who in Science and Technology*.

Of course, economic systems have always existed in human societies. Humans have always exchanged goods within and between tribes and villages. For centuries trading took place in villages and local marketplaces, where people exchanged a morning's eggs for vegetables, seeds and homemade goods. After the Enclosure Acts in Britain and the birth of the Industrial Revolution, Britain's laws set up national systems of rules imposing the "market" and national currency, rather than barter, as the predominant system for exchange and trade. The economic sphere became split off from society as if it were a neutral, free-standing mechanism, when in reality it is inextricably embedded in social systems and their power relationships and value structures.

As the Age of Enlightenment spread through eighteenth century Europe, the great French philosopher Rene Descartes and other scientists and mathematicians led the scientific revolution. When I was writing *Creative Alternative Futures*[2] in the 1970s, I began to focus on the problems inherent in this scientific Cartesian method of studying systems by examining their parts and seeing systems as the sum of those parts. This method leads to familiar errors: Knowledge is fragmented into "silos" and "stovepipes," and dots are not connected. Studying economics separately, instead of as part of a social system, is such an error. Even though the Cartesian method allowed a tremendous flowering of science and technology, it cannot readily be applied to living systems, the parts of which cannot be teased apart as entities independent of the larger system in which they operate. That economics cannot be separated from the power relationships and value systems in which it is embedded became clear to me as I traveled and conducted my research. Even as the same industrial system took root in country after country, each one had its own value system regarding which jobs were to be done for free, which were worth a lot of money, and which were worth only a little. Rather than being decided scientifically, as many economists insist, it is instead all a matter of power relationships and culture.

In 1776, Adam Smith, a Scots economist, published his great work on economics, *An Inquiry Into the Nature and Causes of the Wealth of Nations*, to explain how the free market could self-correct and ultimately serve the welfare of everyone. Analogizing from Isaac Newton's Laws of Motion, Smith believed that societies were self-equilibrating and guided by an "invisible hand" similar to that of the celestial mechanics of Newton. Yet his message, with its strong sense of morality, also held that these markets could only allocate resources efficiently if buyers and sellers had equal power and information and no harmful effects fell on others. Today, these conditions are almost never met.

Over time, modern markets devolved into a misinterpreted view of Charles Darwin's theory, so that "survival of the fittest" (a phrase coined by British economist Herbert Spencer, not Darwin) allowed the few to prosper, expecting wealth to trickle down to the many. The elite in Britain and elsewhere in the West quickly realized that the notion of free markets and competition suited them very well, allowing them to maintain the upper hand, bolstered by "scientific" fact. Within a hundred years after Britain's Enclosure Acts, this economic model had become fully entrenched within national operating systems. Today we see this "enclosure" ideology colonizing ever more natural resources, water, oceans, the atmosphere—even turning biodiversity and DNA into "markets."

Finally, during World War II, Britain needed a method to measure wartime production; so, economists there devised the model of the Gross National Product and the narrower version, Gross Domestic Product, which were later extended and adopted to national production. The United States also adopted this system, as did the United Nations later on, making it the world's official system of national accounts even though it was never intended as the "scorecard" of wealth and progress it became.[3] The GNP and GDP measure all spending in a country, including the cost involved in such activities as cleaning up toxic waste dumps, dealing with crime, or developing military weapons. So, while these costs clearly are inappropriate as measures of national wellbeing, this measurement system depends upon them to keep the economy humming. Measures of well-being—the unpaid work of caring for children and households, civic volunteering, environmental assets—are ignored, despite their being the foundation from which all other activities spring.

In 1992, at the United Nations Conference on Environment and Development—the Earth Summit—in Rio de Janeiro, many of the non-governmental organizations in attendance took a stand on this issue. They demanded that economists, in constructing the GNP and the GDP, deduct environmental costs and add unpaid production, which we know in many countries averages fifty percent of all activity, and is closer to sixty-five or seventy percent in developing nations. The NGOs were not successful in their efforts with the economists, although they did lobby these provisions into Agenda Twenty-One, signed at Rio by 170 governments, and they did bring this issue to worldwide attention. Yet, today, few governments have begun overhauling their national accounts and mass media continue to slavishly report GNP and GDP figures with little comprehension (see my commentary on this topic at www.marketplace.org).

Clearly, economics is not gender-neutral or value-free, as its champions claim, but is in fact patriarchal to the core. If you look at its model of who is "productive" and who isn't, it is clear that women who are working without pay to raise children or care for the household are categorized simply as uneconomic. According to economics, the only rational model is the masculine model—that is, competing against all others in pure self-interested gain and accumulation. In fact, the values behind the economic model are encouraging the Seven Deadly Sins!

Such an entrenched bias reveals the reality of economics: Rather than being a science, it is a political ideology, pure and simple. As I've been saying in one form or another for thirty years, economists are not hired by the poor. They are hired by banks and corporations and governments—mostly wealthy, male-dominated organizations. Like most of us, they are not inclined to bite the hand that feeds them.

I saw this ideology in full force when I was working at the Office of Technology Assessment in Washington between 1974 and 1980, following the years when many environmental and social welfare laws were put into effect for the first time. By 1975, economists had rushed into nearly every agency, saying that every piece of legislation regarding health or education or the environment must be assessed for its economic cost. Unfortunately, since the benefits of educating a child or the value of a tree standing in a forest, for example, cannot be quantified, the economists were able to engineer an intellectual coup that is now deeply entrenched in Washington. Using cost benefit analysis is totally inappropriate in these issues because economists never include avoided costs. As one example, investing in clean energy means avoiding the cost of fighting a war in the Middle East to secure dwindling oil supplies.[4]

Fortunately, some of us are beginning to re-examine our belief systems and the extent to which we may be trapped in the earlier, primitive stages of our development—including the truth about the economic model, which assumes that competition and self-interest are the only rational actions to take. Competition, territoriality, and tribalism are legacies from the fears of our long-ago past; they served us well then and remain key drivers in evolution and all human affairs. In fact, competition produces benefits in society by spurring innovation and efficiency and driving industrialism and economic growth.

But ignoring cooperation, collaboration, and the ability to trust and bond with one another ignores an essential portion of the range of human responses. The cooperation in families and communities remains unpaid, unrewarded, and invisible within economic models, even though it allows for collective action, taxes, and the vital infrastructure for commerce—in short, makes possible the rest of life outside the family.

With the world's political situation and environmental health deteriorating daily, we have to ask: Why do we underestimate our real genius for bonding, cooperation, and altruism? Why do so many still believe, and act as if, the individual has primacy over the community? Why can't we use all the available evidence—and there is a great deal—to seek a balance to also acknowledge society, culture, and the Earth's ecosystems in order that we don't destroy ourselves? I submit that the malfunctioning economic source code still lurking in our minds and the hard drives of many of our institutions is a cause.

Help is coming from an unexpected quarter. A growing body of information from a number of sciences is pointing to the importance and evolution of the human emotional capacity for bonding, cooperation, and altruism. To begin with, quite literally, these nurturing qualities stem from the human hormone oxytocin, which bonds mothers to their babies as it is released during pregnancy and lactation—the time in human life when bonding is at its highest and most necessary point. Other sciences—neuroscience, endocrinology, psychology, physics, thermodynamics, mathematics, anthropology, and archeology—are invalidating the core assumptions underlying economic models now in use. They have also brought about a welcome reappraisal of Charles Darwin's *The Descent of Man* and *The Origin of Species*. Although Darwin clearly saw the human capacity for bonding, cooperation, and altruism as an essential factor in our successful evolution, this side of his work was conveniently ignored by those wishing to promote "Social Darwinism." Without such qualities, how could humans have emerged from tiny, roving bands to create the huge metropolises of today? Early economists seized on Darwin's research about how species survive and evolve through competition—misinterpreting it as they applied it to humans—to buttress their notion of laissez-faire, or the idea that human societies could advance wealth and progress by allowing that "invisible hand" of the market to work its magic. Social Darwinism took on a particularly callous quality in the drive to deregulate global financial markets, promoted in the USA by Ronald Reagan, in Britain by Margaret Thatcher, and echoed by today's neoconservatives.[5]

This lopsided attitude is still very much alive in our business schools, whose methods and curricula continue to encourage managers in the kind of behavior that led to the scandals at Enron, Tyco, Worldcom, and Arthur Anderson. If society is to shift its beliefs in this matter of economics, business schools must begin to teach that our skill in bonding and cooperative behavior is the true foundation of all human organizations and our greatest scientific and technological achievements. Business executives will have to begin admitting what they know to be true: Competition and territoriality are channeled within structures of cooperation and networks of agreements, laws, and contracts. Globalization could not have occurred without this reality of "co-opetition"[6] that permits airlines, communications, and other infrastructure to exist in a cooperative manner, even as they serve competitors.

This kind of skewed belief system also promotes the notion that money is the only source of wealth. This ignores ecological wealth, human and social capital, and knowledge—now our most important factor of production. "Well-being" and "quality-of-life" are well-rounded and true ways of measuring human development and social progress.

Several new indices are part of the effort to develop comprehensive statistics of national well-being that extend beyond traditional macroeconomic indicators such as the GNP. One of these is the United Nations Development Index, which uses three basic measures of human development: a long and healthy life, as measured by life expectancy at birth; knowledge, as determined by the adult literacy rate; and income levels.

The king of Bhutan created another index. While prosperity is important, he says, it is also necessary to ensure that it is shared across society as well as balanced against protecting the environment, maintaining a responsive government, and preserving cultural traditions. Using these measures, the government of this tiny Buddhist country can measure its Gross National Happiness.

Another index is the Calvert-Henderson Quality of Life Indicators, which I helped to create with the Calvert Group, released in 2000. These Indicators use a systems approach to illustrate the dynamic state of our social, economic, and environmental quality of life. The dimensions of life examined include education, employment, energy, environment, health, human rights, income, infrastructure, national security, public safety, recreation, and shelter. These indicators are multidisciplinary and only use money-coefficients where appropriate. They are "un-bundled" for political transparency and public education—rather than weighted by economists and averaged into one unintelligible number, like GDP. They are updated regularly at www.Calvert-Henderson.com.

Additionally, another new kind of environmental analysis makes up for the fact that traditional economics does not include or encourage measures of sustainability. Ecological Footprint Analysis determines relative consumption in order to educate people about their resource use and perhaps encourage them to change their consumption patterns. Ecological Footprint Analysis tells us the amount of ecologically productive land and sea area necessary to sustain a population, manufacture a product, or undertake an activity. It takes into account the use of food, water, energy, building materials, and other consumables, as well as trade flows.

Thousands of companies and corporations around the world have also seen the light.[7] Following are only a few examples. Two thousand companies have signed on to the ten principles of Global Corporate Citizenship of the Global Compact. Launched in 2000 by the UN, this compact covers human rights, workplace safety, justice, ILO standards, the environment, and anti-corruption. Civic groups monitor all the companies to ensure that they are walking their talk. The new auditing standards of the Global Reporting Initiative prescribe Triple Bottom Line accounting, covering not only profits but also people and the planet; 600 global corporations now comply with the GRI in their annual reports. Even the Dow Jones now has a Sustainability Group Index. A number of new indices based on sustainability and social responsibility, such as the Domini Social 400 Index, now regularly outperform Dow Jones and Standard and Poor's 500. Others include London's FTSE4Good, the U.S. Calvert Social Index, and Brazil's BOVESPA. The Grameen Bank in Bangladesh, Women's World Banking, and ACCION, all serving in many countries, and other organizations now deliver micro-credit to poor people, who finally are able to lift their families from dire poverty thanks to loans often of less than $100. The success of micro-credit programs rests on the fact that these poor borrowers, mostly women, pay back their loans more reliably than richer borrowers.

The essential tasks of our generation are: (1) to reintegrate our fragmented knowledge, and (2) to understand once and for all that humanity's success has always rested on cooperation, even as we embrace competition and creativity. Holding us back from eliminating poverty, war, and the rape of the planet is the collective buried fear of scarcity and attack lodged in our ancient reptilian brains, which react without thought. If we are to rethink our view of economics and reshape our world—if we are to survive—we must move from that unthinking, reactive brain to our thoughtful forebrain, to the economics of our hearts and our highest visions for human evolution, together with all life on this planet.

1. See for example Polyani, K. *The Great Transformation*. Beacon Press. (2001).
2. Henderson, H. *Creating Alternative Futures: The End of Economics*. Kumarian Press. Bloomfield Hills, CT (1996).
3. Henderson, H. *Paradigms in Progress: Life Beyond Economics*. Berrett-Koehler. San Francisco, CA (1995).
4. Henderson, H. *The Politics of the Solar Age*. Doubleday. NY (1988).
5. Henderson, H. "21st Century Strategies for Sustainability," FORESIGHT. Cambridge, UK (Feb. 2006).
6. Brandenburger, A.M. and Nalebuff, B.J. *Co-opetition*, Doubleday. NY (1996).
7. All these visionary leaders are interviewed and their new enterprises are documented in my thirteen-part PBS series, "Ethical Markets," available on DVD from www.EthicalMarkets.com.

# PART NINE

# Dancing With the Infinite

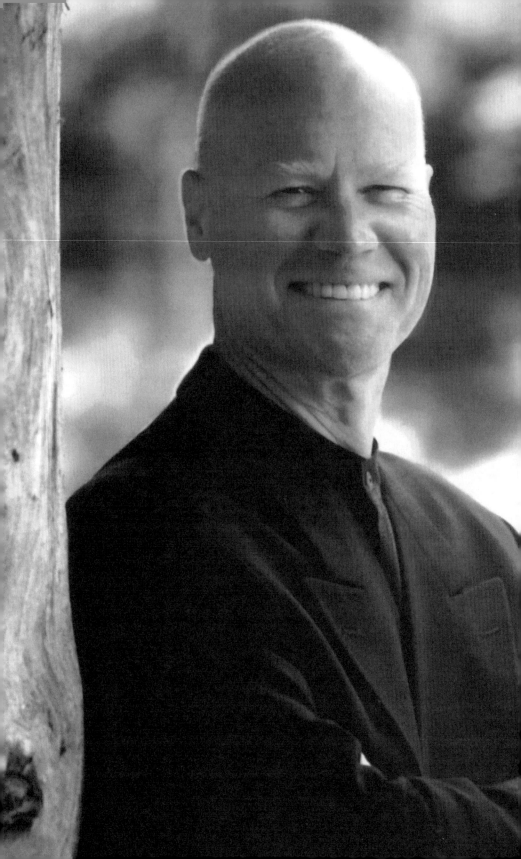

# LANCE SECRETAN:

# Remembering to Dream Again

reams inspire us—both our own and those of others. Dreams offset our contemporary weariness with a BlackBerryed, 24/7, bad-news-streamed-constantly-to-your-desktop world. We are inspired by the stories of people who choose to channel their passions into issues that positively impact our global experience of connection. Some dream about growth, sustainability, and health. Others dream about the way we work, creating organizations that honor the wholeness of our lives. Some, in the entertainment industry, for example, dream and create courageous new conversations. Yet others dream beyond our wildest imaginations to create new models of global philanthropy. These dreamers inspire us and give us hope that our children's children may live in the kind of world we dream and hope for.

A common thread in all dreams is that they are delivered with one or more of six common qualities I refer to as the CASTLE principles: Courage, Authenticity, Service, Truthfulness, Love, and Effectiveness.

This chapter explores our need to dream and how some of today's leaders identify, realize, and sustain their own dreams using the CASTLE Principles. As you read their stories, feel your own dreams stirring within you and imagine what we could create together if we all lived with the passion of our dreams.

Lance Secretan is a cutting-edge thinker in the field of leadership and a pioneer in innovative methods of inspiring people and organizations. He is an award-winning columnist, teacher, philosopher, corporate coach, mentor, and international best-selling author of fourteen books on leadership, including *One: The Art and Practice of Conscious Leadership* (The Secretan Center, Inc., 2006). His clients include 30 of *Fortune* magazine's Most Admired Companies, and 11 of its Best Companies to Work for in America. Lance chaired the 1997 Special Olympics World Winter Games Advisory Board, and is a former Ambassador to the United Nations Environment Program. Visit www.secretan.com.

# CHAPTER THIRTY-EIGHT

# Why Dream?

What is the common, unifying experience among winning teams, great endeavors, and innovative achievements? What uniqueness can be found in groups of people who achieve the extraordinary — creating revolutions, overthrowing despots, founding nations (or fusing them into one), climbing Everest, reinventing organizations, creating breakthroughs, building something never thought of before, or changing the way we live or think, or even how the world works?

The answer is that each of those teams had a dream.

We are deeply connected to our dreams, whether we realize them or not. We spend our lives dreaming — about a perfect partner, our hopes for our children, our career aspirations, our security, and the kind of world we want to live in. When we become separated from those dreams we are sad, and when we are one with them, we are inspired.

*Whenever we experience pain or sadness, it is because we have become separated from what, or whom, we love. And whenever we are inspired and joyful, it is because we are one with what, or whom, we love.*

## The Illusion of Separateness

In a September 2006 edition of NBC's "Meet the Press," Former U.S. President Bill Clinton told interviewer Tim Russert that the biggest problem confronting the world today is "the illusion that our differences matter more than our common humanity".

We live with the illusion that we are separate. We live in a world that relies on complicated, old thinking models that seek to separate, and we have become experts in our ability to view our world and all that makes up our lives as separate. We separate people by their religions, political affiliations, national boundaries, and ethnic backgrounds; we educate by different and separate disciplines; we treat patients not as whole beings but as "cases" separated by their seemingly disconnected illnesses, attended by separate specialists; we treat management and staff as separate, analyzing organizations as separate departments, competitors, and customers; we separate ourselves from our environment and from our authenticity. Our organizations and communities are filled with people experiencing the dysfunctions and unhappiness that separateness creates. Most have fantasies of walking away from their careers or relationships, having long forgotten how to dream. For many, life and work are no longer fun because we have become separated from our passion, inspiration, and hope — we have become separated from what we love.

Over the last 50 years of business theorizing and academic and professional development, we have succeeded in expanding our capacity to quantify, measure, and analyze, but we have stifled our capacity to dream. We may even think that dreaming is too "out there" for a business environment. So we no longer talk about dreams in organizations. Instead, we create stale, forgettable "mission, vision, and values" statements—all too often never reaching the inspiring power and passion that is to be found in a dream.

When we speak about dreams, we are talking about passion—and usually *with* passion. Greatness in leaders comes from their ability to ignite the passion in others that leads to the accomplishment of something extraordinary...such as a dream. Not a two percent increase in market share or a five percent improvement in the employee satisfaction metrics—but a bold, daring, impudent, audacious, outrageous, thrilling, exhilarating, and inspiring *dream*.

Consider some of humanity's most audacious accomplishments. For example, how did we land a man on the moon? Jack Kennedy had a dream, and it was a dream so powerful that thousands of people embraced it, making it their own and making it real. Indeed, it was such a powerful dream that it restored America's self-esteem (Sputnik had just been launched), galvanized Americans, and inspired much of the rest of the world. Dreams are like that—they transcend differences, disagreements, and petty arguments, because the dream unites us at a higher level and engages us in a higher purpose. And it is this elusive oneness for which we are yearning.

Great historical leaders—Christ, Buddha, Lao-Tzu, Confucius, Mohammed, Nelson Mandela, Mother Teresa, and Martin Luther King, Jr., among them—all had a dream. In his famous speech delivered on the steps of the Lincoln Memorial on August 28, 1963, Martin Luther King repeated "I have a dream..." eight times. It was his ability to articulate his dream that united hundreds of thousands of people who ushered in a new era of civil rights and liberties.

Dreams are like that—they have the power within them to change the world.

## Focusing on the Power of our Dreams

In my work with leaders of organizations around the world, I've noticed that our work (called Higher Ground Leadership) results in amazing outcomes. Yet, reflecting on these results, I realized that we had been focused on the processes rather than the outcomes—in other words, we had been attentive to the means rather than to the dream. So, more recently, our work has focused on inviting leaders to describe their dream. We ask them to identify their most extraordinary, outrageous, never-before-achieved aspirations. We ask them to be fearless and imaginative, to think outside the box, to be truly outrageous and boundlessly creative. They come up with some remarkable ideas—hospitals who dream of eliminating all avoidable deaths, banks who dream of increasing market share by 10% in one year, corporations who dream of becoming environmentally friendly, organizations who dream of changing the world. These are not the kinds of ideas that fit easily under a heading of "mission, vision, and values". We need a much larger container to accommodate such magnificent ideas—we need a dream.

And so we ask our clients to believe in the dream, to assume that the dream is realizable and assume that when the energies of their entire organization are harnessed behind that dream, it will be achieved. An organization with 10,000 employees and a dream, and which harnesses this total energy—every employee—behind that dream, stands a great risk of achieving it!

Understanding the power of modern leadership to transform organizations, communities, countries, or the world means understanding how to harness the power of dreams.

In the twenty-first century, and throughout history, leaders can be found in every age, gender, region, or vocation. They emerge by identifying, realizing, and sustaining their dreams. They may challenge our old models and ask new questions (or sometimes, some very old, time-tested ones), and they often explore uncharted or unfamiliar territory. What is consistent for them all, though, is their embodiment of the CASTLE principles, by which they illuminate, tend, and protect our global values and dreams, and by doing so, create a better world for humanity—now and into the future. In short, they inspire us.

## The CASTLE Principles

CASTLE is an acronym for Courage, Authenticity, Service, Truthfulness, Love, and Effectiveness. These six very obvious concepts distinguish the Higher Ground Leader from the old story leader and, when fully lived, are profoundly inspiring to others. These are concepts that are within us already, but yearn to be recalled. It is through the CASTLE principles that we develop, realize, and sustain our dreams, guiding the contribution of brilliance from others.

I discovered these concepts by first asking people what they disliked about their uninspiring leaders. Our research showed that these followers were typically turned off by leaders who were cowardly, inauthentic, self-serving, dishonest, unfeeling, and ineffective. I reasoned that inverting these deficiencies might reveal the proficiencies of great leadership—and so the CASTLE Principles were born! The six CASTLE Principles are:

**C**OURAGE: Being brave enough to reach beyond the boundaries created by our existing, often deeply held, limitations, fears, and beliefs. Initiating change in our lives, of any kind, is only possible when we are courageous enough to take the necessary action.

**A**UTHENTICITY: Committing oneself to showing up and being fully present in all aspects of life. Removing the mask and becoming a real, vulnerable, and intimate human being, a person without self-absorption who is genuine and emotionally and spiritually connected to others.

**S**ERVICE: Focusing on the needs of others by listening to them, identifying their needs, and meeting them. Being inspiring rather than following a self-focused, competitive, fear-based approach.

**T**RUTHFULNESS: Being truthful in all thoughts, words, and actions, and listening openly to the truth of others and refusing to compromise integrity or to deny obvious or universal truths—even when avoiding the truth might, on the face of it, seem easier, especially in testing times.

**L**OVE: Embracing the underlying oneness with others and life. Relating to and inspiring others and touching their hearts in ways that add to who you both are as people.

**E**FFECTIVENESS: Being capable of, and successful in, achieving the physical, material, intellectual, emotional, and spiritual goals we set in life.

The perfection of using the CASTLE Principles to identify, realize, and sustain our dreams is that there is nothing new to learn. These six qualities are within us all, yearning for the opportunity to be remembered and lived to their fullest.

## Becoming a Plate-spinner

Remember your childhood visits to the circus or state fair, and the performers who were "plate spinners"? Typically, after getting about seven or eight plates spinning at the top of their sticks, the first one would start to wobble, and the performer would race back to the first plate, re-spin it, and thus enable it to maintain its momentum.

They repeated this process to keep all of the plates from falling. I think of a leadership team as a team of plate-spinners. Their role is to keep the plates spinning, and the plates represent the inspiration of others. When we do something uninspiring or demoralizing, a plate drops and quickly sucks the passion from the dream. The role of all the leaders in an organization (and for politicians, teachers, ministers, caregivers, parents, spouses, and friends), is to never do anything — I repeat, *never* do anything — that is uninspiring or de-motivating to all of those people who are united in their efforts to achieve the dream. The team that is directly responsible for leading those who are realizing the dream must be fully inspired, too — all of the time — inspired to live their lives in a way that inspires others — all of the time — never dropping a plate.

Note that it doesn't always matter how they get there, but that they do so by simply by shifting their focus, whenever necessary and in an inspiring way, to accomplishing their dream. Wal-Mart identified a need to meet its consumers' concerns about corporate practices and value to its communities. In response, Wal-Mart became actively engaged in first dreaming, and then realizing a new dream, as articulated by CEO, Lee Scott: "I had embraced this idea that the world's climate is changing and that man played a part in that, and that Wal-Mart can play a part in reducing man's impact. We recognized that Wal-Mart had such a footprint in this world, and that we had a corresponding part to play in sustainability." Wal-Mart's dream is to obtain 100 percent of its energy from renewable sources, cut energy use in stores by 30 percent and cut fuel consumption in its truck fleet by 25 percent within two years. They are using their muscle as the world's second largest company to make positive changes that will impact the environment. They are installing solar panels in their stores, insisting that the cosmetics they carry use less packaging, and are fast becoming a huge seller of organic foods in North America — currently they have more than 10 percent of the market.

## Identifying the Dream

Muhammed Yunus is the Founder of Grameen Bank. This former economics professor dreamed of inventing a new model for global capital investment that offered modest (micro) loans to Third World entrepreneurs. During a trip to a Bangladeshi village, he discovered he could help a poor bamboo craftswoman start her own independent business with a loan of just 22 cents. During that one moment of choice, Yunis focused on the needs of others and met them in service by founding Grameen Bank in Bangladesh. He employed all the CASTLE principles and his awareness of oneness by connecting an international network of investors to would-be entrepreneurs looking for micro investments to jump-start their small business ideas. Grameen has since lent more than $5 billion.

Yunus' exciting contributions include his dream to widen the boundaries of capitalism by harnessing it to serve to the diverse needs of our global family. His dream asks us to make way for Social Business Entrepreneurs (SBE) and Social Stock Markets, allowing new definitions of success, profit, and growth to contribute to making the world a better place. As he describes:

They are totally committed to make a difference to the world. They are social-objective driven. They want to give better chance in life to other people. They want to achieve their objective through creating/ supporting sustainable business enterprises. Their businesses may or may not earn profit, but like any other businesses they must not incur losses. They create a new class of business, which we may describe as "non-loss" business. If SBEs exist in the real world, it makes no sense why we should not make room for them in our conceptual framework.

Imagine a world in which Yunus' inspiring dream of Social Business Entrepreneurs was sustained.

Jeff Skoll, Founding President of eBay, identifies his dreams by launching businesses that result in positive social change. In 1999, Jeff created the Skoll Foundation, which takes an entrepreneurial approach to philanthropy by investing in, connecting, and celebrating some of the world's most promising social entrepreneurs in order to effect lasting, positive social change worldwide.

*Participant Productions,* for which Jeff serves as Chair and CEO, is one of his latest passions. It was founded in 2004 with the dream to create a long-term, independent, sustainable media company focused on the public interest. Says Skoll, *"I'm interested in leveraging the power of Hollywood to tell great stories and make a difference in the world."*

In an era in which entertainment often seeks to manipulate the truth more than model it, Skoll's dream is to create and finance movies that refuse to compromise integrity or deny obvious or universal truths. Jeff was Executive Producer of four Participant films: *Good Night, and Good Luck*; *North Country*; *Syriana*; and the documentary *Murderball* — films that collectively garnered 11 Academy Award nominations in 2006. Jeff is also Executive Producer of *An Inconvenient Truth*, a documentary about global warming featuring former Vice President Al Gore, which opened to standing ovations at the 2006 Sundance Film Festival.

In April 2005, in partnership with Silicon Valley entrepreneur Kamran Elahian, Jeff launched The Gandhi Project, which dubbed the epic film *Gandhi* into Arabic in order to screen it throughout the

Palestinian territories. His dream is to work with nongovernmental organization partners to promote Mahatma Gandhi's teachings of non-violent resistance through screenings of the movie, combined with discussion. Plans are under way to expand the project throughout the Arab world.

## Realizing the Dream

Bill and Melinda Gates co-chair The Bill and Melinda Gates Foundation, the largest foundation in the world. Guided by the Gates' belief that every life has equal value, the Foundation's dream is to reduce inequities and improve lives around the world. They dream, too, of infusing business performance metrics into philanthropy. In developing countries, the foundation focuses on improving health, reducing extreme poverty, and increasing access to technology in public libraries. In the United States, the foundation seeks to ensure that all people have access to high quality education and to technology in public libraries. Locally, it focuses on improving the lives of low-income families.

As of June 2006, the foundation employed 270 people, has endowments of $29.2 billion, and has committed $10.5 billion in grants since its inception in 1994. In 2005 it gave $1.36 billion, and in 2006, expects to spend around $1.5 billion. Bill and Melinda have said that almost all their fortune (currently estimated at $50 billion) will go to charity.

Bill and Melinda Gates have used a remarkable dream and the CASTLE Principles, especially that of Effectiveness, to inspire a new world of philanthropy by turning it upside down and introducing the previously unheard of idea that recipients of funds should be businesslike and accountable. Their foundation often requires recipients to prepare business plans, goals and targets and sophisticated metrics, and it then allocates funds according to the incremental achievement of these of targets, ensuring that good management is part of the effectiveness recipe. Jeffrey Skoll calls this "social entrepreneurship" which hew defines as "...people who apply rigorous discipline to social problems. They use many of the tools and techniques of business and apply them to the world of the social sector or the citizen sector... Their work is characterized by innovation, leverage, empowerment, and lasting change. The difference is, their bottom line is not in profits earned, but in lives, communities, and societies transformed." They are achieving their physical, material, intellectual, emotional, and spiritual goals to make the world a better place.

Vinod Khosla has said, "An entrepreneur is someone who dares to dream the dreams and is foolish enough to try to make those dreams come true." Khosla should know. He has spent 25 years building some of Silicon Valley's best-known technology companies—he was co-founder of Sun Microsystems and one of the most influential partners at top venture capital firm Kleiner Perkins Caufield & Byers. Now, as founder of Khosla Ventures, his dream is to work with and learn from fun and knowledgeable entrepreneurs, build impactful companies through the leverage of innovation, and spend time as a partnership making a difference to have a beneficial effect and economic impact on society. He's putting his passion, name, and wealth into finding new ways to produce ethanol, in the hope that it might dramatically reduce America's dependence on foreign oil. Through Khosla Ventures, he has invested tens of millions of dollars in firms that are developing techniques to generate ethanol using vegetation other than corn, such as "cellulosic" ethanol produced by turning agricultural waste into fuel. He's also financing a November 2006 California ballot proposition to increase taxes on statewide oil production for funding alternative energy research and development.

Khosla's dream is being realized in his daily embodiment of courage as he pushes the boundaries of North America's limiting and fear-based beliefs about its need for foreign oil. During an interview with NBC's Dateline anchor Stone Philips, Khosla passionately shared:

What could be better than a greener fuel that's cheaper for consumers, that doesn't feed Mideast terrorism, yet instead fuels rural America? The environmentalists love it because it's greener. The neo-conservatives like it because it ensures energy independence and security for America. The farmers love it because it takes oil dollars and moves it to rural America.

## Sustaining the Dream

Jeffrey Swartz, CEO of Timberland, has been at the helm of this family-built footwear and apparel company since 1998, enjoying sales that have risen 75 percent, a net profit that has nearly tripled, and a stock that is up over 300 percent. Contributing to this success is the bold nature of his dreams. Timberland sustains those dreams with an organizational culture built on authenticity, which integrates personal values into a cause that is lived every day.

Timberland is known for its strong employee volunteer programs, like its decade-old "Path of Service" program that provides employees 40 hours of paid time to contribute to the community during working hours. Swartz's latest dream is developing environmental programs that tap deeply into the vein of corporate authenticity. In early 2006 Timberland announced its new shoebox "nutritional label," detailing where the product was made, how it was produced, and its impact on the environment and communities. He says:

We thought about how closely consumers read nutritional labels on food products and thought, why doesn't this happen in our space? We want to create a broad awareness among consumers so that perhaps eventually they will expect all manufacturers to rise up to this level of detail on how and where a product is made.

Authenticity is often expressed as accepting what is real rather than continuing to deny it, and learning to live with, use, and partner with it. Swartz has used this simple, authentic labeling dream to inspire his organization and its customers. Before he's done, he may inspire an entire industry to share his dream!

# What is Your Dream?

You don't need charts, graphs, matrices, complex theories for this. It's pretty simple: When you think about what's possible, even if it has never been attained before, identify it as your own dream and seek to realize it, and then make the commitment to align an entire team of plate-spinners, even an entire organization, behind doing everything necessary to achieve that dream...then the dream becomes possible. Anchor the dream with healthy doses of Courage, Authenticity, Service, Love, Truthfulness, and Effectiveness and you'll see it sustained.

Martin Luther King shared his dream with the world. So did Jack Kennedy. And the world changed.

Today, leaders like Jeff Skoll, Vinod Khosla, Jeffrey Swartz, Muhammed Yunus, and Bill and Melinda Gates continue to inspire the world with their dreams.

So can you.

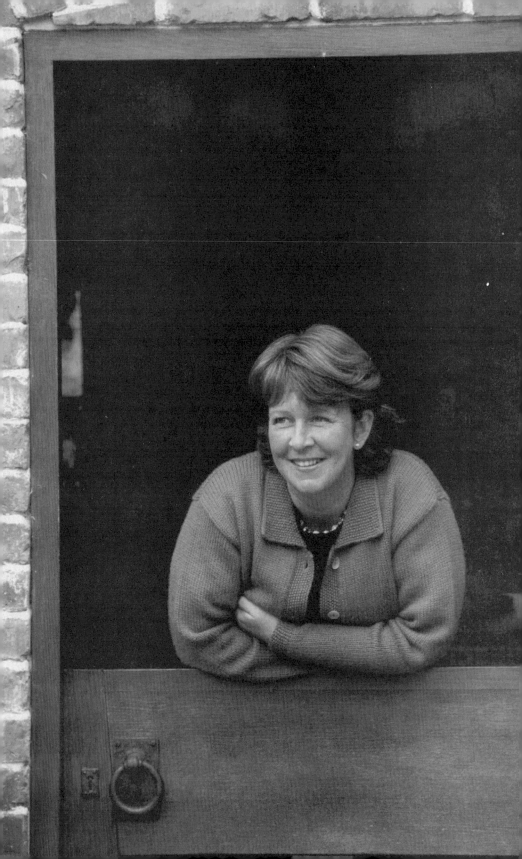

# Mandy Voisey:

# Dreams and Consequences

I learned profound pleasure and a life-long love of plants through gardening alongside my grandmother, Lulu. Working side-by-side, young and old, we were united in trying to tame the profusion of an English country garden, knowing that these were special times that must not be wasted. There I learned the ingredients needed to create a gorgeous garden: Choose seeds and plants that suit both you and the soil, prepare the ground making sure it is clean and free of obstacles, add compost if needed, water and watch over the young tender growth, and finally, trust that Nature will do everything possible to let the plants thrive and flower! Wonderfully enough, this process is perfectly suited to starting a healthy company.

## The Ground

Home was on the other side of the globe in Hong Kong. Out there, you can actually hear a hum—the buzz of business and buildings all concentrated in one electrifyingly busy area, Central. It is like hearing the whirring cogs of effort as millions of people concentrate on finding ways to build a better life. Somehow everyone congregated on the lower slopes, cramming into a tight space at the foot of the mountains. Even if you lived higher up, you still looked out across the sheer mass of humanity, all living in flats, one on top of the other.

Mandy Ellis Voisey grew up in multicultural Hong Kong. She graduated in French and Modern Languages, and subsequently enjoyed a meteoric career in publishing and advertising. Inspired by East and West, she and her former husband founded the enormously successful import company, Junction 18. Mandy has learned that it is unnecessary to limit dreams. She allies creativity to integrity in everything she starts up, from writing and designing gardens and homes to playing music and sport. Mandy shares her home in the west of England with her daughter, numerous pets, and any visiting family or friends. Visit www.AnywherElseOnEarth.co.uk.

Simple pleasures open to other people are beyond the reach of most inhabitants of Hong Kong, pets and gardening being impossible dreams. Even a window box is dangerous; from thirty floors up, falling objects kill. After years on upper floors, we were suddenly allocated a ground floor flat right on top of the Peak…with a garden…which translated into a puppy. The exhilaration we felt for our flat at aptly named Cloudridge never lessened. Like Janus, it had two faces, one of which looked out over a small, pretty garden—but the other! Seventy feet of veranda, edged with grass and railings, framed a jaw-droppingly spectacular panorama over the harbor a thousand feet below. Our view was even better than the one from the Peak Tower, where thousands of tourists mass daily to capture it on film. As a teenager, I would wake early and slip out to sit cross-legged, in total rapture, watching for the moment everything came alive. First the sun boiled up behind the Kowloon Hills, ready to flood the valleys with its searing daily heat. Then the noises would begin, pianissimo at first, but like an orchestra tuning up before a concert, leading to an inevitable crescendo that would last well into the glittering night.

The utter contrast with our long holidays back to England every three years could not have been greater. There, tucked snugly into a Devon valley, was my grandparents' home, gloriously named The Jungle. Calm, with hidden paths and generously planted with huge hydrangeas and camellias, this oasis represented everything that was sane and special to our over-stimulated souls. It was the antithesis of Hong Kong..

## Sowing the Seeds

Hong Kong provided proof that energy and enthusiasm mixed with hard work and clear dreams could make anything possible. The Jungle taught me that only through honouring the earth, being intimate with Nature, and caring deeply for the people you worked with could internal peace and harmony be achieved. I didn't realize then just how these two contrasting environments fused East and West into a variety of seeds that would eventually grow in me.

**Choosing and Saving Seed:** Hunting for signposts to future professions among childhood tendencies and influences is like starting a jigsaw without looking at the picture; patterns and important pieces only stand out later, when you can literally see the bigger picture.

**Seed of Fearlessness:** I travelled all over the world with my parents—their feet lead them to explore countries as others do local shopping malls. This instilled in me a deep sense of ease while being on the move. My fearlessness in exploring countries where I neither spoke nor read the language came from years of knowing that the universal language of smiles, eye contact, intention, and human similarities would always succeed.

**Cross-Pollinated Seed:** Hong Kong was a huge melting pot of nationalities. Visiting school friends' homes, with their widely diverse ethnic backgrounds—Japanese, Cantonese, Thai, Indian, Swiss—I loved the impact these different sensibilities made on me. Years later, I see how these influences flowed together, prompting me to recognize the potential of melding Oriental craftsmanship with Western styles.

**Seed of Diligence:** Hong Kong permeated my consciousness on many levels. All over the island, the Chinese work ethic was evident. Cantonese grandmothers sat assembling silk flowers with children joining in after homework. Job demarcations such as "this is not my responsibility" didn't exist: all in the family were working toward the common goal of prosperity. Memories of this came flooding back as, years later, I watched my parents sitting in the courtyard, polishing carved wooden animals before dispatch.

**Seed of Recognition:** Another vivid Hong Kong business ethic was that shopkeepers recognized and greeted their customers by name—even years later! A cynic could say this makes good business sense, but I know it is more fundamental than that. A customer can feel deep down that she is being respected as a person and not just a passing wallet. Why on Earth should we differentiate in our dealings with people?

# Bud Growth

Blue-chip companies scour English universities to handpick the best of the next crop of scholars. Despite pressure to attend "The Milk Round," such a constrained approach to business felt like factory farming to me. The feeling stuck, and I turned avoiding large companies into an art form. Despite my parents' tempting offer to holiday in Hong Kong after graduation, I asked instead for a summer's breathing space before searching for full-time work.

Looking back, this was undoubtedly one of most important decisions of my life and an instance in which I was guided to honor my inner nature. After just a few weeks, however, I started job-hunting. A listing for "a man with five years' experience in advertising" appealed. Undeterred by my obvious lack of credentials for at least two of the main criteria, I posted my CV. The publisher, a man named Moss Walters, promptly phoned back. Although admiring my audacity, his company really needed a man with experience, not a young girl straight from University. We continued talking for an hour, after which he funded my journey to London, where he put me through all the company's tests and interviews, then argued my case before the board. One week later, I stood outside MacLean Hunter's office in Oxford Street, a job offer of £6,000 in one hand, the keys to a gorgeous new car in the other, and both feet firmly on a business ladder that was to lead me only upwards. The Milk Round had offered starting salaries of £4,000!

Moss was a leader in publishing and advertising, deeply respected by staff and clients alike. Once again I was blessed with the chance to learn alongside someone older and with wonderful experience. We all-too-readily jettison older citizens, pushing them to the fringe, and so miss out on their extensive life knowledge. Working at his side, I realized that this power and respect stemmed from Moss's ability to stay true to himself. Everyone he came into contact with was captivated by his kind, honorable nature. Another future seed this experience planted was that of integrity. He took a natural, unashamed pride in enjoying his work and never used different sets of ethics for his personal or professional life; everyone received courtesy, time, and respect.

## Gardening as a Team

Newly married and wanting my husband Chris to understand Asia in order to understand me, I convinced him to take off backpacking for a year through China, Tibet, Nepal, Burma, Thailand, and onward. These travels forged deep links with Asia, and highlighted the frustration we might feel if trapped in mundane jobs, returning only every few years. We were struck by the kindness and the creativity of people in the Far East, and inspired by the stunning artifacts in their markets. And so, a planting scheme began to take shape: We would combine these elements with our own skills and ground them in our desire and commitment to deal with good people and good products, and to travel for three months of the year. A simple business plan for our new company, called Junction 18, started to form.

Chris has an incredible mind for figures, always recalling conversion rates and product prices. His best and simplest business precept is to overestimate costs and underestimate profits, which greatly reduces unpleasant shocks. Many women, myself included, downplay expenditure, thinking, "It was only £20" when it had really cost £29.99. Almost believing the new price, we experience a nasty moment when we search for the missing £9.99!

# A Sprinkling of Magic

Chris and I united our individual gifts and strengths to start our company from the kitchen table. We were committed to the integrity of everything we tackled, and our exuberance was incredibly infectious. Parents and friends were all sufficiently excited to muck in—literally, on one occasion as, scraping dried muck off the walls, we converted a recently vacated cowshed in the beautifully named Friggle Street.

# Basic Gardening Rules

As the company grew, one of my roles jokingly became that of "Moral Director." It mattered deeply to me that morals and ethics should permeate the whole business. I felt everything could be whipped away if we ever stepped off the path. I now know that worse things can happen. Nearly all my decisions were colored by the basic knowing that we had been blessed in being allowed to use our energies in this way.

**Plants Need Light and Air:** We wanted the team to feel cherished, so when constructing our first offices we chose a site with natural light, gardens, attractive cloakrooms, a games room, and a stunning kitchen where they could prepare their lunches. Such surroundings tangibly inspired staff and visitors alike. Selling beautiful products from seedy surroundings with sordid lavatories just doesn't make sense!

**Gardening Clothes:** Before us, the gift industry in Britain had consisted of large import companies dominated by grey-suited men. After my precocious entry into publishing, I knew women could play a unique role here, too. The majority of small gift retailers were women, or husband-and-wife teams. Well educated and well motivated, they ran their shops as a way of life—which dovetailed beautifully with our own business wish. Our shopkeepers wore smart but casual clothes; we didn't need to coerce or project a false image, so why assume a different persona by donning a suit and wielding a briefcase, as if selling insurance?

**Don't Overplant:** In an ideal world, how should products be presented, invoiced, and so forth? Picturing ourselves as shopkeepers, we presented actual samples. Previously, importers had sold in carton quantities, giving smaller retailers a choice of buying dozens of an item or nothing at all. We let shops buy however much they wanted. Actually that isn't entirely true; we wouldn't let someone order 12 candlesticks if we believed they would only sell six. Should those six sell rapidly, confidence in our company would naturally grow. Selling only by the dozen means that even if six fly out the door, the other six gather dust, tie up cash, and scream "unsold" every time the shopkeeper passes—not a very positive message!

**Caring for Tender Specimens:** Nobody enjoys receiving something dirty or damaged. Existing companies had refused to accept financial or moral responsibility for breakages, so we checked and cleaned products, ready to go straight on the shelves. When our clients alerted us that something had arrived broken, we offered to replace or credit it. No one ever abused this trust, so it would have been foolish to treat people suspiciously.

After long journeys across the seas, some wooden animals arrived injured, swans with clipped wings or partridges with pecked beaks. As we accumulated a veritable hospital of ailing animals, it seemed morally wrong to ditch them—so we cured them. Yes, that particular piglet's ears became smaller than its siblings', but being handmade, further care enhanced their individuality. Many recuperated at my in-law's home in Cambridge, returning soothed and often adorned with amazing new plumage.

**Responsible Gardening:** We shunned hard woods, animal products, and companies that were careless with their employees. In Manila we found some gorgeous metal chairs, but after a two-hour drive to the factory, the hot, atrocious reality met us: The place stank of urine and was dirty and run-down. Worse still, the European owners were arrogant and dismissive of their staff. We knew the chairs would sell successfully, but refused to deal with that company. How could we, with hand-on-heart truthfulness, present something to a customer knowing it carried hidden traces of sadness, greed, urine, and sweat?

**Fertilizing the Soil:** We shared in the excitement of villagers as bus shelters, prayer houses, and airy buildings for craftspeople were built using money we paid for goods. We also shared the joy of getting to know whole families and hold their new babies, admire graduation photos, and attend marriages. Sending cards or flowers to celebrate marriages and births, and sympathize with divorces and deaths, was not a calculating business tool but one human's response to another human's situation.

This whole business continuum made dreams come true for people on both sides of the globe. Several Thai carvers with sweet smiles and long fingernails worked toward funding operations to become young women, or *Katoey*. It was chastening to know that their hard work would pay for such pain so that they could be true to themselves.

Our shops knew the origins and stories behind products, and would pass them forward to their customers. A man buying Gertie, our original wooden swan, probably knew that she had been created in the north of Thailand. Our business cycle was a world removed from the grey-suited, grey thinking of large multinational companies.

**Watering on Time:** Finances are simple if you want them to be. By remembering that currency represents an exchange of energy, we were sincerely motivated to settle accounts. Suppliers sought us out, having heard that we paid promptly. Similarly, we refused to pay corruption money to freight forwarders. The power of the dollar is starkly apparent when one visits a typical Filipino home. Where no free health care or housing exists, bad debts by overseas companies bite hard.

In England our reputation grew. A customer who is informed of delays, rather than being kept in the dark, knows you value their peace of mind. We all feel let down when ignored, so why do many business people tuck basic kindness and honesty up into a bundle, leaving it outside the office door?

**Letting Nature Work:** We never took references at trade shows; using our intuition, we rarely needed extra identification. When I told people that I had already done a credit check, their inevitable response—*how?*—was all the prompting I needed to say that I had looked into their eyes and made the decision to trust them. It is hard to describe the instant, visible lift to a customer's spirit when they realize that you have credited them with honesty and human decency. Not once did this lead to a bounced check.

# Collecting Seed and Germinating New Growth

Instead of negotiating with fat cat middlemen in air-conditioned Bangkok hotels, we spent happy hours trawling markets, finding the actual creator of a particular piece. This literally led us down many interesting roads and into beautiful old Thai homes and villages.

In Chiang Mai's night bazaar, we met a smiling young mother with breathtaking embroidery draped across her small stand. Using my basic Thai and Chris's calculator, we asked how much first for one, then two, then 20, then all her cushion covers—and could she make more? The expression on her face changed from pleasure to worry as she considered the investment needed in cotton and threads to fuel such growth. Her designs were so beautiful that we advanced her money to purchase enough materials to fulfil the first order. The relationship prospered and lasted years.

Like a pagan god, the hungry UK market demanded new products regularly. A cushion embroiderer cannot suddenly produce metalwork, so mindful of the thousands of villagers all sewing, painting, and carving, we often extended a product's natural life by carefully mutating designs, thus using inventiveness to keep sending work their way. The fact that so many people relied on us for their livelihood was a source of both pride and concern.

Think about how you feel in the presence of true works of art, or the energy of children, new lovers, or relatives waiting at the airport for a loved one to arrive. There is something deeply moving about the sheer simplicity of their dedication. Their purpose isn't muddled by extraneous concerns, and their soul is singing its message pure and true. I believe that this clarity allows the universe or Nature to use every power at its disposal, to ensure that the purpose or wish is fulfilled. With our dedication to the integrity of our business—and business relationships—success felt like an organic blessing.

## The Hidden Costs of Harvest

Natural success mostly inspires loyalty and a desire to be somehow involved. A few, however, stand aloof, not understanding, and will not be soothed. It is impossible to please or appease everyone. Maintaining integrity when faced with such resentment or injustice is a tough but integral part of unexpected success. Lottery winners often gain fortunes, but lose loved ones. Success causes pain by highlighting hidden fault lines in relationships. Maybe we should make plans for success as well as business, because while money is terribly quantifiable, kind actions are not. The dream that Chris and I shared caused us unexpected casualties—miscarriages, soured relations with relatives and family friends previously spanning five generations, and ultimately our marriage.

Power from success can most certainly erode and corrode even those with huge potential to shine. Our company grew and grew like Alice in Wonderland, beyond all initial dreams and into uncharted territory. It felt essential to me to keep the company our own, to always honour the ingredients that had led to it being blessed. This belief caused friction with Chris who, seeking further growth, brought in new directors. The chemistry changed; profits grew but the diffusion of views and muddied aims loosened my attachment to the company.

## Growing On

Leaving the company and my marriage were not decisions made lightly. I now view our business as one would a precocious teenager.

Yes, I am proud of its achievements, but I am happy to be detached. I have had no regrets about choosing to leave and continue on, steadfastly clambering over occasional obstacles that stand in my way. I follow serendipitous signposts placed blatantly by guiding hands to shake me out of the earthbound mundane and urge me to remember the sublime. The joy of experiencing this journey is not one I would willingly swap.

With my spirit still hungry to create, the time since has been crammed full of writing, designing gardens, and house renovations. Essential strands linking all these professions, past and present, are integrity and the ability to place things intuitively and see past obstacles without losing my original vision.

I know now that dreams have consequences. Every gift comes with a price tag. Like a white witch who has seen the power of her spells, I make few wishes now, preferring to wait and see what the universe has in store for me.

There is profound wisdom contained in the joke in which the long-married couple, now in their sixties, are visited by a fairy godmother. She tells them that she is able to grant them just one wish each. The wife thinks, then replies "I want to travel around the world with my darling husband." Two tickets for a luxury cruise magically appear in her hand. Her husband looks at her and says, "Sorry, my dear, but my wish is to have a wife thirty years younger than me." The fairy waves her wand and the husband instantly becomes 92!

Imagine a world where you could wish for absolutely anything and fortune would manifest your desire exactly as you had envisioned it.

Now imagine this same world, where you could wish for absolutely anything and fortune would eventually manifest your desire, exactly as you had envisioned — but trailing obligations and implications that, in your naïve enthusiasm, you hadn't ever considered. Jeanne Detourbey writes, "Fortune has its part in human affairs, but conduct is really much more important."

Having business dreams is not enough; various practicalities need to be observed, such as honoring innocence, managing the mundane, and recognizing synchronicity. A true gardener would never scatter seeds onto unprepared ground without checking the requirements of that particular plant. Ensure that your basic spiritual and moral needs are met, sprinkle lightly with water, add magic, and the seeds will grow — not always exactly when or in the way that you had imagined, but they will grow.

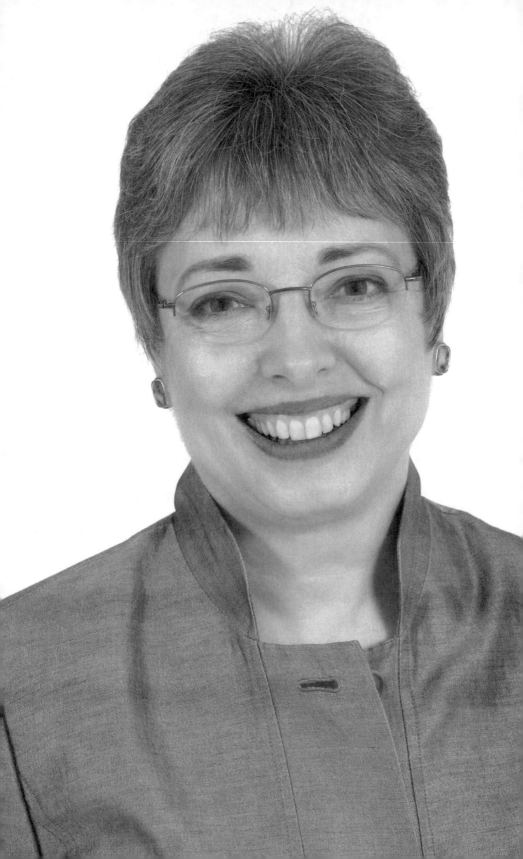

# MADELINE GERWICK: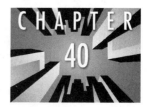

CHAPTER 40

# Nature's Business Guide

W e all seem to appreciate that babies are naturally born when they are ready to arrive. As inconvenient as this might be, we cannot control the timing. Yet, when it comes to our other babies—our projects at work and other creative efforts—we seem to think they should be born according to *our* schedule. Seldom do we consider that the creative process is organic in nature, that it requires us to be open instead of tied to an arbitrary schedule.

Year after year we run frantically through our work lives, often wondering if there isn't a better way to approach business or our work. Indeed there is—and it involves our attitudes, expectations, and use of time. Time is one of those things we tend to "swim in," so we often forget to consider its impact.

Most of us have been given our share of advice about successful attitudes and using time well. Unfortunately, we usually haven't been told that days are not created equal and that there are larger cycles or patterns that underlie each day's potential. In fact, it appears that the Universe has a completely different view of what good time management is!

We would laugh at someone who tried to get a tan at midnight, but many of us make this same mistake with other, less obvious cycles. What we've long forgotten is that there really *is* a time for every purpose under heaven. And astrology, which is essentially the study of time and cycles, contains the key to understanding the best times for our purposes.

Madeline C. Gerwick is an internationally recognized business astrologer, speaker, and author. She has a B.A. degree with honors in economics, and is listed in several Who's Who books, including *Who's Who in the World* and *Who's Who in America*. She annually writes *The Good Timing Guide: An Astrological Business Planner*. Ms. Gerwick is heard frequently on Conscious Talk Radio and her column appears regularly in *Promise Magazine*. Her company, Polaris Business Guides, is a metaphysical business consulting and training firm, which guides organizations to prosper by working in harmony with the universe. Please visit her at www. PolarisBusinessGuides.com.

In business, we expect constant forward progress in sales and growth, our speed to market, our daily performance, and product or service quality. No wonder we're so stressed out! Many of us also experience every minute of every workday completely filled with more work than can be accomplished. And to top it off, even though we've never experienced a year without challenges, delays, or setbacks, there's an unspoken belief that we shouldn't encounter any obstacles or delays if we're competent.

Regardless of how unrealistic these ideas may be, they permeate all aspects of business life. We've developed a nearly religious belief in always accomplishing something and pushing forward at all costs. But the Universe seems to have a different agenda. Instead of constant progress, the Universe is characterized by a well-considered order that closely resembles what we see in nature—and when was the last time you saw constant growth and progress without rest and renewal in the natural world?

Now consider how completely inappropriate our expectations must seem when viewed from the perspective of the Universe. Unlike our goals and expectations, which tend to look like straight lines with an upward slant, our creative and learning processes are *nonlinear*. As in most things, the Universe created regular *cycles* for these processes, instead. What has creativity and learning got to do with business? Just about everything, including the results we achieve.

# The Gestation or Time-Out Period

The Universe set up regular periods for renewal and replenishment as a part of the creative process. In astrology, these periods of time are shown by void-of-course Moons or Time-Outs. The Universe believes there is a need for downtime as part of the creative and learning processes. It thinks we need gestation periods to develop new ideas, gather information, and prepare ourselves for the right time to birth our projects or action plans.

These Time-Out periods are also perfect for renewing our energy and ourselves. They occur from two to four times per week and can last anywhere from a few minutes to nearly two and a half days. The most important thing to understand is that when we push forward with important actions and make key decisions during these times, the Universe rewards us with *nothing*.

Nothing? Yes, if we're lucky we get nothing or nowhere with our actions and decisions. When we're unlucky we get led down a dead-end path with one obstacle after another, and in the end it leads to...*nothing*. The worst examples I have seen over the last 15 years occurred when new products were approved for development during these Time-Out periods. The result: Several hundred thousand or even millions of dollars later, the projects were canceled. That's expensive nothing. Remember, just as in sporting events, *you can't score during a Time-Out.*

The *Wall Street Journal* once published a report of a research project conducted by astrologers. They randomly selected 1,400 bankrupt businesses to review their incorporation charts (using the date, time, and location they were incorporated). It turned out that 100 percent of them were started during Time-Outs. Certainly nothing came of those bankrupt companies. Imagine what happens when we introduce new products, launch websites, hire new employees, sign contracts, or place ads during Time-Outs. Nothing! Or at least nothing positive.

When I was working in the corporate world as a marketing professional for an international test equipment company, we learned about bad timing the hard way. Our division once signed off on a cost-cutting change to a major product line during a Time-Out. We had tested the change and it would save money. But we had somehow missed a major problem. A few months later, we had to internationally recall the products for a safety issue. The recall cost us nearly $900,000 — no savings at all!

When we're in a Time-Out period, we're either missing, or we misunderstand, some critical piece of information. When we make the decision without the correct data or understanding, we march down a dead-end path, going nowhere fast. When we finally get the correct information, we scrap what we did and start over. Can you remember encountering those scenarios? We've all had them. Wouldn't it be more productive to wait for the right information and a better time to push forward?

Consider the time when a small retailer unwittingly chose to hold a big promotion on a day with an all-day Time-Out. They spent $1,400 on advertising and bringing in special products for the event, only to have no one show up. Not one person came.

The purchasing department of the electronic test equipment company once signed an annual contract with one of the major suppliers for accessories during a Time-Out. We had horrendous problems with that contract, including several stop shipments, lots of quality problems, and late shipments. The following year, after I informed the manager about Time-Outs, he selected a good day to sign the contract. In one year, the supplier went from being our worst to being on our best vendor list.

With stories like this, why wouldn't we all want to use good timing? I know, I know... We have deadlines to meet! Even self-employed people have them. How can we work with good timing and still meet our due dates?

I like to tell my own story in answer to that question. One time I was late getting a newsletter written and delivered to the printer. When I finally finished writing it, a 20-hour Time-Out had started. I knew it was a bad idea to take it to the printer then, so I waited. I was completely irritated with myself. I *knew* that Time-Out was coming and I still didn't manage to get the newsletter written before it started.

What followed was an eye-opener, even for me. By the time this period was over, I discovered five mistakes in my newsletter. Even more important, someone sent me a critical piece of information that needed to be incorporated into it. I was overjoyed that I hadn't printed it yet. After integrating those changes, my newsletter was far better and my credibility was preserved. Yes it was mailed out a day later than it would have been, but in the overall scheme of things, that was a better choice.

Since nothing positive comes of actions taken and decisions made during Time-Outs, it seems only logical to stop wasting our energy, money, and time by using these periods more appropriately. These are great times to file paperwork, catch up, and clean up. They're the perfect time to finish anything, read, review, gather information, and do paperwork. Brainstorming for new ideas is also favored. Whenever possible, don't plan anything at all, and just follow your instincts. Meditate, get centered, and renew yourself. Just don't start something new, especially anything important.

Does your company have a department or division that needs better results? Ask that group to try an experiment by using good timing for a year. Just have the group avoid taking important actions and making important decisions during Time-Outs. I'm convinced that if we simply observed the Time-Out periods alone, we would save trillions of dollars annually in business worldwide.

## The Catch-Up and Fix-Up Period

As part of our learning process, the Universe also set up regular times to review, find our errors, catch up, and make corrections. The Universe expects us to learn by looking back, rethinking, and redoing things. This is another reason why our constant desire for forward progress thwarts our goals. We don't want to take the time to look back and rethink our erroneous decisions. Even the old song admonished us, "Don't stop thinking about tomorrow." But until we do, it's hard to make a course adjustment.

For some reason we've all gotten it into our heads that we shouldn't have to make corrections, change our minds after learning more, or make changes to a project mid-stream. But can you think of any long-term project that didn't have or need any changes. If the Universe is right, it's not possible.

The major periods for catching up and fixing our mistakes are known as Mercury retrograde. Basically, when Mercury appears to move backwards from the Earth's perspective, we experience schedule delays and difficulties in communications, transportation, and computers. This occurs three times per year for about three and a half weeks at a time. Anyone who has studied astrology at all has heard of these difficult periods. But we wouldn't experience so much frustration if we used this time more appropriately.

What does the Universe want us to do instead of speeding forward? It thinks we need some time to catch our mistakes, correct our erroneous assumptions and decisions, and fix them. It also thinks we need time to look back, reflect, catch up with people we haven't communicated with in a long time, and get organized. It wants us to have time to learn, and very few of us learn by looking forward. Instead we need to look back, review what has happened, and take the time to understand what went right and wrong.

None of this can happen while we're pushing full speed ahead. So guess what the Universe does with these periods? It fills them with *delays*. Computers and all forms of transportation break down, along with our communications. The UPS strike, for instance, took place during one of these periods. I've always imagined that the planet Mercury changes outfits and shows up as Murphy and his crew, making everything go wrong. And that's usually what happens!

This is a terrible time to sign contracts. One or both parties may misinterpret the agreement or wish they hadn't signed, and contracts frequently contain mistakes. Even more importantly, we all reconsider our needs during this period and we're usually not clear about what they really are until it is over. I've had several clients sign contracts during Mercury retrograde, only to regret doing so later when they discovered that their needs were different than they had thought.

This is definitely not the time to start new projects, since the purpose of this cycle is to catch-up. Project schedules run into "Murphy Time," as mistakes are uncovered and need to be fixed. It's better to schedule some extra time for projects in order to cover the changes needed and delays encountered during these periods. If you do start a project during Mercury retrograde, spend the period rethinking and replanning the project. Things will turn out much better if you do.

Products and services introduced or promoted under this cycle are unsuccessful in terms of actual sales versus forecasts. Sales can be as low as 40 percent of the forecast. Why? Customers misunderstand what is being offered, or miss the offer and fail to buy. Equally often, the product is incomplete or ineffective, especially in terms of documentation or software. The promotion may also miss the mark and fail to create desire for the product.

Generally, when we look back at these failures, we see that we rushed to market, or to complete our project, in time to fail! We took shortcuts that didn't work, or refused to reconsider previous decisions, even when we were warned otherwise. In short, we used the period inappropriately and paid the price. Sometimes we pay dearly.

Once a large company I worked for decided to build a new distribution center. This new center incorporated a major change in software, and a whole new way of picking the products to be shipped. When the time came, the new distribution center was scheduled to open at the beginning of Mercury retrograde. By now warning bells should be going off in your head. Even though everyone on the transition team had reported that they were ready, no one was.

Of course, since no one admitted to not being ready, the transition to the new center was a disaster. Several months and millions of dollars later, they were still sorting it out. This disaster could have been prevented by using this time to work out the bugs before making the transition. Whenever your project introduction coincides with Mercury retrograde, you can be sure you've missed something critical. It's a warning to slow down and fix it.

What's truly amazing about these Mercury retrograde periods is that even though they occur regularly, three times every year, for at least three weeks each time, we still ignore them. We still pretend that we don't need time to correct our mistakes. We still expect that we can do projects without any delays or changes. We still believe that constant forward progress is achievable. No wonder we're frustrated!

But in fact, according to Mother Nature, constant forward progress is not only unachievable, it's undesirable as well. I believe that the Universe is trying to tell us that creativity, learning, and productivity are intimately linked. When we fail to make room for the complete creative and learning processes, our productivity declines. Unable to replenish ourselves or use what we've learned to reconsider our decisions, we burn out and become zombies, chasing the same problems over and over again.

Inherent within the creative process lies the unknown, which is the seed of our mistakes and our learning experiences. But we need these elements of the creative process in order to create something better. Without the unknown, we wouldn't have anything to learn. It's all part of the cycle, a process to be repeated again and again.

How do we know this about the Universe? When we look at all other aspects of nature, we find that there are no examples of constant forward progress. The seasons change. Plants grow and then rest. The Sun rises and sets. The tide comes in and goes out. The Moon grows in light and then gets dark. There is a regular rhythm of increase and decrease throughout the Universe. How can we then expect something completely different for our businesses and the way we manage them?

## Can We Work in Harmony with the Universe?

So what's a person to do when the business world has no comprehension of the natural cycles of the Universe? Since the Universe is not going to change its design, we're left with learning how to match its patterns and cycles. Indeed, the root meaning of the word "consider" is *with* (con) *the stars* (sider). When we contrast that to the root meaning of the word "disaster," which is *against* (dis) *the stars* (aster), we get a clear idea of how we manage to create so many debacles.

What could we expect if we used good timing in business? Both J.P. Morgan and Walt Disney used astrological timing for their businesses. J.P. Morgan used it for his investments and became a billionaire doing so, back when millionaires were rare. Walt Disney used astrological timing for signing contracts, introducing his movies, products, and opening his theme parks. Asians have used good timing for centuries and consult an astrologer for a good date and time to open their business or sign contracts.

Are *you* ready to take a different approach to your work? Are *you* ready to work in harmony with Mother Nature? If so, I challenge you to begin prospering in peace with the use of good timing. Anyone can know what time it really is and plan schedules accordingly. All you have to do is check the daily cycles of any astrological calendar.

When we begin planning our schedules accordingly and consider the potentials for each day, we'll make major headway in the way we do business and how we feel about our work. We'll have fewer losses and better outcomes for our projects, products, and services, and we'll find better ways to be productive while renewing ourselves, too. Best of all, we'll have the wind at our backs. We'll prosper in peace as we work in harmony with the natural rhythms of the Universe.

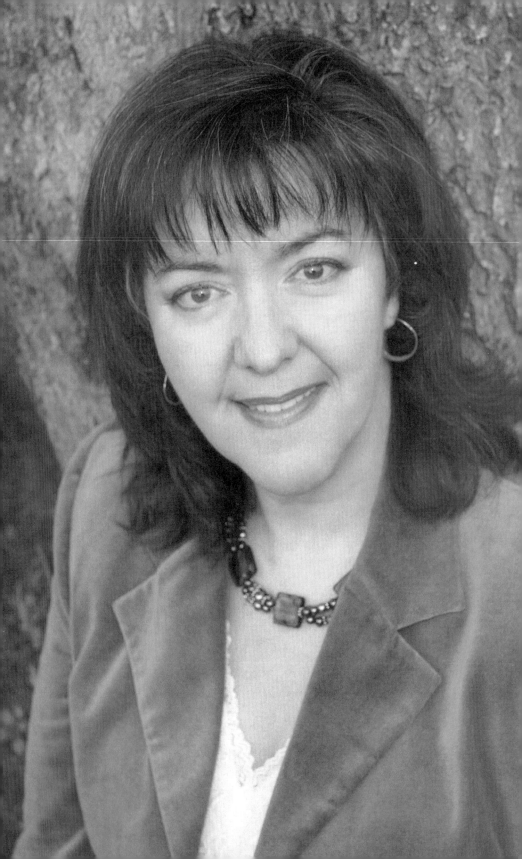

# ISABELLE ST-JEAN:

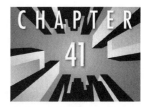

# The Circle Being

We were seated in a semi-circle in a spacious meeting room overlooking the expansive Pacific Northwest coast. The mission statement had been revisited and the core values identified, and we were now putting our minds together to reformulate an engaging vision for the organization. As I guided this group of helping professionals and consultants deeper into the dialog session, they began to be more animated, their eyes gazing upward as they spoke—a sure sign that they were getting into visionary mode.

Something was just starting to take flight, but not everyone was quite ready to join this momentum. "We're not used to thinking this way," Tom said with crossed arms and reluctance in his face. Then he paused and the realization came to him: "I think we've been caught up trying to solve short-term problems." He was right, but before I could address this all heads swiveled in Lisa's direction and the discussion turned to the limitations of the current structure and service delivery models.

The enthusiasm was dropping and we were loosing altitude. But viscerally I understood what was weighing us down. "Can you see what is happening here?" I asked them. "We want to reach a new perspective, to birth a vision of tremendous possibilities, but we've shifted our focus onto perceived limitations and this attention is keeping us stuck in the darkness of the birth canal!" All eyes were riveted on me as I continued. "Your service delivery model works

Isabelle St-Jean, a professional speaker, author, consultant, and NLP life coach, integrates into her work ideas, tools, and skills from the fields of cognitive sciences, organizational learning, ecopsychology, and philosophy. A graduate of the Authentic Leadership program at Naropa University, she is an eloquent communicator and change agent. Through her company, Inspired Momentum, Isabelle facilitates personal, professional, and organizational learning and development. Her book, *Living Forward, Giving Back: The Boomers' Call* (2007) inspires and empowers the Boomer generation to choose joyful, compassionate, and sustainable ways of living in mid-life and retirement. Visit www.InspiredMomentum.com.

well in some ways, but holds you back in others. Ultimately, we're aiming for a dynamic balance between conservation and growth."

I invited the group to take some time to reflect individually on the different needs, intents, goals, and possibilities they could see for their team. When we came back to the circle, the energy had noticeably changed. Jeffrey shared an important insight: "I know that our attachment to structure and status quo is undermining our progress and cutting the wings of our vision. I think we should fly with it instead, keep learning and reflecting and see where it takes us."

"Yes!" I affirmed as the group's energy rose to new heights. It was as if the roof had been swept off from the conversation. Everyone suddenly felt liberated, as if they were finally giving themselves permission to align with the fullness of the possibilities. You could almost feel an invisible current moving through the room, sparking our synapses into flames. And with far greater clarity we could finally see the steps required to close the gap between their present organizational reality and the next great milestone toward the new transformative vision.

What had just happened? Where did this feverish intensity come from to produce the vortex of ideas and energy now swirling at the center of the room? This is the mysterious force of collective intelligence that turns up when the right conditions converge. Described variedly by different people yet hardly describable in words, this force has been explained as a new entity arising suddenly among us. It is an ambient energy, or a liberated field in which extraordinary things happens. However it's described, its essence and its energy liberate our greatness so that we can accomplish together what might otherwise seem impossible.

I became excited and fascinated by this phenomenon after experiencing it on several occasions in group settings in my personal and professional life over the last couple of decades. From the corporate world into the not-for-profit sector, people are increasingly yearning to experience this kind of collaborative energy. It breaks through the isolation many of us feel when we try to come up with solutions or want to work more effectively together or create something that did not exist before. Indeed, the thrill of innovation is one of the gifts that collective intelligence can yield as it lifts us up under its wings.

Out of his passion for collective intelligence, social scientist and Senior Lecturer at the Massachusetts Institute of Technology Dr. C. Otto Scharmer describes the group experience of this energy as the "Circle Being." So, just what values, attitudes, personal qualities, skills, and actions are conducive to the emergence of this collective wisdom? Scharmer suggests that more and more people are experiencing this force because we are individually and collectively evolving into a higher, more purposeful future that seeks to come through us. Scharmer studied this phenomenon in the context of the U-theory, a model for understanding deep learning, and the process of co-creation between the individual, the collective, and the world.

In the interest of engaging the motivation and best productivity of employees, a movement toward real collaboration and cooperation in the workplace has been gathering momentum in the last decades. Since the field of coaching has spread to influence management and leadership styles, hierarchical approaches to leading have been tossed aside into obsolescence. Surely, the emphasis on tapping the power of collaboration has gained further ground. Likewise, recognition is growing of the importance of shared learning, dialogs, and collaboration as ingredients in the complex matrix that is conducive to collective intelligence within organizations.

Although cooperation is an accepted value in most organizations, this doesn't mean that people know how to translate this value into collaborative behavior. In order to yield real benefits, cooperation needs to be spelled out and installed into the organizational culture — which is a process that can take time to achieve. Evidently, we are still subject to the impact of a working society that has favored competition. Gradually, change toward a more healthy balance of these values is accelerating as its results of increased productivity and innovation become more evident.

Meanwhile, on the daily scene in the corporate world, frustration is common in group meetings and a kind of devolution often drags people toward the lowest common denominator. The boardroom is frequently host to a complex mixture of professional agendas and personal unfinished business, most of which tend to be unspoken. At times it feels as if the room is fed by pressurized air, like on an airplane — only there are no oxygen masks available when the system goes haywire.

Boardrooms and conference rooms are the scenes of personality clashes, abrasive comments stemming from ego-driven agendas, and power struggles over who will have the last word in a conflict. Another common pitfall of meetings is the trap of indecisiveness following a dissipated focus. Especially when intentions lack clarity at the onset, the collective energy begins to weaken as the meeting lingers in an unproductive wasteland and people begin to "check out." With less and less willful presence in the room, meetings are sure to deteriorate.

While the experience of collective intelligence may seem foreign to most workplace meetings, a simplified, practical version of it can be reframed as the ability to ask questions and seek answers together. Founder of Axiopole and author of *Managing Collective Intelligence*, Olivier Zara asserts that, when coupled with knowledge management, collective intelligence leads to collective performance that exceeds the sum of individual performances. Looking into the individual capacities of the members of an organization, we can draw the analogy between the best functioning of the human brain and the best functioning in organizations.

From the field of neurology we now know that human intelligence is optimized by the synapses interconnecting neurons, and the connections between the two hemispheres of the brain. Likewise, skillful interpersonal exchanges can generate access to a higher, collective intelligence that is greater than that of any individual. As Richard McDermott of McDermott Consulting says, "Neuron connections are essential to human intelligence; people connections are essential to organizational intelligence." And the merging of two or more brilliant ideas can generate a breakthrough innovation. Think about how nature excels at this everyday in the world: A sperm merges into an ovum and a whole new, unique person is launched into existence.

From an evolutionary perspective, what's apparent is that we have grown from an industrial and commercial society into an information society now moving toward the conceptual age. And while artificial intelligence is advancing at break-neck speed virtually on its own, there's a mounting urgency to tap the higher reaches of our own human intelligence and inner resources. As Daniel Pink explains in *A Whole New Mind: Moving from the Information Age to the Conceptual Age,* most in demand now is the ability to assemble disparate pieces of information into an "arresting new whole." This is what happens when we "get the picture," when we can pull back and see a situation from a bird's eye view. It's the ability to synthesize pieces into an entirely new perspective that can generate deeper meaning, which in turn provokes new insights. This is what Douglas Cohen, Founder of The Leadership Center and Sustainability Leadership Alliance, is referring to when he says:

> When working with deeply experienced and knowledgeable partners, I often encounter in them an outstanding capacity to diagnose a complex organizational situation in seconds. As I bring my almost instantaneous assessment to the same set of observed dynamics, within minutes we are into an in-depth analysis of a corporation or state agency. This allows for a mind-meld focused on our shared diagnosis that translates into a design of our actions as agents of change. Then, as we join the organization's

members in their next meeting, our interventions facilitate fruitful conversations and free up the members to be more collectively effective. It is a thrilling combination of synergetic creativity and of seeing the immediate impact within a matter of hours.

Along with the thrilling occurrence of mind-meld, the shift toward greater organizational intelligence can be accelerated when its people embrace the value of interdependence. In *The Fifth Discipline,* Peter Senge describes the three attitudinal orientations typical with respect to people's self-perception in relation to others and to outer circumstances. "The world is happening to me" is an inner view in which people tend to see themselves at the mercy of outside forces and lacking any sense of control over their own lives. This orientation is typical in people who have relatively low self-esteem and are not aware of their patterns of behavior

-§-

"The ant is a collectively intelligent and individually stupid animal; man is the opposite"
–Karl Von Frisch

-§-

or how they tend to use their personal power indirectly. Because they operate in a reactive or defensive mode, they often crave being "left alone" when confronted with requests that they easily perceive as impositions of demands.

On the other hand, people who are in the creative orientation tend to feel in charge of their lives and their achievements. When this orientation is part of an organization's culture, people are at risk of becoming workaholics as they are urged to "do what it takes" to achieve their goals and advance the success of their company. This viewpoint tends to offer little empathy toward the frailties and shortcomings that are part of our human nature. Typically, creatively oriented people thrive while they feel in control and are confident that they can achieve what they want to benefit themselves and those they selectively care about.

In contrast to this, in the interdependent orientation we see ourselves as part of a greater whole. As we strive to achieve a sense of personal mastery over life, we are conscious of the multitude of factors and forces interacting within and without. From this viewpoint, we aim at striking a balance between exerting a certain influence over events and allowing the emergence of opportunities or circumstances to arise in support of our most heartfelt commitments. This orientation embraces the paradox that, in the ability to be open, attentive, responsive, and flexible, we gain a more authentic sense of personal mastery and strength.

An exquisite example of interdependence in nature was demonstrated in the documentary *The March of the Penguins.* This film showed how the community of male penguins survives in the harsh, cold winter of the Antarctic while the females travel hundreds of miles across landscapes of thin ice to feed themselves from the ocean. As the males wait for months for the females to return, they cuddle together in a large group formation. Each of them carefully holds an egg, containing his progeny, between his feet and the folds of his furry belly. To allow each of the penguins to be sheltered for a time from the bitter cold, they take turns being on the outer circles of the group. Interdependence and collective wisdom come together here in magnificence! It is built into the natural instinct that compels each and every penguin to behave in a way that insures his survival and that of the community as a whole.

When we adopt an orientation that includes the value of interdependence, we're also inclined to come to other character strengths that promote the well-being of the whole. Humility, for example, has been found to be an important character trait in exceptional leaders. In his article entitled "Level 5 Leadership: The Triumph of Humility and Fierce Resolve," Jim Collins affirms that, throughout his research on leaders of corporations, he found that humility is necessary to the ability to lead from an effective core of authenticity. Paradoxically, when humility is combined with fierce resolve, it yields a mighty force that exerts motivating and inspiring energies, igniting a unifying spirit at the center of the organization.

In the context of my own experiences in personal development I have developed a deep respect for the power of openness and humility. Over several years of work with a group devoted to personal growth, I witnessed numerous occasions in which people inadvertently triggered one other into intense emotions. Members of this group often explored the roots of dysfunctional patterns while expressing the emotions that would surface through this process. Over the years, we each developed the ability to sense when a member in process would finally surrender their defensive behaviors and align themselves with the truth emerging from the core of their being. When this happened, a beautiful humility would emanate from the individual and our collective wisdom would take over, lending the most generous support possible.

I recall one unforgettable session, in which a member I'll call Brian relived a very traumatic experience of his childhood and at once discovered the roots of his persistent low self-esteem. As he worked through the pain, he reached a place of profound, almost luminous openness and vulnerability. At one point he turned to group members, face still glistening from tears, and asked them individually if they could accept him as he was in that moment. We were all deeply moved. The energies of empathy and compassion arising from the group were virtually palpable. The spirit of collective wisdom was ignited, in this case, as Brian courageously touched an issue of universal dimension that resonated within each of us: Am I good enough to be truly accepted and loved as I am, even in my barest truth and imperfect human nature?

Perhaps you've been aware of this question being tucked secretly into your dialogs at work. It is no wonder, then, that you would naturally feel at ease when the group allows its openness and humility to shine forth. But our secret yearning for acceptance also places us at risk of unconsciously projecting our disowned unfinished business onto others. What we do not like about ourselves is often exactly what we unconsciously focus on in others. In these moments, acute self-awareness can help us to acknowledge what is happening within. In the spirit of self-empathy, humility clears a path that leads beyond the clashes of differences and personalities. Then we are better able to hold our personal judgments and qualifying comments in the interest of building momentum toward the greater collective purpose. This is not a matter of holding back, but rather of holding oneself still in the authentic experience of what is while being open to what wants to come through from the collective realm.

At times, tension builds because many in the group have strong feelings about something that has happened in the organization. In these cases it is important for members to take responsibility for and skillfully express relevant personal feelings about what has happened. Otherwise, the suppressed emotions tend to drag the energy downward and prevent people from being fully present. I recall times during the professional development sessions that I have led when the tension dissipated once I encouraged people to break through the collusion of silence. When just one person takes that step, it enables others to also drop into their more authentic selves and gain access as a group to the visionary field that may otherwise be out of reach.

In a group dialogue there may also be another kind of silence, pregnant with brilliant ideas within the minds of those who fear speaking and being rejected for their differences. This can be a shadow side of shared values toward a superficial melding of minds in which differences are unintentionally perceived as annoyances or resistance. If there is an unstated value placed on unanimous agreement, the energy in the group is likely to stagnate as people hold back their views. This is why the conscious creation of a group culture that invites new and different ideas is paramount to building the trust that fosters collective wisdom.

As trust is built and a group courageously moves away from the grip of preconceived agendas and roles, another door may open that leads toward the vortex of ambient energy. In "Coming Together," an article published in *What is Enlightenment Magazine* in 2004, Craig Hamilton provides an example of a meeting in which the Circle Being showed up to the amazement of 15 top telecom executives. In this retreat, organized to discuss the future of the industry, two days had been spent going around in plummeting circles. Finally, a dialog facilitator was flown in.

The facilitator stressed the importance of real listening and suspending assumptions, while reminding them of what they had come together to do. At this suggestion, the atmosphere began to shift—and then the CEO of one large wireless company said something that finally instigated real, authentic conversation: "I think we need to stop thinking of our work in purely business terms," he said, then after a pause added, "What if we began to see one another not simply as competitors for market share but as partners in uniting the world through technology?"

More than just conversation, this CEO actually launched a provocative vision that stirred the group out of their guarded sidestepping and stalling. His openness shook up the stagnant pattern of interaction that had formed over the previous two days. After a silence that cleared the way for the renewed, vibrant energy growing in the room, others began to concur with the CEO's statement. "If there's anything this industry needs right now, it's vision," said one executive. Their vibrant dialog went on for hours, a sense of energy, renewed creativity, and space emanating from everyone in the group. At last, they were thinking together rather than against each other.

In this example, it was the shift away from competitive friction and "expert" attitude toward a visionary idea that unlocked the door to a real, collaborative conversation. When everyone engaged around the vision, the most purposeful and creative parts of them stepped forward into the pool of common meaning. They were all inspired to contribute to the vision of what they could be if they truly became partners.

This experience is familiar to a number of consultants and dialog facilitators around the world. Myriam Laberge, Certified Professional Facilitator and Co-founder of Breakthroughs Unlimited, has witnessed this kind of magic firsthand. She says it's as if "the many become one heart, one mind, one spirit releasing extraordinary creativity and power." And she points out that this experience rarely occurs spontaneously. Rather, this creative spirit may be tapped in conjunction with a significant investment of time spent sharing, learning, listening, and discovering. This time together enables the necessary trust to flourish in the group. "A deeply compelling question must catalyze the group's central intention," Laberge insists, "so that people may rise up to what they could be." This is exactly what occurred among the 15 telecom executives who united in dialog around the vision that was so candidly articulated.

At this juncture in the unfolding of our human history—in our Western cultures particularly—people are hungering for a deeper connection at work and in their personal lives. You may have noticed that the opportunities for such connection are turning up more and more. In the midst of writing these last paragraphs, I took a fruitful pause to attend the book launch of a kindred spirit in my community. With new her book, One *Circle,* Maureen Fitzgerald is helping others to develop groups in which people creatively solve problems in their professional or personal lives. Connected in the unified purpose of helping each other, group members in such circles support one another to achieve their goals while taping the power of collective wisdom and intelligence.

Clarity of purpose and intentions, trust, skillful communication, and presence can enable the rise of a large wave of wisdom to swell on the moving waters of group dialogs and yield its transformative energy. Also conducive to increasing that wave's momentum is a willingness to adopt a beginner's mindset and to venture beyond the discursive logic mode of operation that pervades most workplaces. We need to allow fluidity between our personal and professional selves. As Peter Senge and co-authors of *Presence* so eloquently stated: "There is nothing more personal than vision, yet the visions that ultimately prove transformative have nothing to do with us as individuals."

As we harness the power of our imaginative and visionary capacities, we rise to the challenge of what we must become in order to survive, and perhaps even thrive, on our home planet. While we enable the Grand Will to work through us, our multiple streams of endeavor will converge so that we can collectively embrace the evolutionary task that Einstein urged us to take on: to free ourselves from the prison of our illusory separateness, to embrace all living creatures, and to restore our harmony with the whole of nature. We must awaken to this vision as we pursue our own prosperity. Our continuity on the planet depends on this now, as the old "business as usual" threatens to lead us into oblivion. Will you rise to the challenge and invite the Circle Being to ignite a participatory vision within your own organization? Join me in cultivating the ground to allow the spirit of oneness and collective intelligence to lift us to new heights as we serve humanity through our work.

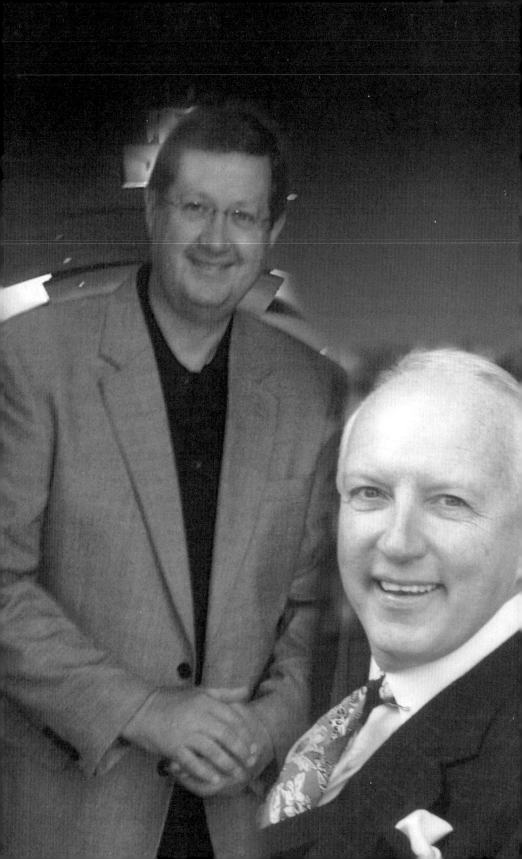

# MARK VICTOR HANSEN & ROBERT ALLEN:

# The Infinite Network

*You can rest assured that if you devote your time and attention to the highest advantage of others, the Universe will support you, always and only in the nick of time.*

*–R. Buckminster Fuller*

Enlightened Millionaires realize that there is a spiritual dimension to wealth. They understand that this unseen world is the source of infinite abundance. When you unite with the source of infinite abundance, you also become infinitely abundant.

How do you tap into this Infinite Network of abundance? Tithing expands, multiplies, and adds value to all that you do.

Another way you tap into the Infinite Network is to simply maintain your integrity. It is this integrity that ensures your long-term success.

Knowing and acknowledging the spiritual dimension makes your life far less stressful. Moreover, as your success gracefully unfolds, a deep sense of gratitude will permeate your being.

Embracing the spiritual component of wealth and recognizing the existence of the Infinite Network is the single most important and most powerful form of leverage.

**Mark Victor Hansen is the co-author of Chicken Soup for the Soul series, one of the best-selling book series in history, with more than 80 million copies currently in print. He has been a public speaker for twenty-five years, is the author of five other books, and has received numerous honorary degrees and awards, including the Horatio Alger Award. Visit www.markvictorhansen.com.**

**Robert G. Allen is the author of some of the most successful financial books in history, including multiple *New York Times* bestsellers such as *Nothing Down* (Simon & Schuster, 1984), which has sold more than 1,250,000 copies. Allen has been featured in the *Wall Street Journal*, *Newsweek*, *Money Magazine*, anwd *Reader's Digest*.**

**Hansen and Allen co-authored *The One Minute Millionaire* (Harmony, 2002). Visit www.OneMinuteMillionaire.com.**

All Enlightened Millionaires humbly acknowledge their reliance on the Infinite Network.

## Tapping into the Power of the Universe

*What senses do we lack that we cannot see or hear another world all around us?*

—From *Dune*, by Frank Herbert

The 1981 Oscar-winning movie *Chariots of Fire* tells the story of two British runners in the 1924 Olympics: Harold Abrahams, a Jew driven to compete by anti-Semitism, and Eric Liddell, a Christian missionary who feels God's presence when he runs. Did you know that the title of the movie was inspired by one of the most remarkable stories from ancient scripture?

In this story, the King of Syria is angry with the Jewish prophet Elisha and sends a great army to capture him. Elisha's servant awakes one morning to find that their city is surrounded with a huge Syrian army "both with horses and chariots." (II Kings 6:15-17).

He runs to tell Elisha. "Alas, my master! What shall we do?"

Elisha responds, "Don't be afraid. Those who are with us are more than those who are with them."

We can only imagine what the servant was thinking when he heard this: *How ridiculous! There are thousands of them and only two of us!* Then Elisha prays and says, "O Lord, open his eyes so he may see." Then the Lord opens the servant's eyes, and he looks and sees the hills full of horses and *chariots of fire* all around Elisha.

If *your* eyes were "opened," what would *you* see?

If you've ever been snorkeling near a tropical reef, you've experienced what it's like to peer into another world. As soon as you put your mask in the water, a brilliant new dimension of bright-colored fish and strange creatures explodes into sight. We're not accustomed to seeing such brilliant color in our normally drab existence, but that doesn't mean it doesn't exist. To use Wayne Dyer's analogy, this physical world is only one room of a thousand-room mansion. There is so much more for us to explore beyond our physical senses.

Call it what you will—the "other side," the "other world," or "the world of spirits"—most of us admit to a system of spiritual beliefs. Is there another world all around us right now—an invisible world? Is there a thin curtain that separates us from this invisible world? Are dozens of unseen beings anxiously waiting to do our bidding, to help us? Are chariots of fire around *you*? And if not chariots, is an angel or two cheering you on?

Yes, this may seem far-fetched, but what if it was true? In the Jewish tradition, every blade of grass has an angel standing over it, encouraging it: Grow! Grow! Wouldn't it be nice to know that you are not alone—that there might be a powerful support system surrounding you?

We believe there is such an invisible world—a world just waiting to help you fulfill your congruent desires—summoned to your side "with horses and chariots of fire".

## Your Infinite Network

*If only God would give me some clear sign! Like making a deposit in my name in a Swiss bank account.*

–Woody Allen

To grow and maximize your leverage, you need to work with several expanding bandwidths from the broadcast station called *you*.

The infinite is infinite. You are the center of the world, metaphorically speaking. Think of your mind and brain as a radio station that outputs your chosen messages. Your imagination creates the broadcast that originates your future. If you send the wrong outbound messages, you get the wrong results. If you broadcast the right messages consistently and persistently, you will get the right results, right here and right now.

First, as we've established, you need a mentor, a guide, and someone to share with you the shortcuts to instant success in an endeavor or enterprise. All successful people whom we have ever encountered have had a great and inspiring mentor with whom they were attuned and who wanted to personally help them become who they were capable of becoming.

The second circle out from your broadcasting station is your Dream Team. It starts with you and at least one other person. Miracles only happen when you have a dedicated Dream Team. Greatness only happens to and through teams.

Third, your alliances and networks will geometrically expand from your association with your Dream Team. It's as if the "brothers of serendipity" arrive just in time with the right people. Your million-dollar Rolodex will source and serve you in ever-expanding ways.

The Universe is forever testing you and giving you feedback. The messages that you have been sending create an echo effect. The problem is that the feedback is not instantaneous, so it is sometimes difficult to observe and understand the cause-and-effect relationship.

Alone, you and your task have a one-to-one relationship; your task will be slow, arduous, and painful drudgery. With your mentor, team, and network in place, your power is greatly multiplied and your Infinite Network comes into serious play. You have witnessed its presence and its superlative results, though it was not previously named or popularized. The Spiritual Internet kicks in when a team has a big purposeful dream, and everyone stays positive about its accomplishment.

It is impossible to obtain these results in any other way.

# PART TEN

❧

# Huge Leverage

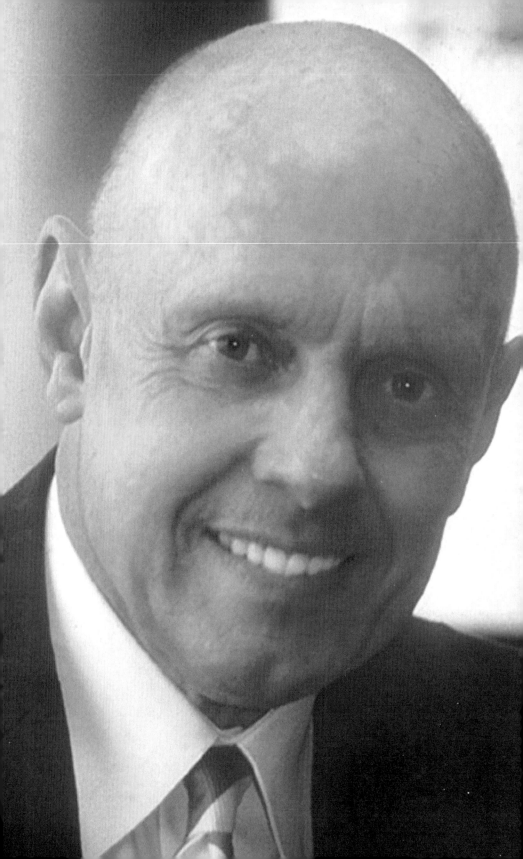

# Stephen Covey:

# Thirty Methods of Influence

Wreall want to have positive influence with certain people in our personal and professional lives. Our motive may be to win new business, keep customers, maintain friendships, change behaviors, or improve marriage and family relationships.

But how do we do it? How do we powerfully and ethically influence the lives of other people? I submit that there are three basic categories of influence: 1) to model by example (others *see*); 2) to build caring relationships (others *feel*); and 3) to mentor by instruction (others *hear*).

The following 30 methods of influence fall into these three categories.

## Example: Who You Are and How You Act

1. **Refrain from saying the unkind or negative thing,** particularly when you are provoked or fatigued. In these circumstances, to not say the unkind or critical thing is a supreme form of self-mastery. Courage is the quality of every quality at its highest testing point. If we have no model of restraint to follow, we will likely take out our frustration on our fellow workers. We may need to find new models, new examples to follow, and learn to win our own battles privately, to get our motives straight, to gain perspective and control, and to back away from impulsively speaking or striking out.

Stephen R. Covey was recognized in 1996 as one of *Time* magazine's 25 most influential Americans. Dr. Covey is the author of the bestselling *The 7 Habits of Highly Effective People* (Free Press, 2004). Other bestsellers authored by Dr. Covey include *First Things First* (Simon & Schuster Ltd, 1999), *Principle-Centered Leadership* (Simon & Schuster, 1999), *The 7 Habits of Highly Effective Families* (Simon & Schuster, 1999) and *The 8th Habit: From Effectiveness to Greatness* (Free Press, 2004). Dr. Covey is co-founder and vice chairman of FranklinCovey, the leading professional services firm, with offices in 123 countries. Visit www.stephencovey.com.

2. **Exercise patience with others.** In times of stress, our impatience surfaces. We may say things we don't really mean or intend to say—all out of proportion to reality. Or we may become sullen, communicating through emotion and attitude rather than words, eloquent messages of criticism, judgment, and rejection. We then harvest hurt feelings and strained relationships. Patience is the practical expression of faith, hope, wisdom, and love. It is a very active emotion. It is not indifference, sullen endurance, or resignation. Patience is emotional diligence. It accepts the reality of step-by-step processes and natural growth cycles. Life provides abundant chances to practice patience—to stretch the emotional fiber—from waiting for a late person or plane to listening quietly to your child's feelings and experiences when other things are pressing.

3. **Distinguish between the person and the behavior or performance.** While we may disapprove of bad behavior and poor performance, we first need to communicate and help build a sense of intrinsic worth and self-esteem totally apart from comparisons and judgments. Doing this will powerfully inspire superior effort. The power to distinguish between person and performance and to communicate intrinsic worth flows naturally out of our own sense of intrinsic worth.

4. **Perform anonymous service.** Whenever we do good for others anonymously, our sense of intrinsic worth and self-respect increases. Moreover, we gain insight into the worth of others by serving them without expectation of publicity or reward. Selfless service has always been one of the most powerful methods of influence.

5. **Choose the proactive response.** Why do so few of us "do" as well as we "know"? Because we neglect a connecting link between what we know and what we do—we don't choose our response. Choosing requires us to gain perspective and then to decide our own actions and reactions. Choosing means to accept responsibility for our attitudes and actions, to refuse to blame others or circumstances. It revolves a real internal struggle, ultimately, between competing motives or conflicting concepts. Unless we exercise our power to choose wisely, our actions will be determined by conditions. Our ultimate freedom is the right and power to decide how anybody or anything outside ourselves will affect us.

6. **Keep the promises you make to others.** By making and keeping our resolves and promises, we win influence with others. To be and do better, we must make promises (resolutions, commitments, oaths, and covenants), but we should never make a promise we will not keep. Using self-knowledge, we can be very selective about the promises we make. Our ability to make and keep promises is one measure of faith in ourselves and of our integrity.

7. **Focus on the circle of influence.** As we focus on doing something positive about the things we can control, we expand our circle of influence. Direct control problems are solved by changing our habits of doing and thinking. Indirect control problems require us to change our methods of influence. For instance, we complain from time to time that "if only the boss could understand my program or my problem..." But few of us take the time to prepare the kind of presentation that the boss would listen to and respect, in his language, with his problems in mind. With no control problems, we can control our reaction to problems, deciding within ourselves how anything or anybody will affect us. As William James said: "We can change our circumstances by a mere change of our attitude."

8. **Live the law of love.** We encourage obedience to the laws of life when we live the laws of love. People are extremely tender inside, particularly those who act as if they are tough and self-sufficient. And if we'll listen to them with the third ear, the heart, they'll tell us so. We can gain even greater influence with them by showing love, particularly unconditional love, as this gives people a sense of intrinsic worth and security unrelated to conforming behavior or comparisons with others. Many borrow their security and strength from external appearances, status symbols, positions, achievements, and associations. But borrowing strength inevitably builds weakness. We all distrust superficial human relations techniques and manipulative success formulas that are separated from sincere love.

# Relationship: Do You Understand and Care?

9. **Assume the best of others.** Assuming good faith produces good fruit. By acting on the assumption others want and mean to do their best, as they see it, you can exert a powerful influence and bring out the best in them. Our efforts to classify and categorize, judge, and measure often emerge from our own insecurities and frustrations in dealing with complex, changing realities. Each person has many dimensions and potentials, some in evidence, most dormant. And they tend to respond to how we treat them and what we believe about them. Some may let us down or take advantage of our trust, considering us naive or gullible. But most will come through, simply because we believe in them. Don't bottleneck the many for fear of a few! Whenever we assume good faith, born of good motives and inner security, we appeal to the good in others.

10. **Seek first to understand.** Seek first to understand, then to be understood. When we're communicating with another, we need to give full attention, to be completely present. Then we need to

empathize—to see from the other's point of view, to "walk in his moccasins" for a while. This takes courage, and patience, and inner sources of security. But until people feel that you understand them, they will not be open to your influence.

11. **Reward open, honest expressions or questions.** Too often we punish honest, open expressions or questions. We upbraid, judge, belittle, embarrass. Others learn to cover up, to protect themselves, to not ask. The greatest single barrier to rich, honest communication is the tendency to criticize and judge.

12. **Give an understanding response.** Using the understanding response (reflecting back feeling), three good things happen: 1) you gain increased understanding and clarity of feelings and problems; 2) you gain new courage and growth in responsible independence; and 3) you build real confidence in the relationship. This response has its greatest value when a person wants to talk about a situation laden with emotions and feelings. But this response is more attitude than technique. It will fail if you try to manipulate; it will work if you deeply want to understand.

13. **If offended, take the initiative.** If someone offends you unknowingly and continues to do so, take the initiative to clear it up. Consider two tragic consequences of not taking the initiative: first, the offended one often broods about the offense until the situation is blown out of proportion; second, the offended one then behaves defensively to avoid further hurt. When taking the initiative, do it in good spirits, not in a spirit of vindication and anger. Also, describe your feelings—when and how the offense took place—rather than judging or labeling the other person. This preserves the dignity and self-respect of the other person, who then can respond and learn without feeling threatened. Our feelings, opinions, and perceptions are not facts. To act on that awareness takes thought control and fosters humility.

14. **Admit your mistakes, apologize, ask for forgiveness.** When we are party to seriously strained relations, we may need to admit that we are at least partly to blame. When one is deeply hurt, he draws back, closes up, and puts us behind prison bars in his own mind. Improving our behavior alone won't release us from this prison. Often the only way out is to admit our mistakes, apologize, and ask forgiveness, making no excuses, explanations, or defenses.

15. **Let arguments fly out open windows.** Give no answer to contentious arguments or irresponsible accusations. Let such things "fly out open windows" until they spend themselves. If you try to answer or reason back, you merely gratify and ignite pent-up hostility and anger. When you go quietly about your business, the other has

to struggle with the natural consequences of irresponsible expression. Don't be drawn into any poisonous, contentious orbit, or you'll find yourself bitten and afflicted similarly. Then the other person's weaknesses will become your own, and all this will sow a seed bed of future misunderstandings, accusations, and wrangling. The power to let arguments fly out open windows flows out of an inward peace that frees you from the compulsive need to answer and justify. The source of this peace is living responsibly, obediently to conscience.

16. **Go one on one.** An executive might be very involved and dedicated to his or her work, to church and community projects, and to many people's lives, yet not have a deep, meaningful relationship with his or her own spouse. It takes more nobility of character, more humility, more patience, to develop such a relationship with one's spouse than it would take to give continued dedicated service to the many. We often justify neglecting the one to take care of the many because we receive many expressions of esteem and gratitude. Yet we know that we need to set aside time and give ourselves completely to one special person. With our children, we may need to schedule one-on-one visits—a time when we can give them our full attention and listen to them without censoring, lecturing, or comparing.

17. **Renew your commitment to things you have in common.** Continually renew your basic commitment to the things that unite you with your friends, family, and fellow workers. Their deepest loyalties and strongest feelings attach to these things rather than to the problems or issues around which differences often emerge. Differences are not ignored; they are subordinated. The issue or one's point is never as important as the relationship.

18. **Be influenced by them first.** We have influence with others to the degree they feel they have influence with us. As the saying goes, "I don't care how much you know until I know how much you care." When another feels you genuinely care about him and that you understand his unique problems and feelings, he also feels he has influenced you. He will then become amazingly open. We take the prescription because it is based on the diagnosis.

19. **Accept the person and the situation.** The first step in changing or improving another is to accept him as he is. Nothing reinforces defensive behavior more than judgment, comparison, or rejection. A feeling of acceptance and worth frees a person from the need to defend and helps release the natural growth tendency to improve. Acceptance is not condoning a weakness or agreeing with an opinion. Rather, it is affirming the intrinsic worth of another by acknowledging that he does feel or think a particular way.

# CHAPTER FORTY-THREE

# Instruction: What You Tell Me

20. **Prepare your mind and heart before you prepare your speech.** What we say may be less important than how we say it. So, before your children return from school full of their own needs, stop and get control. Plumb your resources. Set your mind and heart. Choose pleasantness and cheerfulness. Choose to give full attention to their needs. Or sit a moment in the car before coming in from work and do the same. Ask yourself, "How can I bless my wife (or husband) and children tonight?" Plumb your resources. Choosing to be your best self will arrest fatigue and renew your best resolves.

21. **Avoid fight or flight—talk through differences.** Many people either fight or flee when they disagree. Fighting takes many forms, ranging from violence and open expressions of anger and hate to subtle sarcasm, sharp answers, clever comebacks, belittling humor, judgments, and reactions. Fleeing also takes various forms. One is simply to withdraw, feeling sorry for oneself. Such sulking often feeds the fires of revenge and future retaliation. People also flee by growing cold and indifferent, by escaping involvement and responsibility.

22. **Recognize and take time to teach.** With differences come supreme teaching moments. But there's a time to teach and a time not to teach. It's time to teach when 1) people are not threatened (efforts to teach when people feel threatened will only increase resentment, so wait for or create a new situation in which the person feels more secure and receptive); 2) you're not angry or frustrated, when you have feelings of affection, respect, and inward security; and 3) when the other person needs help and support (to rush in with success formulas when someone is emotionally low or fatigued or under a lot of pressure is comparable to trying to teach a drowning man to swim). Remember: We are teaching one thing or another all of the time, because we are constantly radiating what we are.

23. **Agree on the limits, rules, expectations, and consequences.** These must be clearly established, agreed upon, understood, and enforced. Personal security is largely born of a sense of justice— knowing what is expected, what the limits, rules, and consequences are. Life can be thrown out of kilter with uncertain expectations, shifting limits, or arbitrary rules: one day this, the next day that. No wonder many grow up learning to depend only on their own ability to manipulate people and life. When life becomes a game to be manipulated, the only sin is getting caught.

24. **Don't give up, and don't give in.** It is unkind to shield people from the consequences of their own behavior. In doing so, we teach them they are inadequate and weak. When we give in to irresponsible

behavior by excusing it or sympathizing with it, we condone and foster spoiled, law-unto-self behavior. And if we give up — by ignoring people or tearing into them — we undermine their motivation to try. The discipline of *Don't give up, and don't give in,* tempered with love, comes from responsible, disciplined living. Otherwise we take the course of least resistance — giving in when we care or giving up when we don't.

25. **Be there at the crossroads.** None of us want the people we care most about to make decisions that have important long-range consequences on the basis of short-range emotional perspectives and moods, personal insecurity, and self-doubt. How can we influence them? First, think before you react. Don't be controlled by your own short-range emotional moods and do something that injures whatever relationship and influence you now have. Second, understand that people tend to act in terms of how they feel instead of what they know. Motivation is more a function of the heart than the head. When we sense that our reason and logic aren't communicating with their sentiment and emotion, we should try to understand their language as we would a foreign tongue, without condemning it or rejecting them. This effort communicates respect and acceptance, lowers defenses, diminishes the need to fight, and restores the desire to do what is right.

26. **Speak the languages of logic and emotion.** The language of logic and the language of emotion are as different as English and French. When we realize we don't have a common language, we may need to communicate in one of four other ways: 1) Give time, for when we cheerfully give time, we transfer its worth to another; 2) Be patient, as patience also communicates worth and says "I'll go at your speed; I'm happy to wait for you; you're worth it"; 3) Seek to understand, because an honest effort to understand eliminates the need to fight and to defend; and 4) Openly express our feelings and be congruent with our nonverbal expressions.

27. **Delegate effectively.** Effective delegation takes emotional courage as we allow, to one degree or another, others to make mistakes on our time, money, and good name. This courage consists of patience, self-control, faith in the potential of others, and respect for individual differences. Effective delegation must be two-way: responsibility given, responsibility received. There are three phases. First, the initial agreement. People have a clear understanding of what is expected and what the resources, authority, latitude, and guidelines are. Second, sustaining the delegatees. The supervisor becomes a source of help, the advocate, not the feared adversary. He provides resources, removes obstacles, sustains actions and decisions,

gives vision, provides training, and shares feedback. Third, the accountability process. This is largely one of self-evaluation, since delegatees are supervised by results, by actual performance.

28. **Involve people in meaningful projects.** Meaningful projects have a healing influence on people. However, what is meaningful to a manager may be meaningless to a subordinate. Projects take on meaning when people are involved in the planning and thinking processes. We all need to be engaged in a good cause. Without such projects, life loses its meaning; in fact, the life span is short for people who retire, looking for a tensionless state. Life is sustained by tension between where we are now and where we want to be—some goal worth struggling for.

29. **Train them in the law of the harvest.** We teach the "agricultural principles" of preparing the soil, seeding, cultivating, watering, weeding, and harvesting. We focus on natural processes. We align the systems, especially compensation, to reflect and reinforce the idea that we reap what we sow.

30. **Let natural consequences teach responsible behavior.** One of the kindest things we can do is to let the natural or logical consequences of people's actions teach them responsible behavior. They may not like it or us, but popularity is a fickle standard by which to measure character development. Insisting on justice demands more true love, not less. We care enough for their growth and security to suffer their displeasure.

## Overcoming Three Big Mistakes

In our attempts to influence others, we commonly make three mistakes, all related either to ignoring or short-cutting these three categories of influence.

**Mistake #1: Advise before understand.** Before we try to tell others what to do, we need to establish an understanding relationship. The key to your influence with me is your understanding of me. Unless you understand me and my unique situation and feelings, you won't know how to advise or counsel me. Unless you're influenced by my uniqueness, I'm not going to be influenced by your advice. Cure: Empathy—seek first to understand, then to be understood.

**Mistake #2: Attempt to build/rebuild relationships without changing conduct or attitude.** We try to build or rebuild a relationship without making any fundamental change in our conduct or attitude. If our example is pockmarked with inconsistency and insincerity, no amount of "win friends" technique will work. As Emerson so aptly put it, "What you are shouts so loudly in my ears I can't hear what you say." Cure: Show consistency and sincerity.

**Mistake #3: Assume that good example and relationship are sufficient.** We assume that a good example and a good relationship are sufficient, that we don't need to teach people explicitly. Just as vision without love contains no motivation, so also love without vision contains no goals, no guidelines, no standards, no lifting power. Cure: Teach and talk about vision, mission, roles, goals, guidelines, and standards.

In the last analysis, what we are communicates far more eloquently and persuasively than what we say or even what we do.

# Indivisible Life

In a very real sense there is no such thing as organizational behavior. There is only individual behavior. Everything else flows out of that.

The main sticking point between Sigmund Freud and Carl Jung dealt with conscience. Freud believed the conscience or superego was basically a social product. Jung believed it primarily to be part of the collective unconscious, transcending the mortal overlay of culture, race, religion, gender, or nationality.

I believe Jung was right and Freud was wrong. In working with thousands of organizations and individuals around the world in preparing mission or value statements — assuming four conditions are present, namely 1) enough people; 2) interacting freely; 3) well informed about the realities of their situation; 4) feeling safe to express themselves without fear of censure, ridicule, or embarrassment — then the values or principles part of the mission statement all basically say the same thing, even though different words are used, regardless of nationality, culture, religion, or race.

Gandhi emphasized: "A person cannot do right in one department whilst attempting to do wrong in another department: Life is one indivisible whole." John Wesley's mother taught her son, "Whatever weakens your reason, impairs the tenderness of your conscience, obscures your sense of God, takes off your relish for spiritual things, whatever increases the authority of the body over the mind, that thing is sin to you, however innocent it may seem in itself."

Further, I believe God is the true name and source of the collective unconscious and is therefore the ultimate moral authority in the universe. The daily prayerful study of His revealed word is the single most important and powerful discipline in life because it points our lives, like a compass, to "true north" — our divine destiny.

It also sets us on a life of service, and I fear, unless enough of us capture the spirit of the following conviction of George Bernard Shaw, that the social problems of today will overwhelm the economic machine and discombobulate all of society.

"This is the true joy in life, being used for a purpose recognized by yourself as a mighty one.

"Being a force of nature instead of a feverish, selfish little clod of ailments and grievances complaining that the world will not devote itself to making you happy.

"I am of the opinion that my life belongs to the whole community and as I live it is my privilege—my *privilege* to do for it whatever I can.

"I want to be thoroughly used up when I die, for the harder I work the more I love. I rejoice in life for its own sake. Life is no brief candle to me; it is a sort of splendid torch which I've got a hold of for the moment and I want to make it burn as brightly as possible before handing it on to future generations."

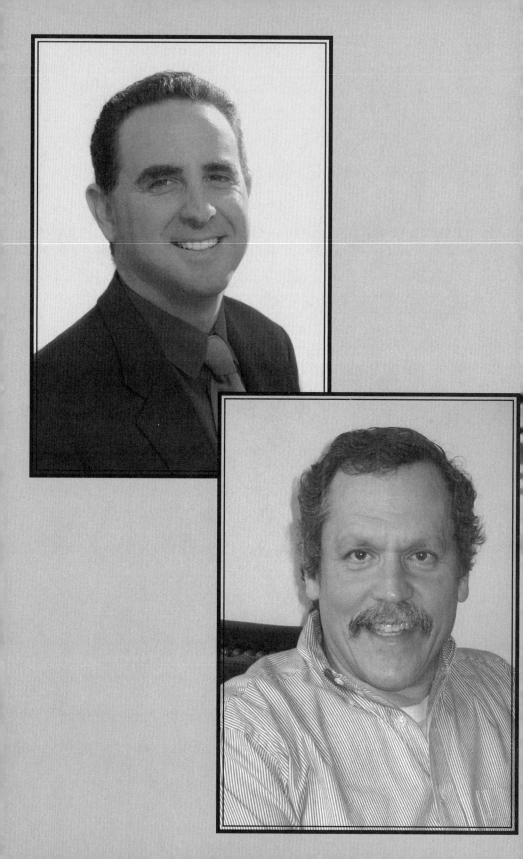

# David Rock & Jeffrey Schwartz:

# The Neuroscience of Leadership

**M**ike is the CEO of a multinational pharmaceutical company, and he's in trouble. With the patents on several key drugs due to expire soon, his business desperately needs to become more entrepreneurial, particularly in its ability to form internal and external partnerships to reduce time-to-market. Yet his organization has a silo mentality, with highly competitive teams secretly working against one another. How can Mike change the way thousands of people at his company think and behave every day?

Businesses everywhere face this kind of problem: Success isn't possible without changing the day-to-day behavior of people throughout the company. But changing behavior is hard, even for individuals, and even when new habits can mean the difference between life and death. In many studies of patients who have undergone coronary bypass surgery, only one in nine people, on average, adopts healthier day-to-day habits. The others' lives are at significantly greater risk unless they exercise and lose weight, and they clearly see the value of changing their behavior. But they don't follow through. So what about changing the way a whole organization behaves? The consistently poor track record in this area tells us it's a challenging aspiration at best.

**David Rock is the author of *Quiet Leadership: Six Steps to Transforming Performance at Work* (Collins, 2006) and *Personal Best* (Simon & Schuster, 2001), and the co-creator of the management coaching curriculum at New York University's School of Continuing and Professional Studies. As the CEO of Results Coaching Systems, he has trained hundreds of coaches. He can be reached at davidrock@workplacecoaching.com.**

**Jeffrey Schwartz, M.D., is a research psychiatrist at the School of Medicine at the University of California at Los Angeles. A seminal thinker in the area of self-directed neuroplasticity, Dr. Schwartz has authored some 100 scientific papers and several books, including *The Mind and the Brain* (with Sharon Begley, Regan Books, 2002) and the bestseller *Brain Lock: Free Yourself from Obsessive-Compulsive Behavior* (Regan Books, 1997). His research interests include brain imaging and cognitive-behavioral therapy. He can be reached at jmschwar@ucla.edu.**

During the last two decades, scientists have gained a new, far more accurate view of human nature and behavior change because of the integration of psychology (the study of the human mind and human behavior) and neuroscience (the study of the anatomy and physiology of the brain). Imaging technologies such as functional magnetic resonance imaging (fMRI) and positron emission tomography (PET), along with brain wave analysis technologies such as quantitative electroencephalography (QEEG), have revealed hitherto unseen neural connections in the living human brain. Advanced computer analysis of these connections has helped researchers develop an increasing body of theoretical work linking the brain (the physical organ) with the mind (the human consciousness that thinks, feels, acts, and perceives).

The implications of this new research are particularly relevant for organizational leaders. It is now clear that human behavior in the workplace doesn't work the way many executives think it does. That in turn helps explain why many leadership efforts and organizational change initiatives fall flat. And it also helps explain the success of companies like Toyota and Springfield Remanufacturing Corporation, whose shop-floor or meeting-room practices resonate deeply with the innate predispositions of the human brain.

Managers who understand the recent breakthroughs in cognitive science can lead and influence mindful change: organizational transformation that takes into account the physiological nature of the brain, and the ways in which it predisposes people to resist some forms of leadership and accept others. This does not imply that management — of change or anything else — is a science. There is a great deal of art and craft in it. But several conclusions about organizational change can be drawn that make the art and craft far more effective. These conclusions would have been considered counterintuitive or downright wrong only a few years ago. For example:

§ **Change is pain.** Organizational change is unexpectedly difficult because it provokes sensations of physiological discomfort.

§ **Behaviorism doesn't work.** Change efforts based on incentive and threat (the carrot and the stick) rarely succeed in the long run.

§ **Humanism is overrated.** In practice, the conventional empathic approach of connection and persuasion doesn't sufficiently engage people.

§ **Focus is power.** The act of paying attention creates chemical and physical changes in the brain.

§ **Expectation shapes reality.** People's preconceptions have a significant impact on what they perceive.

§ **Attention density shapes identity.** Repeated, purposeful, and focused attention can lead to long-lasting personal evolution.

# Change is Pain

"Why do people resist change so stubbornly, even when it's in their own interest?" wonder CEOs like Mike. Changing the way others go about their work is harder than he has expected. New advances in neuroscience provide insight into why change can be so difficult, and there are several key findings.

The first has to do with the nature of human memory and its relationship to conscious attention. Working memory — the brain's "holding area," where perceptions and ideas can first be compared to other information — is frequently engaged when people encounter something new. When you see a new product on a supermarket shelf and rationally compare its benefits to a product you already use, it's your working memory that takes in the new information and matches it against the old. This kind of memory activates the prefrontal cortex, an energy-intensive part of the brain.

The basal ganglia, on the other hand, are invoked by routine, familiar activity, like putting an often-purchased product into a supermarket cart without consciously paying attention, and perhaps without later remembering having picked it out. This part of the brain, located near the core, is where neural circuits of long-standing habit are formed and held. It requires much less energy to function than working memory does, in part because it seamlessly links simple behaviors from brain modules that have already been shaped by extensive training and experience.

The basal ganglia can function exceedingly well without conscious thought in any routine activity. In contrast, working memory fatigues easily and can hold only a limited amount of information "on line" at any one time. Therefore, any activity conducted repetitively (to the point of becoming a habit) will tend to get pushed down into the basal ganglia, the habit-center part of the brain. This frees up the processing resources of the prefrontal cortex.

After just a few months of learning to drive a car, people can typically drive "without thinking." If they then try to drive on the other side of the road, say in another country, the act of driving suddenly becomes much more difficult. The prefrontal cortex must now be used to keep track of the action.

The same cognitive dynamics come into play when people face other types of stressful experiences, including any strategic or organizational change. Much of what managers do in the workplace

— how they sell ideas, run meetings, manage others, and communicate — is so well routinized that the basal ganglia are running the show. Trying to change any hardwired habit requires a lot of effort, in the form of attention. This often leads to a feeling that many people find uncomfortable. So they do what they can to avoid change.

The second reason change is hard relates to basic brain functioning. Human brains have evolved a particularly strong capacity to detect what neuroscientists call "errors": perceived differences between expectation and actuality. When a child (or an adult, for that matter) is promised a sweet-tasting treat and then discovers it tastes salty or bitter, the brain emits strong signals that use a lot of energy, showing up in imaging technology as dramatic bursts of light. Edmund Rolls first illustrated this at Oxford University in the early 1980s, with a study involving monkeys. Dr. Rolls found that "errors" in the environment produced intense bursts of neural firing, markedly stronger than the firing caused by familiar stimuli. Trying to change a routine behavior sends out strong messages in the brain that something is not right. These messages grab the individual's attention, and they can readily overpower rational thought.

It takes a strong will to push past such mental activity — and the same is true on the level of organizational change. Try to change another person's behavior, even with the best possible justification, and he or she will experience discomfort. The brain sends out powerful messages that something is wrong, and the capacity for higher thought is decreased. Change itself thus amplifies stress and discomfort; and managers (who may not, from their position in the hierarchy, perceive the same events in the same way that subordinates perceive them) tend to underestimate the challenges inherent in implementation.

## Behaviorism Doesn't Work

Many existing models for changing people's behavior are drawn from a field called *behaviorism*. The field emerged in the 1930s and was led by psychologist B.F. Skinner and advertising executive John B. Watson, building on Ivan Pavlov's famous concept of the conditioned response: Associate the ringing of a bell with food, and a dog can be made to salivate at the sound. The behaviorists generalized this observation to people, and established an approach to change that has sometimes been caricatured as: "Lay out the M&Ms." For each person, there is one set of incentives — one combination of candy colors — that makes the best motivator. Present the right incentives, and the desired change will naturally occur. If change doesn't occur, then the mix of M&M colors must be adjusted.

Yet there is plenty of evidence from both clinical research and workplace observation that change efforts based on typical incentives and threats (the carrot and the stick) rarely succeed in the long run. For example, when people routinely come late to meetings, a manager may reprimand them. This may chasten latecomers in the short run, but it also draws their attention away from work and back to the problems that led to lateness in the first place. Another manager might choose to reward people who show up on time with public recognition or better assignments; for those who are late, this too raises anxiety and reinforces the neural patterns associated with the habitual problem. Yet despite all the evidence that it doesn't work, the behaviorist model is still the dominant paradigm in many organizations. The carrot and stick are alive and well.

## Humanism is Overrated

The next big field to emerge in psychology after behaviorism was the humanist movement of the 1950s and 1960s. Also called the person-centered approach, the field was inspired by such thinkers as Carl Rogers and Abraham Maslow. This school of thought assumed that self-esteem, emotional needs, and values could provide leverage for changing behavior. The prevailing model of humanist psychology involved helping people reach their potential through self-actualization — bringing forth hidden capacities and aspirations. Therapists and trainers left behind the carrot and stick and focused on empathy. They listened to people's problems, attempted to understand them on their own terms, and allowed a holistic solution to emerge.

In theory, an effective solution might well emerge from the person-centered approach. But there is rarely time to go through this process with employees, and no guarantee that it will produce the desired results. True self-actualization might simply lead someone to quit his or her job. Moreover, in practice, the humanist approach leads to an emphasis on persuasion. The implicit goal is to "get people on board" by establishing trust and rapport, and then to convince them of the value of a change. Performance management training manuals on administering annual appraisals often counsel managers to "deliver constructive performance feedback." This assumes that if people receive correct information about what they are doing wrong, and the right incentives are in place, they will automatically change.

But the human brain can behave like a 2-year-old: Tell it what to do and it automatically pushes back. Partly this phenomenon is a function of homeostasis (the natural movement of any organism toward equilibrium and away from change), but it also reflects the fact that brains are pattern-making organs with an innate desire to create novel connections. When people solve a problem themselves, the brain releases a rush of neurotransmitters like adrenaline. This phenomenon provides a scientific basis for some of the practices of leadership coaching. Rather than lecturing and providing solutions, effective coaches ask pertinent questions and support their clients in working out solutions on their own.

## Focus is Power

Some of the biggest leaps in science and industry have emerged from the integration of separate fields. When the study of electricity and of magnetism coalesced to become the science of electromagnetism, the field gave us the electric motor and generator, which in turn sparked the Industrial Revolution. To understand how to better drive organizational change, we turn to another nexus, this time between neuroscience and contemporary physics.

Neurons communicate with each other through a type of electrochemical signaling that is driven by the movement of ions such as sodium, potassium, and calcium. These ions travel through channels within the brain that are, at their narrowest point, only a little more than a single ion wide. This means that the brain is a quantum environment, and is therefore subject to all the surprising laws of quantum mechanics. One of these laws is the Quantum Zeno Effect (QZE). The QZE was described in 1977 by the physicist George Sudarshan at the University of Texas at Austin, and has been experimentally verified many times since.

The QZE is related to the established observer effect of quantum physics: The behavior and position of any atom-sized entity, such as an atom, an electron, or an ion, appears to change when that entity is observed. This in turn is linked to the probabilistic nature of such entities. The quantum laws that govern the observed behaviors of subatomic particles, and also the observed behaviors of all larger systems built out of them, are expressed in terms of probability waves, which are affected in specific ways by observations made upon the system. In the Quantum Zeno Effect, when any system is observed in a sufficiently rapid, repetitive fashion, the rate at which that system changes is reduced. One classic experiment involved observing beryllium atoms that could decay from a high-energy to a low-energy state. As the number of measurements per unit time increased, the probability of the energy transition fell off: The beryllium atom stayed longer in its excited state, because the scientists, in effect, repeatedly asked, "Have you decayed yet?" In quantum physics, as in the rest of life, a watched pot never boils. We now also know that the brain changes as a function of where an individual puts his or her attention. The power is in the focus.

Attention continually reshapes the patterns of the brain. Among the implications: People who practice a specialty every day literally think differently, through different sets of connections, than do people who don't practice the specialty. In business, professionals in different functions — finance, operations, legal, research and development, marketing, design, and human resources — have physiological differences that prevent them from seeing the world the same way.

## Expectation Shapes Reality

Cognitive scientists are finding that people's mental maps, their theories, expectations, and attitudes, play a more central role in human perception than was previously understood. This can be well demonstrated by the placebo effect. Tell people they have been administered a pain-reducing agent and they experience a marked and systematic reduction in pain, despite the fact that they have received a completely inert substance, a sugar pill. One study in 2005 by Robert C. Coghill and others found that "expectations for decreased pain produce a reduction in perceived pain (28.4%) that rivals the effects of a clearly analgesic dose of morphine." Donald Price of the University of Florida has shown that the mental expectation of pain relief accounts for the change in pain perception. People experience what they expect to experience.

The fact that our expectations, whether conscious or buried in our deeper brain centers, can play such a large role in perception has significant implications. Two individuals working on the same customer service telephone line could hold different mental maps of the same customers. The first, seeing customers only as troubled children, would hear only complaints that needed to be allayed; the second, seeing them as busy but intelligent professionals, would hear valuable suggestions for improving a product or service.

How, then, would you go about facilitating change? The impact of mental maps suggests that one way to start is by cultivating moments of insight. Large-scale behavior change requires a large-scale change in mental maps. This in turn requires some kind of event or experience that allows people to provoke themselves, in effect, to change their attitudes and expectations more quickly and dramatically than they normally would.

Mark Jung-Beeman of Northwestern University's Institute for Neuroscience and others have recently used fMRI and EEG technologies to study moments of insight. One study found sudden bursts of high-frequency 40 Hz oscillations (gamma waves) in the brain appearing just prior to moments of insight. This oscillation is conducive to creating links across many parts of the brain. The same study found the right anterior superior temporal gyrus being activated. This part of the brain is involved in perceiving and processing music, spatial and structural relations (such as those in a building or painting), and other complex aspects of the environment. The findings suggest that at a moment of insight, a complex set of new connections is being created. These connections have the potential to enhance our mental resources and overcome the brain's resistance to change. But to achieve this result, given the brain's limited working memory, we need to make a deliberate effort to hardwire an insight by paying it repeated attention.

That is why employees need to "own" any kind of change initiative for it to be successful. The help-desk clerk who sees customers as children won't change the way he or she listens without a moment of insight in which his or her mental maps shift to seeing customers as experts. Leaders wanting to change the way people think or behave should learn to recognize, encourage, and deepen their team's insights.

## Attention Density Shapes Identity

For insights to be useful, they need to be generated from within, not given to individuals as conclusions. This is true for several reasons. First, people will experience the adrenaline-like rush of insight only if they go through the process of making connections themselves. The moment of insight is well known to be a positive and energizing experience. This rush of energy may be central to facilitating change: It helps fight against the internal (and external) forces trying to keep change from occurring, including the fear response of the amygdala.

Second, neural networks are influenced moment to moment by genes, experiences, and varying patterns of attention. Although all people have some broad functions in common, in truth everyone has a unique brain architecture. Human brains are so complex and individual that there is little point in trying to work out how another person ought to reorganize his or her thinking. It is far more effective and efficient to help others come to their own insights. Accomplishing this feat requires self-observation. Adam Smith, in his 1759 masterpiece *The Theory of Moral Sentiments*, referred to this as being "the spectators of our own behaviour."

The term *attention density* is increasingly used to define the amount of attention paid to a particular mental experience over a specific time. The greater the concentration on a specific idea or mental experience, the higher the attention density. In quantum physics terms, attention density brings the QZE into play and causes new brain circuitry to be stabilized and thus developed. With enough attention density, individual thoughts and acts of the mind can become an intrinsic part of an individual's identity: who one is, how one perceives the world, and how one's brain works. The neuroscientist's term for this is *self-directed neuroplasticity*.

You've probably had the experience of going to a training program and getting excited about new ways of thinking, only to realize later that you can't remember what the new ways of thinking were. Were the ideas no good in the first place? Or did you just not pay enough attention? A 1997 study of 31 public-sector managers by Baruch College researchers Gerald Olivero, K. Denise Bane, and Richard E. Kopelman found that a training program alone increased productivity 28 percent, but the addition of follow-up coaching to the training increased productivity 88 percent. Perhaps any behavior change brought about by leaders, managers, therapists, trainers, or coaches is primarily a function of their ability to induce others to focus their attention on specific ideas, closely enough, often enough, and for a long enough time.

## Mindful Change in Practice

How, then, can leaders effectively change their own or other people's behavior?

Start by leaving problem behaviors in the past; focus on identifying and creating new behaviors. Over time, these may shape the dominant pathways in the brain. This is achieved through a solution-focused questioning approach that facilitates self-insight, rather than through advice-giving.

Let's go back to Mike, our pharmaceutical CEO. One of Mike's direct reports, Rob, has hired only three of his targeted six new team members this year. If Mike asks Rob why he didn't reach the goal, he will focus Rob's attention on the nonperformance. As a result of this attention, Rob might make new cognitive connections (also known as reasons) as to why he didn't find the new people. For example, "All the really good people are taken by other companies," or "I don't have time to do the kind of recruiting we need." Although these reasons that people were not hired might be true, they do little to support or foster any change.

A more useful place to focus Rob's attention is on the new circuits he needs to create to achieve his objectives in the future. Mike could ask Rob, "What do you need to do to resolve challenges like this?" Mike's questioning might provoke Rob to have an insight that he needs to remind himself of his annual objectives more regularly, to keep his eyes on the prize. If Mike regularly asked Rob about his progress, it would remind Rob to give this new thought more attention.

In a world with so many distractions, and with new mental maps potentially being created every second in the brain, one of the biggest challenges is being able to focus enough attention on any one idea. Leaders can make a big difference by gently reminding others about their useful insights, and thus eliciting attention that otherwise would not be paid.

At the organizational level, Mike wants to change the way thousands of people think. A common approach would be to identify the current attitudes across the group through some sort of cultural survey. The hope would be that identifying the source of the problem would help solve it. Based on what we now know about the brain, a better alternative would be for Mike to paint a broad picture of being more entrepreneurial, without specifically identifying the changes that individuals will need to make. Mike's goal should be for his people to picture the new behaviors in their own minds, and in the process develop energizing new mental maps that have the potential to become hardwired circuitry. Mike would then get his team to focus their attention on their own insights, by facilitating discussions and activities that involve being entrepreneurial. After that, Mike's job would be to regularly provide "gentle reminders" so that the entrepreneurial maps become the dominant pathways along which information, ideas, and energy flow. He also needs to catch the team when they get sidetracked and gently bring them back. The power truly is in the focus, and in the attention that is paid.

Few managers are comfortable putting these principles into practice, however. Our management models are based on the premise that knowledge is power. This "transmission" approach to exchanging information (exemplified by lectures and textbooks, where knowledge is "transmitted" to a passive receiver) has always been the prevailing teaching method in academia, including the business schools that many managers attend. Since many executives assume that the teaching methods they endured are the only teaching methods that work, it's no small matter to consider trying a different approach in our workplaces. For many executives, leading others in such a new way may be a bigger change, and therefore challenge, than driving on the other side of the road. Perhaps these findings about the brain can start to pull back the curtain on a new world of productivity improvement: in our ability to bring about positive, lasting change in ourselves, in our families, in our workplaces, and in society itself.

# Resources

Leslie Brothers, M.D., *Friday's Footprint: How Society Shapes the Human Mind* (Oxford University Press, 1997): Social impact on brain development.

Tetsuo Koyama, John G. McHaffie, Paul J. Laurienti, and Robert C. Coghill, "The Subjective Experience of Pain: Where Expectations Become Reality," Proceedings of the National Academy of Sciences, vol. 102, no. 36, Sept. 6, 2005. Abstract available at www.pnas.org/cgi/content/abstract/ 102/36/12950: Documents the role of expectations in the placebo effect; summarized in Bruce Bower, "Thinking the Hurt Away," *Science News*, September 10, 2005: www.sciencenews.org/articles/20050910/fob5.asp

Gerald Olivero, K. Denise Bane, Richard E. Kopelman, "Executive Coaching as a Transfer of Training Tool: Effects on Productivity in a Public Agency," *Public Personnel Management*, vol. 26, no. 4 (Winter 1997): Research on the value of follow-up in coaching.

John J. Ratey, M.D., *A User's Guide to the Brain: Perception, Attention, and the Four Theaters of the Brain* (Pantheon, 2001): Readable summary of thinking about the biology of thought, change, and learning.

David Rock, *Quiet Leadership: Six Steps to Transforming Performance at Work* (Collins, 2006): Essentials of coaching by one author of this article.

Jeffrey Schwartz, M.D., *Brain Lock: Free Yourself from Obsessive-Compulsive Behavior* (Regan Books, 1997): OCD function and cure turn out to illuminate many leadership issues.

Jeffrey Schwartz, M.D., and Sharon Begley, *The Mind and the Brain: Neuroplasticity and the Power of Mental Force* (Regan Books, 2002): Rewiring connections and the underlying neuroscience.

Jeffrey M. Schwartz, M.D., Henry P. Stapp, and Mario Beauregard, "Quantum Physics in Neuroscience and Psychology: A Neurophysical Model of the Mind-Brain Interaction," Philosophical Transactions of the Royal Society B: *Biological Sciences*, vol. 360, no. 1458, June 29, 2005: Emerging quantum brain theory.

Martin Seligman, *Learned Optimism: How to Change Your Mind and Your Life* (1990; Free Press, 1998) and *Authentic Happiness: Using the New Positive Psychology to Realize Your Potential for Lasting Fulfillment* (Free Press, 2002): Research-based popular books on the habit of optimism as an attention-focusing process. See also one of Dr. Seligman's Web sites, www.authentichappiness.com.

Adam Smith, *The Theory of Moral Sentiments* (1759; Cambridge University Press, 2002): Smith's masterwork uses self-awareness as a vehicle for developing moral conscience.

Jack Stack, *The Great Game of Business* (Doubleday, 1992): Explains Springfield Remanufacturing's focused use of financial literacy.

Mark Jung-Beeman's Web site, www.psych.northwestern.edu/~mjungbee/ mjungbeeindex.html: Moments of insight and creative cognition.

Edmund Rolls's Web site, http://emotion-research.net/Members/UOXF: Descriptions of his current work and links to his books on the brain mechanisms of emotion.

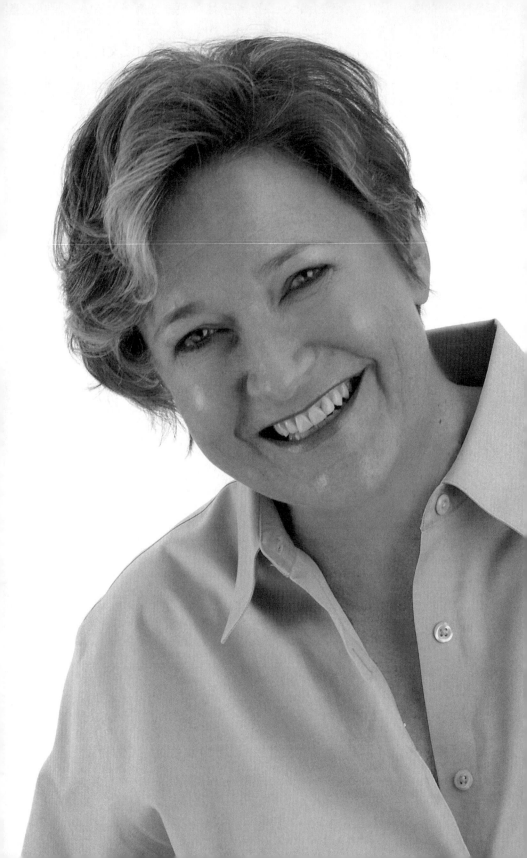

# GABRIELE HILBERG:

# Creative Solutions Under Pressure

**M**oments of sudden inspiration typically occur when you are *not thinking* about the problem. In the shower or at the gym, a solution can come seemingly out of nowhere. Yet, some people frequently have brilliant, perception-altering ideas and seem to be able to rely on their ability to produce cognitive leaps. How do they do that?

Paradoxically, too much thinking and analysis can drive you even further into paralysis. Under pressure, people tend to think in established mental concepts and familiar categories they are comfortable with. The solutions are most likely a reflection of what has worked in the past. How do you avoid imposing old frameworks on present realities? How do you examine your assumptions and go beyond your perceptions of the problem? How do you know whether you are looking at the right problem? How do you come up with a solution when two parties are locked in a total stalemate?

## How to Stop Thinking

In August 2005, we were faced with exactly this kind of situation. A colleague and I had submitted a proposal for a speaking engagement about the "Quantum Process" at the Stanford Linear Accelerator, Stanford University. Our excitement over the acceptance of the talk quickly turned into a frenzy of questions. How should we present

Gabriele Hilberg, Ph.D., MFT, is a psychotherapist, organizational consultant, and international seminar leader. She has led seminars in the U.S., Europe, Russia, Australia, and Central America, maintained a private practice, and served as a consultant to Fortune 500 companies as well as start-ups. Her work is focused on empowering people to go beyond self-imposed limits to experience a greater intelligence and creativity. She is the founder of Thought Horizons, Inc., a consulting organization that offers individuals and businesses practical tools for identifying and changing conscious and non-conscious beliefs, attitudes, and perceptions. Learn more at www.thoughthorizons.com. Photo by Craig Smith.

the material to the scientists? How much detail should we give about the scientific explanation behind the approach? Would they be open to the application of quantum mechanics at the macroscopic level? How could we get all that information covered in the time available? We were caught up in a flurry of rewriting notes and researching textbooks in preparation for the presentation.

Suddenly, we hit on the idea—why not use the Quantum Process to solve this problem? We agreed to step into the future reality of the car trip *back from* our presentation.

"Wasn't it a great idea to start the talk with a demonstration?" The words flew out of my mouth the instant we stood in our virtual future.

Nothing had prepared me for this idea—there had been no hint that I was even thinking about it. Yet, we both know immediately that this was the answer we had been looking for.

This kind of sudden outburst is an intuitive flash, a spontaneous creative expression that is generated by something other than the rational mind. An intuitive flash is accompanied by an instant recognition that the solution will work. You can sense the rightness in a direct, palpable way. This sudden insight shifts you out of your existing cognitive framework and allows you to see the problem from a new perspective. In other words, your brain activity shifts to the right hemisphere, the center for creative, holographic processing of ideas and images, and gives you a snapshot of a possible outcome for the problem. Though you might not immediately find the right language to exactly describe your intuitive impressions, you now have a complete picture to work with. Had you limited your thinking to the left hemisphere of the brain, which controls reason, logic, and deduction, you would have generated only solutions based on past experiences and familiar frameworks.

-§-
Our best thinking got us here—why do you think that more thinking will bring the solution?
–David Bohm
-§-

After studying the conditions under which we typically experience these blinding flashes of the obvious, this Quantum Process was designed to replicate those conditions and to produce innovative solutions—in the office and on schedule. Think about what could be possible if you didn't have to wait for happy accidents in the shower or at the gym!

# Case Study

My client Katherine, a director of a City Team in Silicon Valley, was exasperated with her administrative staff. After a recent reorganization, her eight team members were up in arms about the new division of the workload. Frustrations had mounted over the past three weeks, and she was considering moving several staff members to different departments.

After she described the situation, I asked Katherine to step with me across the room into a future time, when the problem was solved and she was happy with the outcome. Standing in the future and looking back to see herself dismayed with the rebellious staff, she was able to relax and open her mind to seeing the situation from a new perspective. It was easy for Katherine to resolve the problem by generating this "virtual hindsight." As she put it:

> Looking at the situation from the future, I suddenly started laughing when I realized that the "I" was the source of the problem! I went back to my group and shared with them what I had seen, and asked if they were willing to wipe the slate clean and approach the situation anew. They enthusiastically agreed and we are now in the process of building a powerful team where everyone contributes and feels free to voice their thoughts.

Katherine was able to access her own creative, intuitive side to produce the needed breakthrough in a minimal amount of time. She was amazed that only 30 minutes prior to working the Quantum Process she had felt frustrated, stressed, and out of options. It was particularly inspiring to her that she had discovered the solution for herself, which strengthened her trust in her own creative potential and capacity to be a good manager.

-§-
The intuitive mind is a sacred gift,
The rational mind is a faithful servant.
We have created a society that honors the servant
And has forgotten the gift.
–Albert Einstein
-§-

Success often requires that you step outside of your habitual ways of thinking and reacting. The Quantum Process enables you to recognize your assumptions and beliefs, which underlie your perception of the problem. Once these assumptions are made transparent, you will be in a better position to resolve problems or conflicts.

Katherine resolved her issues quickly because she was willing to consider that she had been wrong. This does not come easily for many people in business. Once people have established their position and have a personal investment in being right about an issue, it is extremely difficult to find innovative solutions to resolve the conflict. To be creative and innovative, you cannot at the same time be convinced that you already know the answer.

The successful use of the Quantum Process hinges on the willingness of the individuals to consider the possibility that their truth is only a personal, biased perception. Here, a basic understanding of the quantum paradigm allows you to see your own view of reality for what it truly is: your subjective experience of truth. This understanding of subjective truth is at the core of the Quantum paradigm.

## Perceptions versus Objective Reality

We are living during a great paradigm shift from the Newtonian worldview to the quantum perspective of the nature of reality. This shift has drastically changed the foundation of science over the past 80 years, and quantum mechanics has revolutionized technology and innovation. Scientists, after initial disbelief and struggle, are now embracing the shift and going beyond it. Quantum mechanics has taught us a new way of interpreting the world around us.

We are learning that the world shows up for each of us as we expect it to. When scientists discovered that if you look at light as a wave, you will see light as a wave function, and when you look at light as particles, you will observe light as a function of particles, this new understanding defied our old belief in an objective reality as separate from and outside of ourselves. We can no longer deny that our reality is subjective. This paradigm shift is now infiltrating our perception of reality in other segments of our lives, as it has far-reaching implications in fields such as medicine, law, and business.

-§-
We deceive ourselves by assuming that our view represents truth when it is really just an interpretation, a lens through which we choose to see the world.
–Loehr and Schwartz,
*The Power of Full Engagement*
-§-

In everyday living, this shift becomes evident when we deal with the question: What is really happening here? From the Newtonian point of view, you would answer the question by looking for the objective, measurable reality based on data and a linear reasoning process. This approach is rooted in the belief that reality exists independent and outside of you and can be described by standardized methods of measurements.

Quantum mechanics showed us that the observer influences the observed outcome. What was first discovered on a microscopic level has been found to be true on the macroscopic level, also. The reality we perceive depends upon our personal lens of perception — which makes reality highly subjective.

Once a problem begins to fester, it becomes more and more difficult to recognize your own assumptions and beliefs about an issue. Although you attempt to be objective, your perception of the problem is highly affected by your conscious and non-conscious beliefs about the origin and nature of the problem.

In vertical time, all possibilities occur simultaneously. Your thoughts are attractors, which collapse the field and generate the reality you perceive. The Quantum Process challenges you to question your assumption that your view is accurate. It allows you to recognize those false, often unconscious beliefs and assumptions that keep you from resolving the problem.

## Case Study

My client Paul, a pioneer and celebrated author in the field of software engineering, was referred to me by his brother. According to the brother's description, Paul had moped around for months, tinkering all day long with model airplanes and leaving him to run their business single-handedly.

Paul wanted me to know that building model airplanes was his great hobby, the thing that gave him the greatest pleasure. But it wasn't until I began probing about the time years before, when his first and second book had come out, that his eyes lit up and he became alive and animated. Paul told me that he had a third book in his head, but that he could see no chance of it ever being accepted by his peers in the industry.

He gave a lengthy and detailed explanation of why investors and leaders in the industry would reject his innovative ideas based on their inability to face the end of an area. Paul went on to say that he would be hit with great resistance because he did not have a college degree and had taught himself everything he knew in his field. As an aside, he mentioned that, several years ago, Bill Gates had personally asked him to join Microsoft after purchasing one of Paul's software products.

I listened intently and, when he paused, I said, "This is a very fascinating analysis of your dilemma. I almost started to believe your story." Paul was startled for a moment—and then burst out in a roaring laughter. "You got me, I am telling my old story again. The amazing thing is that I really believe that it is true when I tell it to myself!" We were off to a good start.

Paul's problem was that of being the expert. Fortunately, he was willing to consider that at the brink of publicly expressing his newly forming ideas, he experienced recurring attacks of old low self-esteem based on his being a high school dropout. What was harder for him to see was that his view of venture capital investors and industry leaders could also be a biased perception.

*The most insidious belief is that we see reality as it really is.*

Paul described two incidences in the recent past when venture capital investors had been unwilling to consider his new concept because they lacked the courage to see new horizons. As a result of these experiences, he had given up and thrown himself into building his model airplanes.

"You took your marbles and went home," I observed.

My analogy brought a big grin to Paul's face. "Well, they just don't get it that you can be smart without a degree."

It became obvious that this deep-seated belief kept Paul stuck in the perception that he and his innovative concepts would be rejected. He looked dismayed and extremely frustrated.

I asked Paul to step with me across the room and into a future time, when his third book had been written and was very well received. I asked him to look back at himself, in the "present," feeling frustrated and stuck. He took a quick glance at his miserable self and spouted: "He acts like a pompous S.O.B. and, on top of it, he is impressed by his own pity party." We both burst into laughter—I could have not said it better!

I challenged him to look at the benefits he was getting from holding on to his negative view of the situation. He squirmed a bit, but then offered that he was really afraid of being wrong about his new ideas. He began to see that it was very convenient to see possible investors and supporters as incapable of understanding his creative ideas, because it got him off the hook in terms of developing and testing his ideas further.

"He is acting overly confident and boasting because he's covering up his fear that his new concepts might belong in the garbage," Paul realized. "And, he is really going to piss people off with his attitude before they are ready to get it."

He felt drained and exhilarated at the same time; yet when he returned to the present, he was changed.

"It is amazing what I can see about myself from over there—maybe there is hope for me and my project. My big ego is really preventing me from moving ahead."

Within one hour Paul had shifted his perception and gone from seeing an external problem to recognizing that his block was really internal. He felt renewed energy and hope when he saw his old construct of the problem crumbling, and was empowered by his more truthful view of the situation.

Again and again, I am fascinated by how boldly my clients

confront their core issues when standing in the future and looking back. It seems particularly important that they speak to themselves in a language that hits the mark in a personal way.

## Righteousness versus Resolution

There is nothing more delicious than being right. But while there are times when you *are* right, self-righteousness might be exactly what gets in the way of solving your problem. A problem always exists between two or more people. A win/lose solution cannot bring a lasting resolution to any conflict, because it invites retaliation and further conflict. You might win the battle, but you will have lost the probability for future cooperation.

There are also times when you are convinced that you are right, but in actuality you have misinterpreted information or based your opinion on assumptions that left out relevant data. The danger of expertise lies in the very knowledge that makes you an authority, as your confidence in your particular perspective can blind you to other relevant data.

More often, because we have advanced to an expert status in one area, we falsely assume or are given authority and expertise in other areas. A classic example is Margaret Mead, who was an outstanding and highly accomplished anthropologist. When she became a Representative in the English Parliament, her speeches were so absolutely horrible that people frequently left the room when she spoke.

So, how can you be sure that you know what is right and what is wrong?

Within the Newtonian paradigm, there is assumed to be one right answer, which seemingly exists independent and separate from you out there in the world. This creates the illusion that one right answer can be found. Whoever finds that answer is the winner.

Within the Quantum paradigm, however, the "right" answer is understood to be a subjective interpretation of truth as seen through your personal lens of perception. While your answer is right from your point of view, another right answer also exists from a different perspective. Both answers are subjectively correct.

It is easy to loose this new Quantum understanding in the middle of a conflict, when you are strongly attached to the belief that you are right. People confuse the intensity of their feelings with truth; the more strongly we feel that we are right, the more we think our belief is true.

# Chapter Forty-Five

*Feelings don't tell you the truth; feelings only tell you what you feel.*

Often, by the time individuals come to work with the Quantum Process, they are beyond their attachment to being right. Typically, the struggle and conflict has brought them so much frustration and suffering that they are willing to find a solution and get on with life. When working with a business team or department, however, it is harder to assess how willing individuals are to let go of being right. In these situations, people can tend to give lip service to the idea of finding a win/win solution, while subconsciously holding on to their need to be right.

Before engaging a team in the Quantum Process, I challenge people to question their assumptions that their own view is accurate and contrary views are wrong and biased. I show the team several video clips that were originally used in a Harvard study on Inattentive Blindness. The team members are instructed to pay attention to specific activities in the video clips. The more their attention is focused on the given task, the less capable they are of noticing the unexpected object in each of the videos. This creates a direct, personal experience of being blind to what is in front of them. And worse, they discover that trying harder does not increase the odds of seeing things more quickly the next time.

This is often a very surprising and unsettling experience, particularly for intelligent, successful individuals who are unaccustomed to questioning their perceptions. However, this moment of bewilderment can open a door and allow team members to consider the possibility that they have been wrong or have missed important cues in the problem at hand.

When we translate the team's experiences to the business environment, it becomes obvious that the longer we struggle with a problem the less capable we are of noticing those unexpected elements that could point us to a creative solution. This recognition sets the stage for a successful outcome in working with the Quantum Process.

## Business Applications of the Quantum Process

The Quantum Process is highly effective in any situation in which hard work, commitment, and determination have not resolved a critical issue. When you have become frustrated, jaded, or cynical and it is increasingly difficult to approach the topic of discussion, the Quantum Process offers you a tool to generate new possibilities, options, and avenues to success within a short period of time.

*If you keep doing what you have been doing, you'll keep getting what you've been getting.*

Success in business is ensured when the assumptions you make about business strategies, innovative concepts, and customers are accurate. However, if your assumptions and beliefs are off the mark, no amount of effort, determination, or positive spin will bring you the desired outcome.

The Quantum Process is a practical tool that helps you to challenge yourself and your team to fundamentally rethink your framework and concepts. By accessing your gut instincts and verbalizing your intuitive hunches, you tap into intelligence beyond the rational, analytic mind. This allows you to generate cognitive leaps, to think outside the box, and to come up with creative, innovative solutions — even under extreme pressures.

The Quantum Process helps you to resolve critical, long-standing business issues, refocus your energy, and drastically improve your performance in the following areas:

§ Strategic Thinking and Re-Evaluating Business Strategies

§ Interpersonal Conflict Resolution and Team Building

§ Reorganization and Merger of Cultures

§ Customer Service and Quality Assurance

§ Product Development and Trouble Shooting

§ Mediation and Legal Stalemates

The Quantum Process enables you to honestly face difficult issues and look beneath the surface. It allows you to develop your capacity to question your perceptions and generate solutions that really work — which gives you the ultimate business advantage.

You and I are participating in the most exciting global paradigm shift since medieval times — equal to or larger in proportion than the discovery that the world is round and not flat. Quantum physics, with its shift toward a fundamentally different way of understanding the nature of reality, has opened the doors to rethinking separation and interconnectedness at all levels of humanity.

We have exhausted our past concepts and are outgrowing familiar methodologies and approaches to life. We are beginning to sense the death of an era. Tweaking the old ways of thinking will not work because, as Einstein proclaimed, we cannot solve problems by way of the same level of thinking that created them.

We stand today at the same revolutionary brink at which scientists found themselves over 80 years ago. At that time, the new understanding of reality encountered major opposition and turmoil rocked the scientific communities. Even Einstein struggled with and in the end resisted the conclusions of his own scientific breakthroughs. Yet the scientists have come back from the abyss and told us that the new ways of thinking about interconnectedness have opened up hopeful horizons and vistas.

What might be possible if we applied quantum thinking in everyday life? How would such a shift change our world? I believe that our collective future on this planet depends upon our ability to see the world through innovative and creative eyes. We need to rethink our approach to local and global challenges. We need to invent new concepts and processes outside of the existing frameworks of the past. We need to transform our thinking and ourselves. In order to deal with the inescapable global challenges we now face, we must learn to go beyond our linear, analytic mind and stop worshipping rational thinking as the highest form of intelligence. We have outgrown the Newtonian paradigm of seeing things as separate and isolated.

Through Quantum thinking, we can transform our views and perceptions to see the interconnectedness of all beings and events. This also means that we must transform our view of who we are as individuals by taking a fresh look at our ego-based perceptions of separation and isolation and exploring beyond the linear developmental model of psychological growth, personality, and identity. This is not a challenge for the faint of heart, but if we are to ride the paradigm shift already underway and find workable solutions to the problems we face as businesspeople and members of the human race, then we must rise to the occasion. If we can re-vision our personal realities, then we can change the way we do business; and if we can change the way we do business, then the shift will ripple into all of our potential future realities.

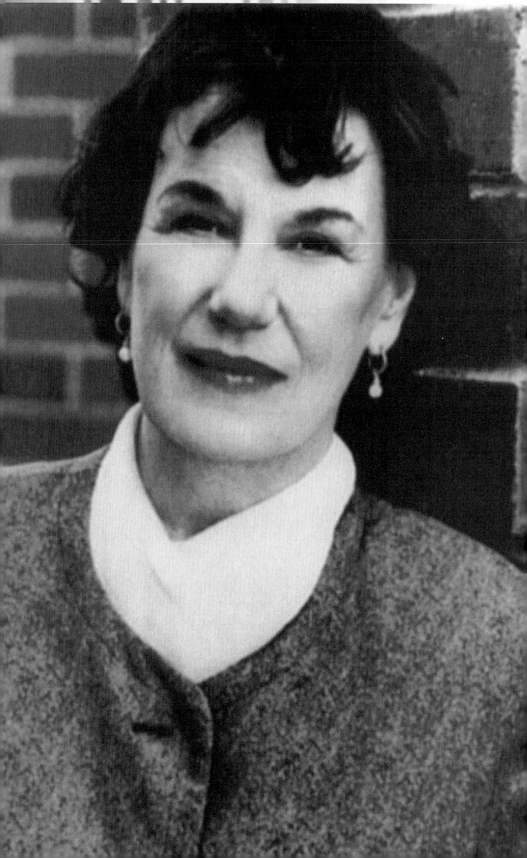

# Sandra Seagal:

# Harnessing Human Differences

In 1995, David Marsing was Vice-President, General Manager of the Technology Manufacturing Group at Intel Corporation. Two years previously, he had been given a huge responsibility: to oversee the building, ramp up, and operation of the largest wafer factory that had ever been built, covering one million square feet and providing jobs to over 3,500 permanent employees and an additional 1,500 contractors.

Not long before, in his mid-thirties, David had suffered a severe and nearly fatal heart attack. He fully understood that this event had been the result of stress; but though his doctor warned him not to return to his old work environment, David chose to do so. He wanted to try a different approach to achieving organizational success. In addition to assuring that the people under his leadership received all the necessary technical training, which was in any case a given at Intel, the focus of training would be on the employees' development *as people*—both as individuals and in their interactions with one another. In fact, his vision was to regard the *purpose* of business practice to be the development of people, with the expectation that this emphasis would not only create a healthier, more fulfilling, more enjoyable (and thereby less stressful) environment in which to work, but also, as an inevitable byproduct, that it would result in greater business success.

As the cornerstone of this new training approach, David chose a basic four-day Human Dynamics Program for Personal,

Sandra Seagal, Ph.D., originated the field of investigation called Human Dynamics in 1979. She co-authored *Human Dynamics* (Pegasus, 1997) with her husband and partner, David Horne. Since 1984, they have worked together to develop programs for applying this work internationally in the fields of business, education, parenting, healthcare, and cross-cultural understanding. Her work has been lauded by such luminaries as the late Buckminster Fuller, who nominated her for a MacArthur Fellowship, and is currently supported in part by the Kellogg Foundation. She is president of Human Dynamics International and founder of the Human Dynamics Institute. Visit www.HumanDynamics.com.

Interpersonal, and Team Development, which would be provided for the entire workforce, from senior management to machinists on the factory floor—thousands of men and women of varied ethnicities, backgrounds, and skills. The results of this strategy? To quote David Marsing:

*[Intel] saw the fastest rate at which teams of people achieved maturity — that is, got to know not only themselves but the other people on their team, and were able to take on more and more difficult projects… We were able to not only greatly accelerate the start-up and ramp of the factory, but bring it in record time to a world benchmark level of performance. And the result of that was that we were able to save…on the order of one factory, which means somewhere between one and two billion dollars investment! We do not think that we could have achieved this had we not taken the vast majority of the people through the Human Dynamics program.*

## What is Human Dynamics?

Human Dynamics is a body of work derived from twenty-seven years of continuous investigation, involving over 80,000 people, that identifies fundamental inherent distinctions in people's functioning as whole systems of mental-emotional-physical interplay. These distinctions seem to be so foundational in the human make-up that they can be seen the world over, characterize males and females equally, and are evident at every age level. They can be identified even among infants! In other words, they are more fundamental than age, race, culture, and gender.

We have discovered that while everyone has mental, emotional, and physical properties, some people are what we term "mentally centered," some are "emotionally centered," and others are "physically centered". Among other things, this centering determines how one naturally processes information. To give the briefest of descriptions, mentally-centered people process information in an orderly, linear, logical, sequential way. They are also characterized by an innate detachment. The emotionally-centered process information in a non-linear, associative way, often in interaction with others. They are by nature relational. And the physically-centered naturally process information systemically, perceiving the inter-relationships of parts within wholes, and collecting and connecting large amounts of data to form operational systems. They are typically highly pragmatic.

There are three variations on each of these major themes (emotional-mental, emotional-emotional, emotional-physical, for example) making nine "personality dynamics" in all. Five of these, however, are by far the most numerous, and these are the major focus of Human Dynamics training programs. Representatives of any or all of these five very different "ways of being" constitute the membership of any Board, management or project team, office staff, or family. They are present in every classroom at every age level in every school. Each is characterized by a natural, specific, and differentiating set of processes of "experiencing experience," of taking in and assimilating information, of learning, communicating, relating, undertaking tasks, and solving problems. Each personality dynamic group takes leadership in characteristic ways; each contributes specific gifts and processes to groups or teams; each functions best and maintains wellness under particular conditions; and each tends to become stressed under particular circumstances. Most importantly, each is characterized by a distinctive path of personal, interpersonal, and transpersonal development.

The characteristic processes of each of these human sub-sets appear to be hard wired. In fact, our research indicates that they are present at birth and remain constant throughout each individual's lifetime. But this does not imply limitation. Understanding an individual's personality dynamic is a key to unlocking his or her potential for unlimited personal and professional development—and the first step is to gain understanding and appreciation of one's own specific human "instrument".

When these inherent and natural differences, *which are equal in value though different in function*, are not recognized, respected, and taken into account, the result is frequent misunderstanding and misinterpretation, miscommunication, strained relationships, less-than-optimum teamwork, and, in classrooms and training rooms, inhibition and even failure for those whose natural learning processes happen not to match those of the teacher. When the differences are recognized, acknowledged, and understood, however, people are able to appreciate their diverse ways of functioning, to understand and accommodate one another's needs, and to relate, manage, and teach in ways that enable all to function at their best. People can *consciously* leverage their own and one another's distinctive gifts and processes to achieve optimal individual and group performance.

## The Beginning: Sandra's Story

In 1979, when I was working as a psychotherapist in private practice, one of my clients asked me to see her daughter, who was having difficulty in school.

Caroline was nine years old, articulate, and very self-aware for her age. As we began to talk, it became clear that she was not so interested in engaging in a dialogue as in having me listen to her.

459

She talked about her experiences in school, I listened...and then something unusual began to happen.

For a brief yet seemingly timeless period, my consciousness shifted. I was no longer aware of Caroline's words, but instead heard her voice simply as sound. Within this stream of sound, I became aware of three distinct frequencies: a high, fast frequency; a low, slow frequency; and a middle frequency in between. I noticed that while one frequency seemed to be clear, the other two were somewhat discordant.

Simultaneously with my awareness of the three frequencies, I also realized that I had access to information that I hadn't consciously known before:

§ Science had linked frequencies in sound and light to the human body, the highest frequencies being associated with the head, and the lowest with the limbs.

§ A new way of assessing and developing balance and harmony in and among people was to be developed, based upon the three frequencies I was hearing in the child's voice.

§ It would be possible to "diagnose" or evaluate people's natural ways of functioning through a sensitive listening process.

§ While all three frequencies were present in all people, one was particularly connected in each individual to a deeper, transpersonal, more spiritual aspect of identity.

When the session ended, I sat quietly for a long time to reflect upon my experience, which had seemed to come from outside myself yet to be meant specifically for me. All I knew for certain was that the experience was real, not a dream or fantasy, and that it had extraordinary significance. I had no idea what the three frequencies represented, but I was left with the compelling certainty that I had to find out.

During the following six weeks I was extraordinarily energized. Fully awake for twenty-two hours a day, my attention was riveted on the sounds of people's voices, which I continued to hear in a new way. I listened to all kinds of people: babies babbling, men, women, and children of all ages and ethnic backgrounds speaking familiar and foreign languages. Always, the frequencies were apparent. The next four years were spent in continuous learning, in relationship, I felt, with something unseen, unheard, but operationally meaningful. I knew that books, for example, about the psycho-acoustics of sound, had nothing to offer me. Rather, I was learning about the properties of the human voice and their significance through my own direct experience.

The first major breakthrough came with the recognition that the high, fast frequency was related to mental functioning, the middle frequency to emotional functioning, and the lowest and slowest frequency to physical (operational) functioning. I then became increasingly aware that the three frequencies combined in people's voices to form distinct *patterns* of sound, like different kinds of music, and that these specific patterns also seemed to exist universally. There were nine such distinct "voice patterns" in all, but five greatly predominated, and each seemed to be related to a specific pattern of mental-emotional-physical organization and functioning. This realization was the second major breakthrough.

In 1981, I was contacted by Dr. June Shoup, who was at that time chairperson of the Department of Communication Arts and Sciences at the University of Southern California, and director of the Speech Communications Research Laboratory in Los Angeles. Together with Dr. Harb Hayre from the University of Texas, we began to use their technology for voice spectrum analysis to objectively record the distinctions in voices that I was able to hear.

Over the course of a year they made and analyzed high-quality recordings of the voices of infants, children, and adults representing the five primary groups. Spectrographic data confirmed that there were indeed correlations within and distinctions among each group. Dr. Shoup and Dr. Hayre were ecstatic and eager to continue the research, but I felt divided. I was intellectually in awe of the potential scientific breakthrough, but my heart was uneasy and I didn't know why. After a few days, I realized that I was reluctant to continue this line of technical research and publish results until I understood more clearly the distinctions in human functioning that were evidently related to the voice distinctions—and the implications of these new discoveries as they affected people. The researchers were obviously disappointed, but graciously accepted my decision.

During this period I had attracted a group of about thirty people of varying backgrounds who were interested in exploring the meaning of the distinctions in voices that I was identifying. As it happened, all of the five primary personality dynamics were multiply represented in the group, so that these people themselves became the "living systems" through whom we could begin to understand the distinctions in experience and functioning associated with the different voice-patterns, simultaneously using this knowledge to further our own development, both as individuals and as a group.

The group was bound not only by the excitement of new discovery but by a sense of reverence in the undertaking. As we worked together every Thursday evening over a period of five years, we came to realize that the mental, emotional, and physical energies, which I first experienced as vibrations that manifested in the voice, had both a personal significance and a more numinous significance related to what I termed a "deeper identity."

At the personal level, we all have developmental work to do: mentally, in seeing and thinking more clearly; emotionally, in being more aware of and managing our own feelings, and becoming more aware of and respecting the feelings of others; and physically in being able to bring ideas to manifestation and take appropriate actions. But we realized that there is yet another level of human possibility, the transpersonal expression of the three basic elements, with the mental being expressed (at least) as a capacity for high vision, the emotional as deep compassion, and the physical as actions that express both, motivated always by the selfless desire to serve.

I had been using meditation techniques for my own spiritual development for several years, and in our sessions we explored ways to nuance these and other practices specifically for mental, emotional, and physical development and integration at the transpersonal level. At the same time we created a variety of practices for personal and interpersonal development and integration, all based upon our growing understanding of the processes and needs of the different personality dynamics.

Despite our successes, however, I was unable to teach others to hear what I was registering in the voices. Then, one day, someone suggested that we videotape the different kinds of people. We invited representatives of each of the five groups to a series of potluck dinners and let the cameras roll. As we subsequently watched the many hours of unedited videotape, it became apparent that these different human systems could be recognized through many signals other than the voice, such as: gestures (or the lack thereof); the degree of personalization with which people interacted; their choices of words and the pace, rhythm and content of their conversation; the degree of mobility in their bodies and faces; and the expressiveness of their communication. It was apparent in the particular focusing of the eyes—whether distant, quite close, or in between, and whether specific or diffuse. There were even clues in the selection of food each group chose to bring and how they laid it out! I realized then that my discernment of the distinctions in voices was simply a key to deciphering the fundamental distinctions in the human make-up that could now be taught in many ways.

In 1984 I received a phone call that turned out to be momentous. Fred Herr, a vice-president at Ford Motor Company, had come across a journal article about these new discoveries. Intrigued, he invited me to Detroit to help his management team work together more effectively. I had always known that the work would contribute broadly to the realization of human potential, and that it was obviously applicable in such people-oriented fields as education, parenting, psychology, and healthcare; but I had not anticipated that it would be of equal value in the business arena. But it was a natural application, of course. Business involves people trying to communicate and learn and work together effectively.

Though we did not know it at the time, the work at Ford initiated an entirely new phase of the Human Dynamics enterprise, in which the discoveries would be given form and taken out to serve in the world. By the time we began our collaboration with David Marsing twelve years later, my husband, David Horne, and I, along with our close colleague Linda O'Toole, had developed a variety of training programs and materials for personal and organizational transformation, as well as for teacher training, parenting, relationship-based healthcare, and cross-cultural bridging and collaboration. We had conducted these programs, and trained others to conduct them, in many countries around the world, each experience providing us with deeper understanding of the personality dynamics and their interactions, and greater awareness of how to make this expanding knowledge serviceable in the different arenas.

It was from this position of broad experience and expertise that we developed our training strategy with David Marsing for the Intel project.

# CHAPTER FORTY-SIX

# Teamwork

David knew that if his employees felt appreciated and understood—not only in terms of the jobs they did, but also as unique individuals—they would be more productive and happier at work. One of his top priorities for the new factory's training program was to create an environment of camaraderie and creative problem-solving, in which people felt empowered both as individuals and as team members, a goal totally compatible with the Human Dynamics approach to group development. The results were better than he had ever expected. As he put it:

*Human Dynamics goes way beyond the tools we used before. It has had the most profound impact on team performance... Individuals learn about their unique capabilities and strengths, tendencies of processing information, communicating, learning, and solving problems. Most importantly, they get an appreciation of how other people do it. It's not that one way is better than another, they're just different...there are different "languages." Different processes are happening. People approach things and relate to work in very different ways.*

*[As a] result of doing the Human Dynamics work, we realized that we needed to start looking anew at the way we deal with each other, and our whole construct of what people are capable of doing and what their potential really is. [Now] we intentionally use diverse teams of people. We find that we get a better outcome from having mixed groups – not only in terms of gender and cultural background but also with respect to their personality dynamics. Human Dynamics training helps people communicate and collaborate across all of these distinctions. When we have mixed groups [that are] conscious of their personality dynamic distinctions, the level of creativity is only bounded by the time and energy put into any activity...*

The analogy I like to use is that it becomes like improvisational jazz. There's an underlying structure, there's a sense of what has to happen, but people begin to play with who comes in, who does a duet together, who starts, who finishes, who should do a solo for a while. And they get so adept at this that after a time it becomes automatic.

# Individual and Group Development

With select groups, David Marsing wasn't afraid to include a module offering exercises for transpersonal development.

It had become increasingly clear to us that the personality dynamics are in fact distinct energy systems, the major locus of energy of mentally-centered people being literally at or above the head; of emotionally-centered people at the level of the heart; and of physically-centered people at the level of what the Japanese term the *hara* (below the navel) — though, of course, all three centers are always active more or less qualitatively and in greater or lesser degree.

One of our exercises based on this recognition is worth mentioning for its sheer practicality. It involves finding solutions to difficult situations by consciously relaxing the body, quieting the mind and the emotions, and adopting in turn mental, emotional, and physical "positions" in relation to the situation: above the head; at the level of the heart; and at the level of the hara. By registering how the situation *presents itself* from each perspective, and then allowing a co-creative solution to emerge without interference from the customary mental, emotional, and physical "noise," insights and options become apparent that would not be available through the usual problem-solving process.

Thus through a variety of methods, the employees learned to more fully engage in their own personal and group professional development. As David Marsing put it:

[Employees] use the new awareness…that Human Dynamics provides to assess their own personal, interpersonal and transpersonal functioning, and then use Human Dynamics tools and practices to achieve further integration and growth.

And David took another innovative step. Recognizing the implications of the work for harmonious family life, he elected to reap the maximum benefit for both the staff members and the organization as a whole by offering at least the basic program for spouses and many community leaders.

## A Contrast in Two Factories

Business was booming for Intel Corporation, and within two years a second factory — with *exactly* the same facilities, structure, and technologies — was built in the vicinity of the one in which the Human Dynamics training was begun. In fact, the only difference between the two was the philosophies with which they were managed; the directors of the new factory placed no emphasis on personal or group development training. This created such an intriguing opportunity for research and assessment that M.I.T. set up not one but two studies, the findings from which were unequivocal. As David Marsing explains:

*They showed that the first factory developed in its staff a collective intelligence and capacity for innovation and systemic improvement that the other factory never achieved. Moreover, the staff of the first factory enjoyed their work. Factory number two never matched the performance of the first, and the retention of staff was extraordinarily different — many senior people in factory one actually refused promotion that would involve a move to other facilities, because their current work environment was so agreeable and fulfilling.*

*The goal in factory one was not just to make products and fulfill quotas (which they did par excellence). It was to develop the people, and in so doing create "the best place in the world to work."*

## Cross-cultural Bridging

Intel is a multi-national organization that spans the globe. The fact that Human Dynamics training helps people communicate with, collaborate with, and appreciate one another at a level deeper than cultural or racial identity has helped Intel personnel to work more effectively together — both inner- and interculturally. In particular, our finding that, unlike in the West where people tend to be emotionally centered, the majority of people in Asia are physically centered, has greatly helped workers at Intel in the East and the West to better understand one another's "languages," and so communicate and collaborate with greater ease and harmony.

## Optimizing Learning

Human Dynamics identifies the different ways that people are inherently wired to learn. Teaching or training that does not accommodate these differences will result in less effective learning — if not outright failure. We recognized the need for more diversified training approaches when we began to work with one of Intel's sites in Penang, Malaysia.

A major problem at the site was that about 30 percent of newly hired operators were dropping out during their initial training, or leaving soon thereafter. We found that the training curriculum, which was quite rigorous, was being conducted in a highly structured way that matched the natural learning processes of one of the personality dynamics (physical-mental), but not the ways in which the majority of the trainees naturally learned. Not only were many of the operators actually failing at various stages of the course, but many who succeeded sufficiently to continue in the program often developed such self-doubt or experienced such discomfort that Intel no longer seemed an attractive place to work. They left, feeling bad about the company, and bad about themselves.

We selected key trainers who were themselves representative of the different personality dynamics, and first helped them to become conscious of their own learning processes. We then asked them to work together to formulate ways in which the delivery of the curriculum could be adjusted to meet *their* different needs, since in so doing the learning needs and processes of all of the trainees would be accommodated. The goal was not to change the content of the curriculum, which was fine, but how it was delivered.

A year later the results were assessed according to three parameters: the trainees' retention of learning; the retention of the operators in the work force; and the incidence of absenteeism during the training period. There were dramatic improvements in every area. In fact, there were no dropouts at all during that year, and the trainers reported that both they and their students experienced greater joy in the training process.

The survival of our species depends in the end on our ability to understand ourselves and develop our individual and collective capacities. This should be the main agenda in our homes, our classrooms, in our daily lives, and not the least in the context of the workplace.

As Einstein's work revealed the functioning of the external universe, so Human Dynamics contributes a new framework for understanding the functioning of human beings and provides invaluable tools and practices based upon this new understanding. In mastering five languages we can move beyond the "confusion of tongues"; in developing conscious empathy, we can surmount divisive barriers of race, color, creed, and station; and in acknowledging and honoring a transpersonal depth in ourselves and one another, we can move toward realizing the true greatness of our human potential and fulfilling our human destiny.

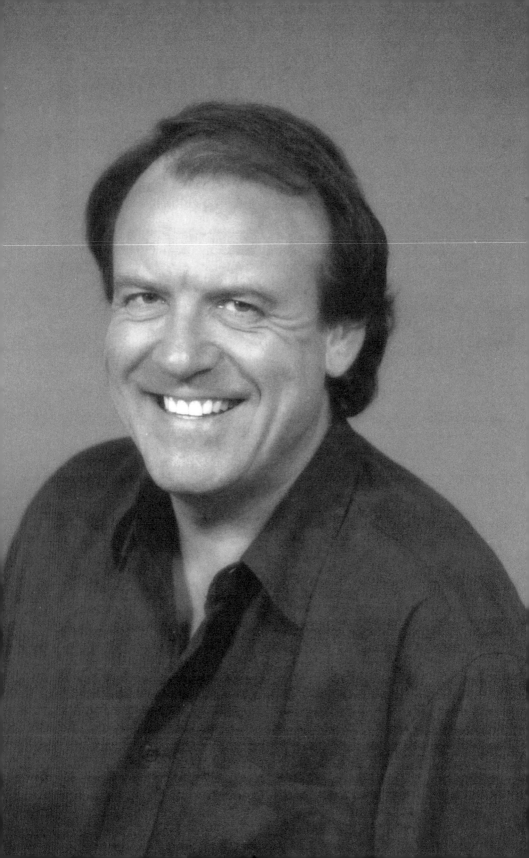

# Dawson Church:

# CHAPTER 47

# Leapfrogging:
## How Species, Companies, and Nations
## Jump Over Their Contemporaries

Duke Wilhelm-Ernst of Sachsen-Weimar, one of the most cultured and distinguished nobles of his era, sat in state on Palm Sunday, March 25, 1714, in his Castle Chapel. Enthralled, he and his courtiers listened to the new cantata, "King of Heaven, Be Thou Welcome," composed by his genius Concertmaster, Johann Sebastian Bach.

Bach wrote most of his music for the wealthy nobles — temporal and spiritual — of his day. Even in the nineteenth century, orchestral music, which required performers and composers, was so expensive that it could be afforded only by the nobility, or by the wealthiest members of the middle class. All that changed when recorded music came along. Suddenly, anyone who could afford a Victrola and some disks had access, on demand, to the music that previously was available only to the wealthiest, and only on certain occasions.

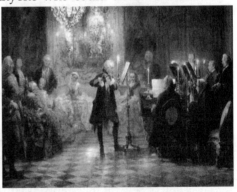

Today it's not just individual songs that can be summoned on demand. Teenagers load entire libraries, thousands of numbers, from each other's iPods at whim,

---

Dawson Church, Ph.D., has edited over 200 books. He is a co-founder of Aslan Publishing, a former CEO of Atrium Publisher's Group, and current publisher of Elite Books. During a long publishing career he has worked with many best-selling authors, as well as developing the careers of unknowns (www.AuthorsPublishing.com). He is passionately interested in emerging psychological and medical techniques that can yield fast and radical cures, recently authoring *The Genie in Your Genes* (Elite, 2007, www.GenieInYourGenes.com), teaching stress-reduction techniques based on these breakthroughs through Soul Medicine Institute (www.SoulMedicineInstitute.org), and drafting a book on leapfrogging.

usually without payment. The recorded music to which any global villager today has access for free dwarfs the entire listening career of the Duke of Weimar. Today's teenager, with a minimum wage job, moody gaze, pierced lips, black ZZ tattoos, and baggy pants, has exponentially greater resources than even the wealthiest baroque-period patron of the arts.

I call this idea *leapfrogging*. A species, nation, or business that leaps over the heads of its neighbors, making their best adaptations or behaviors obsolete in a comparatively brief instant, enjoys a huge advantage for a prolonged period of time.

The history of automotive engineering is replete with ideas that leapfrogged the competition. Henry Ford is famous for putting production of the Model T Ford onto a production line. As each car moved down the line, specialized workers installed just one

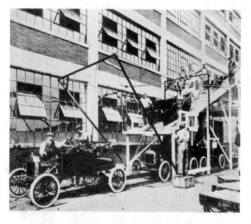

component onto the unit, till it rolled off the line fully assembled. Yet an even more startling innovation was required in order for assembly lines to function. What truly allowed Ford to leapfrog the competition was the idea of interchangeable parts.

Before then, each part of a car was machined individually. Perhaps a magneto was bolted onto the engine block with three bolts. During assembly, an engineer would drill the holes individually, and that particular magneto would fit that particular car. But because each part was custom drilled, the bolt pattern would be slightly different on each car—which meant that you couldn't take the magneto off one car and bolt it to another. This seemed like the obvious way to do things until the assembly line came along. Suddenly, every magneto had to fit any Model T Ford, and interchangeable parts were essential. The idea was one of several that allowed Ford to leapfrog the competition and profitably build a low-cost, mass-market automobile.

What does leapfrogging look like? What conditions encourage and support leapfrogging? How can you leapfrog over the problems that present intractable obstacles to your contemporaries, in life and in business? How can you turn leapfrogging from an occasional lucky accident into a routine event?

# The Comfortable Illusion of Linear Change

Human beings are comfortable with linear change. Chemists measure the rate at which the temperature of a substance rises as heat is applied. Economists measure the annual growth rate of economies. Social scientists track the growth or shrinkage of populations, and of subgroups within those populations. Atmospheric scientists measure global warming.

Linear, incremental change is present in nature. We witness our houseplants growing gradually if we water and feed them, and declining gradually if we neglect them. Our bodies grow incrementally through the end of our teen years. We progress, grade by grade, through school.

The problem with this linear mindset is that much change is sudden and discontinuous. When water reaches 100 degrees centigrade, it *boils,* and when a balloon being filled with air at a regular rate becomes too big, it *pops* — these are sudden, discontinuous changes of state. Every year thousands of medical patients report sudden miraculous cures, after the medical establishment has given up on their recovery. The dinosaurs became extinct suddenly, after they had dominated the biological spectrum for 165 million years — three times as long as primates have been around. Some kids from the ghetto work hard to become attorneys or surgeons, leapfrogging the living standards of their contemporaries in a single decade.

> -§-
> "Everything that can be invented has been invented."
> —Charles Duell, U.S. commissioner of Patents, 1899
> -§-

It's comforting to think of a world in which we can predict the future with some certainty. Yet if we take the rate of change of yesteryears and extrapolate it into the future, there is only one thing of which we can be certain: We will be wrong.

Sometimes societies leapfrog over other societies, just as the kid from the ghetto can quickly attain a much better life than her peers. In the mid 1850s, people in Latin America had a higher per capita income than their contemporaries in the United States.[1] Border cities such as El Paso/Juarez, and San Diego/Tijuana are today's living evidence of the importance that social, financial and political institutions can make.

Consider the European Union countries: With a growth rate of around 3 percent, the population doubles its wealth every 35 years.[2]

Consider China: With a 12 percent growth rate, the population doubles its wealth every six years.

Consider Zimbabwe: With a negative growth rate and terrible governance, its population is about twice as poor today as it was 20 years ago.

Every day, societies are making choices that either create or destroy wealth for their citizens. Certain choices can lead to a country leapfrogging over its neighbors in a time span less than single generation. In 2005, the Gross Domestic Product (measured by purchasing power parity) of emerging economies exceeded that of developed countries for the first time.[3]

Yet raw unbridled economic growth is unsustainable. If China's and India's current growth continues, for instance, they will gobble up the world's entire paper supply in 50 years. So as countries leapfrog ahead in economic growth, they must stimulate innovations that leapfrog current materials and technologies as well.

## Species Leapfrogging

Evolutionary scientists used to perceive natural selection as a long, slow process by which Mother Nature selected certain traits over hundreds of generations whilst weeding out others. But the fossil record and modern dating techniques have shoved that linear model aside for more dramatic leaps. "Punctuated Equilibrium," or "punk eek" in the trade, reveals that species and ecosystems appear to go through long periods of stability, perhaps millions of years long, punctuated by periods of rapid, discontinuous change.

The opposable thumb is a prime example of a single anatomical change that enabled one species, *Homo sapiens sapiens,* to leapfrog over all the other lines of primates then competing for space in that ecological stratum. Having a thumb that rotated out and around allowed early humans to grasp and manipulate items in new ways. They could thus use tools, and with those tools construct other tools, to the point where they began to dominate whole ecosystems in a way that was not possible for primates without opposable thumbs.

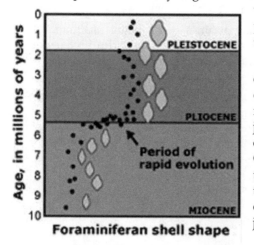

Foraminiferan shell shape

Going back to the other end of the evolutionary scale, one particular variety of micro-organisms did a good job of surviving the planetary catastrophe of the late Cretaceous period that made the dinosaurs extinct. At that time there were many varieties of single-celled plankton, but just one of them survived in large numbers. This lucky variety was the diatoms. Scientists have speculated that the reason that diatoms survived the calamity that claimed so many other species is that they are able to form a protective cyst around themselves. They do this whenever the water they live in dries up.

This adaptation has nothing to do with surviving a catastrophic planetary event. Yet it allowed them to leapfrog over all the other varieties, like radiolaria and coccoliths, by going dormant while the mass extinction went on around them. Once conditions returned to normal, they broke out of their cysts and got on with living their diatomaceous lives; their increased numbers allowed them to rapidly re-inhabit their environmental niche.[4]

Science itself is subject to punk eek. It goes through sudden, disorienting spurts of discovery, with prescient disruptive insights followed by long periods of incremental development in which theories are tested and extended.

## Social Leapfrogging

The separation of powers is a recent, and remarkable, social innovation, one that has enabled societies where it exists to leapfrog over those in which the bad decision of one leader can drag the whole nation into decline. Today's Africa is a laboratory of experiments in governance; those in which functioning democracies have separate power centers have generally prospered, while those countries ruled by the *Monoikos*, or "strong man," have fared well or ill according to his mix of talents.

-§-
"Airplanes are interesting toys, but of no military value."
—Marshall Foch, WWI French Commander, 1911
-§-

Another example of a social innovation that allows societies and individuals to prosper is the land title. Countries which give clear title to land encourage landowners to put the land to productive use. By comparison, experiments in abolishing land titles, such as Vladimir Lenin's declaration in October 1917 that, in Bolshevik Russia, "Private ownership of land shall be abolished forever," are usually a great leap backward; the collective farms of the Soviet era were notoriously inefficient. Other ill-judged attempts to undermine land title, most recently in Zimbabwe, and in the 1980s in some South and Central American countries, have backfired, as occupants without title to the land have little incentive to improve it or use it productively.

The separation of church and state is a principle that allows societies to progress. Public policymaking is a difficult and error-prone business, in which populist sentiments are all too likely to hold more sway than farsighted judgment. But when religious imperatives that are completely extraneous to the policy goals are added to the mix, the chances of sound decision-making diminish even further. Societies that have a separation of church and state can leapfrog those that remain bound in a theocratic straightjacket. So can those that observe the rule of law.

## Commodities Leapfrogging

One of the most passionate public arguments of the current decade is the discussion of whether or not we are at (or past) "Peak

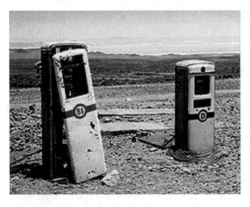

Oil" — the point at which the world's oil production has reached its peak. Some say that we already reached this point in the late 1980s, others say that Peak Oil is still a long way off.

While this lively discussion provides bags of entertainment, history is likely to throw the whole topic into its uncaring shredder long before the controversy is resolved. Why? Sheik Zaki Yamani, Oil Minister of Saudi Arabia, the world's largest oil producer, said in the 1970s, "The Stone Age did not end for lack of stone, and the Oil Age will end long before the world runs out of oil." What he wanted to impress upon his contemporaries was that every technology has its run — and that run comes to an end. From plasma conversion of industrial waste, to cheap ethanol from junk biomass, to hydrogen conversion, to breakthroughs in solar power, history is knocking on oil's door. A new technology will come along and leapfrog oil, as surely and as quickly as steamships put the windjammer into the scrap yard.

## Technological Leapfrogging

Apple Computer has been able to leapfrog its competition not once, but twice. The first time was with the Macintosh computer in 1984. In a world accustomed to the incremental improvement of PCs, Apple suddenly found itself with a 10-year technological lead. It squandered that lead by pricing its products uncompetitively, and with a host of other blunders — but that's another story. And almost two decades later, it again leapfrogged the competition with the iPod digital personal music player.

The Soviet Union leapfrogged over the United States by putting Yuri Gagarin into orbit in 1961. At the time, many in the East and the West—including U.S. President Dwight Eisenhower—believed that the central planning model of the Soviet Union was so efficient that it would lead to greater economic growth than its competitors. Eisenhower warned his contemporaries not to succumb to the greater material prosperity offered by communism. The two countries then proceeded with furious attempts to leapfrog each other in arms and global prestige, until the social fabric of the Soviet Union, and the country itself, fell apart.

In 1906, Great Britain launched a new battleship, HMS Dreadnought. Faster than any other large ship on the seas, with a heavier weight of ordnance, with all her guns housed in rotating turrets, she made every other battleship in the world obsolete at a stroke.

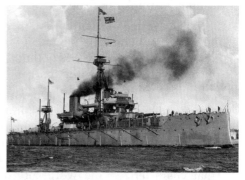

Fifty years after the Dreadnought was launched, Malcom McLean, the boss of a trucking company, had an idea that produced a similar discontinuous change in maritime transportation. McLean's brainwave was to load a collection of goods that would normally have traveled in the hold of a freighter, pack them into 58 metal containers, and strap them onto the deck of the Ideal-X, a World War II surplus oil tanker. The invention of the shipping container leapfrogged other methods of transportation at a stroke.

Businesses rise and fall with remarkable speed. Google celebrates its tenth birthday in 2008, but it has around *10 times* the market capitalization (the combined value of all its stock) of General Motors, which celebrates its *centenary* in 2008. The Dow Jones Industrial Average indexed the stock value of 30 companies, which are added or dropped from the Dow periodically. Remember Corn Products Refining? Remember Woolworth? Both of these companies were components of the Dow in 1950. Like so many others, these companies that comprised the Dow in earlier decades have been surpassed and gone belly-up, or been so chopped and diced into pieces that they are no longer recognizable.

# CHAPTER FORTY-SEVEN

# Consciousness Leapfrogging

Consciousness is a defining trait of human beings and many other animals. The society that first learns to harness the power of consciousness to produce change will leapfrog every other.

As consciousness changes, the world changes. For most of human history, and as late as the 19th century, few people objected to slavery, aside from the slaves themselves. Today it is difficult to find an individual in Western societies who does not believe slavery to be wrong. In the space of just two centuries, there has been a 180-degree change in consciousness. Societies who are at the leading edge of consciousness change can accomplish things that other societies cannot. Examples include:

**The Hunger Project.** Though this bold social initiative of the 1970s did not eradicate hunger, it was the first large-scale attempt to collectively imagine a world without hunger, a project of consciousness inconceivable just a century earlier.

-§-
Computers in the future
may only weigh 1.5 tons.
–Popular Mechanics, 1949
-§-

**Quantum Physics.** The world of quantum physics, in which every possibility exists in the quantum field, while just one result precipitates out of the range of possibilities, leapfrogged the sense of empirical certainty that characterized the world of Newtonian mechanics. Quantum physics points to the importance of attention as a key factor determining the shape of the world around us.

Today, string theory postulates that atomic particles are simply vibrating strings of energy. Echoing Einstein's famous equation with mass on one side and energy on the other, when you increase the energy of a string (the rate of vibration) it shows up as increased mass. Heavy particles like protons have a higher vibrational frequency than "light" particles like electrons. And in a spectacular display of quantum leapfrogging, electrons themselves can jump out of phase in our universe, perhaps, and into phase in another, without any time elapsing between the events.

**Globalization.** Those countries that embrace the reality of a global economy will leapfrog those that resist it. The Chinese Emperor Quinlong was approached by England in 1793 with a request to open a trading relationship. At the time, China's income per head was much greater than that of Europe. Yet Lord George Macartney, the emissary to the Chinese court, returned to King George III with this rebuke from the Chinese emperor: "We have not the slightest need of your country's manufactures." The result was two centuries of economic stagnation for China as the West leapfrogged ahead. In the years up to 1950, Chinese incomes fell by a quarter, while those of Britons rose fivefold.[5] Acknowledging the global economy as a reality, and maintaining a consciousness that seeks ways to function in that context, primes individuals, organizations, and countries for success.

**Human Rights.** In the late 1970s, when U.S. President Jimmy Carter pronounced respect for human rights to be a component of the country's relationship with other countries, he was widely mocked for elevating an intangible moral value to the level of the gold, guns, and glory of the world of *realpolitik*. Yet this was a moral watershed for humanity, as no world leader had ever made such values into policy before, and few other leaders could even wrap their minds around such a concept. This consciousness has grown to the point that today, even though the world may have little practical leverage over genocidal regimes, their actions are universally censured—a moral leapfrogging over previous eras, which turned a blind eye toward atrocities.

-§-
"You can no more win a war than you can win an earthquake."
–Jeannette Rankin
-§-

Around the world, one thousand innocent people die each day through gun violence.[6] Another expression of moral leapfrogging is arms embargoes, gun control, and other government actions that limit the proliferation of firearms.

Britain is famous as a relatively civil society, football hooligans aside. One reason for its low murder rate is the almost-complete unavailability of firearms. If you want to own a gun, you can—as long as it's locked in the gun cabinet of a registered hunting association. In Agatha Christie's mid-century murder mysteries, the premature departure of the deceased was accomplished by ingenious devices that took a long time to think up and stage, like poison and fake accidents. Britons can't just walk into a store, purchase a gun, and keep it in the glove compartment of their car.

The founding fathers of America declared that its citizens have "the right to bear arms." Congress interprets the definition of arms as meaning everything up to and including semi-automatic assault rifles. As a result, when road rage escalates, there are plenty of pistols in glove compartments to stoke the social danger. Societies that ban firearms, as Britain has done, may one day be regarded as having morally leapfrogged over those that have not.

**Success.** The definition of "success" to Paleolithic humans meant simply physical survival. Success to 20th-century suburbanites meant something different: the accumulation of financial wealth. A leapfrogged definition of success for the 21st century and beyond includes happiness, environmental beauty, economic sustainability rather than unchecked growth, caring relationships, and attention to spiritual and emotional needs.

**Spirituality.** The old model believed that consciousness was an epiphenomenon of matter. Scientists held the idea that life progressed from simple forms to more complex forms, and eventually the most complex forms evolved consciousness in order to help them understand and organize their environments.

-§-
"If you want to awaken all of humanity, then awaken all of yourself. If you want to eliminate the suffering in the world, then eliminate all that is dark and negative in yourself. Truly, the greatest gift you have to give is that of your own self-transformation."
–Lao Tzu
-§-

The most recent research turns this order on its head. Scientists have observed consciousness affecting matter, such as the rate of decay of beryllium atoms. A recent study of AIDS patients showed that a single belief held in particpants' consciousness provided the most striking correlation with the rate of progress of the disease. In those who believed in a punishing God, biomarkers of the disease advanced four times faster than in those who believed in a benevolent Deity.[7] Beliefs held in consciousness can literally kill or heal.

Societies and organizations that feed the spiritual well-being of their people can leapfrog those that do not. Spirituality and a rich social network have been shown to reduce hospital stays,[8] increase general health,[9] and boost longevity by several years.[10] A healthy society is a more productive and innovative society, and a society that honors the spirituality of individuals is a healthier society.

# Some Frogs to Watch

Some fascinating examples of potential leapfrogging are evident today:

1. **African Telecommunications and Energy.** A century and a half after first message was sent across an underwater telegraph cable between Britain and America ("Glory to God in the highest, and on earth, peace, good will to men" — August 16, 1858), Africa is leapfrogging over the telecommunications revolution by adopting cell phones. While it took a hundred years of capital-intensive investment for Western countries to wire themselves up, Subsaharan Africa, though a collection of the world's poorest countries, has leapfrogged this entire telecommunications infrastructure. In China, India, and Africa, the number of cellular handsets now exceeds the number of land-line handsets. Next, it is likely that Africa will

leapfrog the electrical grid of Western nations by harnessing its abundant solar energy to power efficient LED devices. This could contribute to rapid rates of growth in some African countries, despite their lack of transparent governance, development infrastructure, and technological skill base.

2. **Nanotechnology.** Nanotechnology provides the promise of changing, by huge orders of magnitude, some of our core assumptions about the efficiencies of common processes.

Conventional computers store every bit of information as either a one or a zero on magnetic media such as a hard drive, using the laws of Newtonian physics. Quantum computers store information as an atomic particle with a known spin. Theoretically, they can process information at a speed many orders of magnitude greater than a conventional computer. 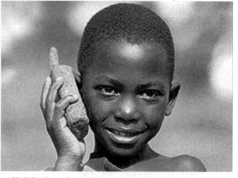 Your laptop today still follows the basic design of the ENIAC computer of 1945, though fortunately it doesn't weigh 30 tons and have 19,000 vacuum tubes, as the first electronic digital computer did. Nanotech quantum computers can be made small enough to fit into a single thread in a garment; in the coming century computers will likely shrink to the point where they are invisibly implanted into many of the common artifacts of everyday life, rather than being bulky specialized machines.

Nanotechnology will leapfrog contemporary medical treatments by combining technology with biology. Simple artificial red blood cells, which are now being tested, store oxygen and then release it, just like the red cells in your blood—but with enormously greater efficiency. Modeling shows that if you were to replace 10 percent of your red blood cells with their nanotechnological equivalents, you could "do an Olympic sprint for 15 minutes without taking a breath, or sit at the bottom of your pool for four hours."[11] Societies and organizations with a lead in nanotechnology will leapfrog those that neglect it.

3. **Energy Psychology.** Energy medicine and Energy Psychology, which treat the electromagnetic field of a patient rather than directly manipulating organs with drugs and surgery, are demonstrating the ability to produce rapid, discontinuous, and sometimes immediate psychological and physical healing. The electrical charge of a healthy human cell is stable at about 90 millivolts. The charge of an inflamed

cell rises to 120 millivolts, then drops to 30 millivolts as the cell degenerates.[12]

Our bodies are sensitive to extremely small fluctuations in the electrical and magnetic fields that surround us. Making minute changes in these fields can stimulate our cells to behave in different ways.

Pulsed Electromagnetic Fields are showing themselves effective in treating depressed patients who have proved resistant to drugs and psychotherapy.[13] Low-intensity currents have been shown to promote the healing of broken bones, and are a growing feature of orthopedic medicine. Tiny piezoelectric charges generated by simply rubbing or tapping certain points on the skin with our fingertips appear to travel through our body's connective tissue, which is a semiconductor, and when administered by a skilled practitioner, can reduce anxiety, depression, and stress. The low-tech methods of Energy Psychology have had astounding results even when dealing with the stress of conflict and war, in places such as Kosovo and Rwanda.

-§-
"We are in a school for gods, wherein in slow motion we learn the consequences of thought."
–Brugh Joy
-§-

Energy Psychology and energy medicine have leapfrogged drugs and surgery for many individual patients. They are safe and noninvasive, and early research shows that they may have far greater healing effects for many conditions than conventional medical alternatives. As a result, they may become the front line of treatment, leapfrogging risky and invasive procedures that are the standard of care today.

4. **Gene Chip Consciousness Experiments.** DNA was once thought to be an unalterable blueprint governing every aspect of human structure and function. The new science of epigenetics is now highlighting the reality that genes must be *read* by the cell (or *expressed,* in the lingo), in order to have an effect, and that the signals that govern gene expression — telling the cell to read the gene blueprint and use it to build proteins — come from outside the cell.

One of the places in which these epigenetic signals originate is human consciousness. With proper funding and well-designed experiments, within a decade we will begin to map which aspects of consciousness affect particular patterns of gene expression.

Gene chips put hundreds of strands of DNA on a single chip, and allow researchers to determine which genes are being expressed during the course of an experiment. Staggering though it may sound, science is jus a few experiments away from linking particular thoughts, emotions, and beliefs with changes in the genes expressed, as determined by DNA chips.

Every one of us is already changing our gene expression by our thoughts, feelings, and beliefs every day—a form of unconscious genetic engineering. Proper experiments will allow us to understand the cause and effect links between them, and start to do *conscious* genetic engineering, creating health and longevity interventions that are safe, noninvasive, and that work in harmony with every system of our unique body. These interventions will

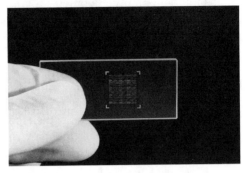

leapfrog many of the medical interventions common today, making invasive and risky treatments like drugs and surgery look like the crude instruments of medieval barber-surgeons.

5. **The Long Tail.** Companies with a large number of products for which there is small demand can compete via the Internet with companies that have a small number of products for which there is large demand. The publisher of a book in a niche subject that will sell just 100 copies a year will, if that publisher has 1,000 titles, realize the same income as a publisher with a bestseller that moves 100,000 units a year. Books today stay in print, as print-on-demand products or ebooks, at much lower sales thresholds than publishers used to require to maintain a book in print using conventional techniques. In this way, the internet, with its endless virtual shelf space, gives such producers an advantage over limited brick-and-mortar retailers, and promotes the availability of specialized niche information. Blockbuster hits now share the limelight with niche products riding the long tail of an extended virtual market, shifting the balance away from a preponderance of bestsellers toward a variety of information and allowing specialist providers to leapfrog into a market position that was the former exclusive domain of well-heeled market leaders.

6. **Societies that Empower Women.** Women first gained the right to vote in national elections in New Zealand in 1893, with Britain following in 1918. Barriers to women's entry into the workforce began to crumble wholesale during the civilian labor crunch of World War II. In a century, the participation of women in the workforce has changed. This is one reason why the societies in which men and women work as equals have leapfrogged those who keep half of their creative capacity online by denying women economic or

political rights. Giving women the vote, and moving toward full participation of women in the workforce, is an immensely potent social innovation. Societies that deny women full participation in effect cut off the creative resources of half their population, allowing those that empower women's involvement to leap ahead.

-§-

"The world is dangerous not because of those who do harm, but because of those who look at it without doing anything."
–Albert Einstein

-§-

**7. Societies that Utilize Seniors.** In the United States in 1950, 46 percent of men over the age of 65 were in the workforce; today, just 19 percent are.[14] This means that a huge percentage of human beings full of rich experience and creativity have gone offline. This century, the societies that engage their seniors have a staggeringly large resource they can use in leapfrogging ahead.

## The Cultivation of Champion Frogs

Leapfrogging is sometimes pure accident, like the encysted diatoms. Sometimes, though, it can be induced. We have all heard of organizations like Apple, and people like Einstein, who find the leading edge more reliably than their contemporaries. How can you turn leapfrogging from an occasional fortuitous accident to a source of ongoing creativity in your life and your organization? Nurturing an emotional, spiritual, and intellectual environment that creates the conditions for leapfrogging takes a focused consciousness, but it can be done. Here are some suggestions for setting up such a creative environment:

§ Be acutely awake to signs of leapfrogging in the news and the people around you.

§ Expose yourself to ideas outside your field of expertise.

§ Allow mistakes in yourself and your organization.

§ Nurture a culture that rewards novelty and creativity.

§ Brainstorm every problem.

§ Meditate, reflect, contemplate, pray, and find your favorite way of tuning into higher sources of wisdom.

§ Cultivate emotional calmness and a healthy emotional climate.

§ Nourish whole human beings, not just parts.

§ Be open to the unexpected and unexplained.

§ See the opportunities lurking in the disguise of a crisis.

§ Use expansive language and avoid limited language.

§ Notice when you're approaching a situation the same old way.

§ Give yourself quiet, unstructured time.

§ Investigate best practices other organizations use to nurture creativity.

§ Stay close to nature.

§ Nourish spiritual values in yourself and others.

§ Fill your life with kindness, philanthropy, and altruism.

Leapfrogging will lead to discontinuous (and sometimes disorienting) change throughout the next couple of centuries. In a few decades, we will read today's arguments over peak oil, gun control, global warming, globalization, public education, corporate governance, and the distribution of wealth with the same fascination as we now read the archaic arguments of phrenologists, anti-suffragettes, anti-abolitionists, Marxists, and antisublapsarianists.

Large changes don't take a majority of people, or even a large number. The Renaissance took about 25 years, and engaged a very small number of individuals—around 1,000 people. Yet it completely altered the shape of Western civilization. Afterwards, science, art, education, mathematics, science, literature, and social values were quite different from what they had been before. We are in the midst of another such large-scale, discontinuous jump today. The balloon is about to pop. Those who turn their faces to the bracing winds of change will leapfrog ahead of those who cling to yesterday's linear certainties.

1.  de la Escosura, Leandro Prados, (2004). "When Did Latin America Fall Behind? Evidence from Long-run International Inequality." (Universidad Carlos III, Madrid. presented at the Inter-American Seminar on Economics 2004 NBER Mexico), December 2-4.
2.  Bernstam, M.D. & Rabushka, A. (2005). "China vs. Russia: Wealth Creation vs. Poverty Reduction." *The Financial Times,* April 14.
3.  *The Economist,* (2006). "The New Titans," Sept. 16.
4.  Gould, Stephen Jay (1994). "The evolution of life on earth." *Scientific American,* October.
5.  *Economist* (2006) p. 28
6.  BBC, World News Tonight, (2006). Oct. 26.
7.  Donnelly, Matt (2006). "Faith boosts cognitive management of HIV and cancer." *Science & Theology News,* May, p. 16.
8.  Koenig, H.G., Larson, D.B., (1998). "Use of hospital services, religious attendance, and religious affiliation." *Southern Medical Journal,* 91:925-932.
9.  McBride, J.L., Arthur, G., Brooks, R., Pilkington, L. (1998). "The relationship between a patient's spirituality and health experiences." *Family Medicine* Feb., 30(2), p 122.
10. Powell, L.H., Shahabi, L., Thoresen, C.E., (2003). "Religion and spirituality: linkages to physical health." *American Psychologist,* Jan. 2003. 58(1), p 36.
11. Kurzweil, R. (2006). "The 'golden era' of nanotechnology." *Science and Theology News,* April, p. 8.
12. Liboff, A.R. (2004). "Toward an electromagnetic paradigm for biology and medicine." *Journal of Alternative and Complementary Medicine,* Vo. 10, No. 1, pp. 41-47.
13. *United Press International* (2006). Magnetic stimulator tested for depression. Jan. 31.
14. Hobbs, F. (2005). "65+ in the United States." U.S. Bureau of the Census, Current Population Reports (Washington: U.S. Government Printing Office), pp. 23-190.